Stedman's

DERMATOLOGY & IMMUNOLOGY WORDS

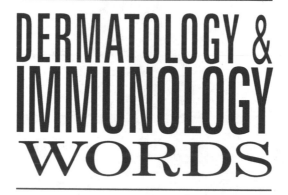

Edited by
Darla Haberer, CMT

Janet Vaughn

Stedman's

DERMATOLOGY & IMMUNOLOGY
WORDS

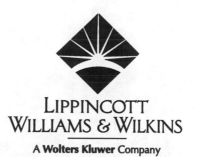

LIPPINCOTT
WILLIAMS & WILKINS

A **Wolters Kluwer** Company

Series Editor: Elizabeth B. Randolph
Associate Managing Editor: Maureen Barlow Pugh
Editor: Darla Haberer, CMT
Production Coordinator: Marette Magargle-Smith
Cover Design: Reuter & Associates

Printed in the United States of America

Library of Congress Cataloging-in-Publication Data

Stedman's dermatology & immunology words / edited by Darla Haberer.
    p.   cm — (Stedman's word book series)
    Includes bibliographical references.
    ISBN 0-683-40080-0
    1. Dermatology—Terminology.   2. Immunology—Terminology.   3. Allergy—Terminology. 4. Rheumatology—Terminology. 5. Communicable diseases—Terminology I. Haberer, Darla. II. Series: Stedman's word books.
    [DNLM: 1. Dermatology—terminology. 2. Allergy and Immunology—terminology. WR 15 S812 1997]
RL41.S74   1997
616.07'9'014—dc21
DNLM/DLC
for Library of Congress   96–36759
                                                    CIP

Developed from the database of Stedman's medical dictionary and supplemented by terminology found in the current medical literature.
    Includes bibliographical references.

Contents

Acknowledgments

An important part of our editorial process is the involvement of medical transcriptionists—as advisors, reviewers and/or editors.

Special thanks are due Darla Haberer, CMT, for editing and proofing the manuscript (and doing the necessary research involved with that large task) as well as helping to compile the appendices. We also would like to extend our thanks to Christa Scott, CMT, who edited the manuscript, and helped resolve many difficult content questions.

Thanks also to our *Stedman's Dermatology & Immunology Words* MT Editorial Advisory Board, consisting of Ellen Atwood; Julia Kathleen Branch; Pat Collins, CMT; Robin A. Koza; and LeVerne Randol, CMT. These medical transcriptionists served as editors and advisors, and spent hours perusing texts, journals, and manufacturers' information to compile the latest terms in the specialties of dermatology, allergy, immunology, rheumatology and infectious disease. In addition, both Ellen Atwood and Pat Collins, CMT, were instrumental in the creation of the appendices for this book.

Other important contributors to this edition include: Colleen Breuer, Debbie Frank, and Gail Lane, all of whom gathered new words and/or provided invaluable suggestions. Barb Ferretti played an integral role in the process by reviewing the content files for format, updating the database and providing a final quality check.

As with all our *Stedman's* word references, we have benefitted from the suggestions and expertise of our many contacts in the medical transcriptionist community. Thanks to all our advisory board participants, reviewers and editors, AAMT meeting attendees, and others who have written in with requests and comments—keep talking, and we'll keep listening.

Preface

They listened, they pondered, they provided! Many of us medical transcriptionists had asked for word books for the specialties of dermatology, allergy, rheumatology, and infectious disease. Once again the Williams & Wilkins staff has heard our pleas, and has given us a concise, easily used reference.

Deciding which word books to publish, and then which terms to include and which to exclude from each book is difficult. Because many of these disease processes overlap, the decision was made to include dermatology, allergy, rheumatology, and infectious disease words in one word book, and to call it *Stedman's Dermatology & Immunology Words*. Combining these different specialties into one volume means that all the information we need about these specialties is in a handy one-stop reference.

This new reference book will provide assistance in the complex, growing, changing world of being a medical language specialist. With the boom in the change from working as a group to working alone, often physically isolated from others, we need reference books such as this one to help us work as much as we can, as accurately as we can, and as fast as possible.

Take a moment (I know they are hard to find) and familiarize yourself with the appendices and the helpful tools in this reference. Did you discover the appendices? Take a close look at the book itself. The "thumb guides" on the right edge are a fast way to get to the beginning or ending of the C's for example. Did you notice you don't have to juggle the book or place a heavy object on it to keep it open at the page you need? Did you find the space for notes on each bottom right page? These are just a few of the requests listened to, pondered and provided. Thank you is not enough to express our appreciation to Maureen Barlow Pugh and the other editors involved in bringing this book to us. It is an honor to work with such dedicated, motivated, and wonderful people.

It is my pleasure to help provide you with this tool and may your yearning for learning forever keep burning.

Darla Haberer, CMT

Publisher's Preface

Stedman's Dermatology & Immunology Words offers an authoritative assurance of quality and exactness to the wordsmiths of the health care professions—medical transcriptionists, medical editors and copy editors, health information management personnel, court reporters, and the many other users and producers of medical documentation.

For years we have received request upon request for word books covering the specialties included in this word book, none of which had a large enough nomenclature to sustain an entire word book. By combining terminology from these separate yet interrelated medical specialties, it is our hope that *Stedman's Dermatology & Immunology Words* will be a useful and unique resource for medical language specialists.

Stedman's Dermatology & Immunology Words, can be used to validate both the spelling and the accuracy of terminology specific to dermatology, immunology, allergy, rheumatology, and infectious disease. Dermatology-related terms include problems like acne, contact dermatitis, alopecia, eczematous dermatoses, and auto-immune bullous diseases. Immunology-related terms encompass allergies, allergic asthma, rheumatologic disorders (such as connective tissue disorders, psoriatic arthritis, fibromyalgia, lupus, and arthritis) as well as infectious diseases like Lyme disease and HIV-AIDS. In addition, the user will find terminology on environmental illnesses, public health, chronic fatigue syndrome, rehabilitation, and related endocrinology.

The user will find listed thousands of bacteria, fungal diseases, drugs, diagnostic and therapeutic procedures, new techniques and maneuvers, lab tests, and equipment, instrument and prosthesis names. Abbreviations and acronyms are also included. For quick reference, anatomy illustrations, a list of dermatology drug names by indication, a list of related combining forms, and a list of common allergens appear in the appendices at the back of the book.

Because our goal has been to provide a comprehensive yet streamlined reference tool, we have omitted terminology that is not specific to these specialties. Thus, some terms (such as anatomy and physiology terms) that are often dictated in these specialties are not included in this text, as they can be found in general medical dictionaries.

This compilation of over 41,000 entries, fully cross-indexed for quick access, was built from a base vocabulary of over 24,600 medical words, phrases, abbreviations and acronyms. The extensive A-Z list was developed from the database of *Stedman's Medical Dictionary* and supplemented by terminology found in current medical literature (please see the list of References on page xvi).

We at Lippincott Williams & Wilkins strive to provide you with the most up-to-date and accurate word references available. Your use of this word book will prompt new editions, which will be published as often make this *Stedman's* product more useful to you. Please use the postpaid card at the back of this book and send your recommendations care of "Stedman's" at Lippincott Williams & Wilkins.

Explanatory Notes

Medical transcription is an art as well as a science. Both are needed to correctly interpret a physician's dictation, whose language is a product of education, training, and experience. This variety in medical language means that there are several acceptable ways to express certain terms, including jargon. *Stedman's Dermatology & Immunology Words* provides variant spellings and phrasings for many terms. This, in addition to complete cross-indexing, makes *Stedman's Dermatology & Immunology Words* a valuable resource for determining the validity of terms as they are encountered.

Alphabetical Organization

Alphabetization of entries is letter by letter as spelled, ignoring punctuation, spaces, prefixed numbers, Greek letters, or other characters. For example:

acid-fast staining methods

acid formaldehyde hematin

α-acid glycoprotein

acid hematin

In subentries, the abbreviated singular form or the spelled-out plural form of the noun main entry word is ignored in alphabetization.

Format and Style

All main entries are in **boldface** to speed up location of a sought-after entry, to enhance distinction between main entries and subentries, and to relieve the textual density of the pages.

Irregular plurals and variant spellings are shown on the same line as the singular or preferred form of the word. For example:

scolex pl. **scoleces**

curette, curet

Hyphenation

As a rule of style, multiple eponyms (e.g., Green-Kenyon corneal marker) are hyphenated. Also, hyphens have been added between a manufacturer and one or more eponyms (e.g., Vital-Metzenbaum dissecting scissors). Please note that hyphenation is a question of style, not of accuracy, and thus is a matter of choice.

Possessives

Possessive forms have been dropped in this reference for the sake of consistency and to conform to the guidelines outlined by the American Association for Medical Transcription (AAMT) and other groups. Please note, however, that retaining the possessive is a question of style, not of accuracy, and thus is a matter of choice. To form the possessive of a word, simply add the apostrophe or apostrophe "s" to the end of the word.

Cross-indexing

The word list is in an index-like main entry-subentry format that contains two combined alphabetical listings:

(1) A *noun* main entry-subentry organization typical of the A-Z section of medical dictionaries like **Stedman's:**

dermatosis
    acantholytic d.
    acquired d.
    ashy d.
    bullous d.

nail
    brittle n.
    convex n.
    parrot-beak n.
    reedy n.

(2) An *adjective* main entry-subentry organization, which lists words and phrases as you hear them. The main entries are the adjectives or modifiers in a multi-word term. The subentries are the nouns around which the terms are constructed and to which the adjectives or modifiers pertain:

congenital
    c. ectodermal defects
    c. erythropoietic porphyria
    c. ichthyosiform erythroderma
    c. syphilis

nevus
    n. comedonicus
    n. fibrosus
    n. flammeus
    n. pigmentosus

This format provides the user with more than one way to locate and identify a multi-word term. For example:

dissemination
  skin d.
disease
  Quincke d.
  Raynaud d.

skin
  s. dissemination
Quincke
  Q. disease
  Q. edema

It also allows the user to see together all terms that contain a particular descriptor as well as all types, kinds, or variations of a noun entity. For example:

balloon
  b. laser angioplasty
  b. occlusion
  Blue Max b.
  Brandt cytology b.
  Express b.

angioplasty
  balloon laser a.
  complex a.
  a. guiding catheter
  high-risk a.
  transluminal coronary a.

Wherever possible, abbreviations are separately defined and cross-referenced. For example:

FUO
  fever of unknown origin
fever
  f. of unknown origin (FUO)
origin
  fever of unknown o. (FUO)

References

In addition to the manufacturers' literature we gather at various medical meetings, scientific reports from hospitals, and our MT Editorial Advisory Board members' lists (from their daily transcription work), we used the following sources for new words for *Stedman's Dermatology & Immunology Words:*

Books

Carter RL. A dictionary of dermatologic terms, 4th ed. Baltimore: Williams & Wilkins, 1992.

Kelley WN, Harris Jr. ED, Ruddy S, Sledge CB. Textbook of rheumatology, 4th ed. Philadelphia: WB Saunders Company, 1993.

Lance LL. Quick look drug book. Baltimore: Williams & Wilkins, 1996.

Leider M, Rosenblum Manual of allergy and immunology. McGraw-Hill 1968.

Mandell GL, Bennett JE, Dolin R. Principles and practice of infectious diseases, 4th ed. New York: Churchill Livingstone, 1995.

McCarty DJ, Koopman WJ, Arthritis and allied conditions: a textbook of rheumatology, 12th ed. Baltimore: Williams & Wilkins, 1993.

Middleton Jr. E, et al. Allergy: Principles and practice, 4th ed. St. Louis: Mosby-Yearbook, Inc., 1993.

Rietschel RL, Fowler Jr. JF. Fisher's contact dermatitis, 4th ed. Baltimore: Williams & Wilkins, 1995.

Pyle V. Current medical terminology, 5th ed. Modesto: Health Professions Institute, 1994.

Sams Jr. WM, Lynch PJ. Principles & Practice of Dermatology, 2nd ed. New York: Churchill Livingstone, 1996.

Sanders CV, Nesbitt Jr., LT. The skin and infection. Baltimore, Williams & Wilkins, 1995.

Sloane SB. The medical word book, 3rd ed. Philadelphia: WB Saunders Company, 1991.

Stedman's medical dictionary. 26th ed. Baltimore: Williams & Wilkins, 1995.

Stedman's medical & surgical equipment words. Baltimore: Williams & Wilkins, 1996.

Journals

Journal of Clinical Rheumatology, Baltimore, Williams & Wilkins, 1995–1996.

Clinical Pulmonary Medicine, Baltimore: Williams & Wilkins, 1994–1996.

Infectious Diseases in Clinical Practice, Baltimore: Williams & Wilkins, 1995–1996.

Internal Medicine. Montvale, NJ: Medical Economics, 1995–1996.

Journal of the American Association for Medical Transcription. Modesto: American Association for Medical Transcription, 1995–1996.

The Latest Word. Philadelphia: WB Saunders Company, 1994–1996.

MT Monthly. Gladstone, MO: Computer Systems Management, 1994–1996.

The Pediatric Infectious Disease Journal, Baltimore: Williams & Wilkins, 1995–1996.

Perspectives on the Medical Transcription Profession. Modesto: Health Professions Institute, 1993–1996.

A

A
A and D Ointment
A 2M

A
angstrom
Å unit

5a8
monoclonal antibody to CD4, 5a8

A-200 Pyrinate

AA
arachidonic acid
AA amyloidosis

AAP
American Academy of Pediatrics

AAV
adeno-associated virus

Ab
antibody

abalone

ABE
acute bacterial endocarditis

Abelcet

Abelson murine leukemia virus

ABG
arterial blood gas

abigne
erythema a.

abiotrophy

ablastin

ablative

abnormal DNA repair

abnormality
biochemical a.
calcinosis cutis, osteoma cutis, poikiloderma, and skeletal a.'s (COPS)
dental a.
a.'s of genitalia, retardation of growth, and deafness
immunochemical a.
microvascular a.
nail fold capillary loop a.
oral cavity a.
pigmentary a.
skeletal a.

abnutzung pigment

ABO
A. antigens
A. incompatibility

abortive
a. neurofibromatosis
a. transduction

abortus
Bacillus a.

ABPA
allergic bronchopulmonary aspergillosis
ABPA panel

abrade

abrasion
brush burn a.
mechanical a.
pleural a.

abrasive

Abrikosov tumor

abscess
brain a.
Brodie a.
cold a.
conglobate a.
cutaneous a.
eosinophilic a.
follicular a.
intraepidermal a.
mixed aerobic/anaerobic a.
Munro a.
mycobacterial a.
parafrenal a.
Pautrier a.
recurrent cutaneous a.
staphylococcal a.
stellate a.
sterile a.
subepidermal a.
subungual a.
sudoriparous a.
tuberculous a.

abscessus
Mycobacterium a.

absent
a. dermal component
a. tonsil

Absidia

absorbent gelling material (AGM)

Absorbine
A. Jock Itch
A. Jr. Antifungal

absorptiometry
dual-beam photon a.

1

absorptiometry *(continued)*
  dual-energy x-ray a. (DEXA)
  photon a.
absorption
  cutaneous a.
  external a.
  fluorescent treponemal
    antibody a. (FTA-ABS)
  nonspecific a.
  parenteral a.
  percutaneous a.
abtropfung
ACA
  anticardiolipin antibody
acacia
  a. tree
ACADERM patch test
Acanthamoeba
  A. astronyxis
  A. castellani
  A. culbertsoni
  A. glebae
  A. hatchetti
  A. palestinensis
  A. polyphaga
  A. rhysodes
Acanthaster
  A. planci
acanthoid
acantholysis
acantholytic
  a. dermatosis
  a. dyskeratoma
  a. dyskeratosis
acanthoma, pl. **acanthomata,**
  acanthomas
  a. adenoides cysticum
  clear cell a.
  Degos a.
  epidermolytic a.
  a. fissuratum
  intraepidermal a.
  pilar sheath a.
acanthorrhexis
acanthosis
  a. nigricans (AN)
acanthotic
  a. epidermal proliferation
acarian
acariasis
  demodectic a.
  psoroptic a.
  sarcoptic a.

acaricide
acarid
acaridiasis
Acarina
acarine dermatosis
acarinosis
acarodermatitis
  a. urticarioides
acarophobia
Acarus
  A. balatus
  A. folliculorum
  A. siro
acatalasia
accelerated
  a. reaction
  a. rejection
Accents system
accentuation
  follicular a.
  perifollicular a.
accessory
  a. auricle
  a. molecule
  a. muscle
  a. tragus
accident
  serum a.
accidental host
acclimatization
Accolate
AccuProbe system
Accutane
ACE
  Aerosol Cloud Enhancer
  angiotensin-converting enzyme
Ace bandage
Acedapsone
Acel-Imune
acellular pannus tissue
Acephen
acephylline
aceracear
Aceta
acetabuli
  protrusio a.
acetaminophen
  chlorpheniramine and a.
  chlorpheniramine,
    phenylpropanolamine, and a.
  a., chlorpheniramine, and
    pseudoephedrine
  a. and diphenhydramine

a. and isometheptene mucate
a. and phenyltoloxamine
phenyltoloxamine,
phenylpropanolamine, and a.
Acetasol HC Otic
acetate
aluminum a.
cortisone a.
cyproterone a.
dexamethasone a.
Florinef A.
fludrocortisone a.
hydrocortisone a.
Hydrocortone A.
mafenide a.
m-cresyl a.
megestrol a.
methylprednisolone a.
paramethasone a.
pirbuterol a.
sermorelin a.
acetazolamide
acetic
a. acid
a. acid, propanediol diacetate,
and hydrocortisone
acetone-insoluble antigen
acetonide
fluocinolone a.
triamcinolone a.
acetylation
a. of cellular protein
a. of serum protein
acetylcholine
a. depletion
acetylcholinesterase deficiency
acetylcysteine
acetylsalicylic acid (ASA)
acetyltransferase
chloramphenicol a. (CAT)
Achard-Thiers syndrome
Achenbach syndrome
Aches-N-Pain
Achilles tendon
Acholeplasma laidlawii
Achorion schoenleinii
achromasia

achromatosis
achromia
a. parasitica
a. unguium
achromians
incontinentia pigmenti a.
Achromobacter
A. *xylosoxidans*
achromoderma
achromotrichia
Achromycin
A. Ophthalmic
A. V Oral
acid
acetic a.
acetylsalicylic a. (ASA)
adenylic a.
a. agglutination
all-*trans*-retinoic a.
aluminum acetate and acetic a.
amino a.
aminobenzoic a.
δ-aminolevulinic a. (ALA)
amoxicillin and clavulanic a.
arachidonic a. (AA)
azelaic a.
battery a.
benzoic acid and salicylic a.
boric a.
cantharic a.
13-*cis*-retinoic a.
clavulanic a.
coal tar and salicylic a.
cytidine monophospho-N-acetyl
neuraminic a. (CMP-NANA)
deoxyribonucleic a. (DNA)
eicosapentaenoic a.
enteric-coated acetylsalicylic a.
(ECASA)
flufenamic a.
folic a.
folinic a.
fusidic a.
gamma-aminobutyric a.
(GABA)
glucuronic a.
guanylic a.

NOTES

3

acid *(continued)*
  hyaluronic a.
  hydrochloric a.
  hydroperoxyeicosatetraenoic a.
  α-hydroxy a.
  hydroxyeicosatetraenoic a.
  5-hydroxyindoleacetic a.
  iduronic a.
  infectious nucleic a.
  inosinic a.
  linoleic a.
  a. maltase
  mefenamic a.
  N-acetylneuraminic a.
  nalidixic a.
  octulosonic a.
  omega-3 fatty a.
  omega-6 fatty a.
  para-aminobenzoic a. (PABA)
  para-aminosalicylic a.
  phytanic a.
  plicatic a.
  retinoic a.
  ribonucleic a. (RNA)
  salicylic a. (SA)
  salicylic acid and lactic a.
  sodium citrate and citric a.
  sulfuric a.
  sulfur and salicylic a.
  Tc-dimercaptosuccinic a.
   (DMSA)
  ticarcillin and clavulanic a.
  tranexamic a.
  trichloroacetic a.
  undecylenic a.
  uric a.
Acidaminococcus fermentans
acidase
  antideoxyribonculeic a.
acid-fast
  a.-f. bacillus (AFB)
acidophilus
  Lactobacillus a.
  a. milk
acidosis
  lactic a.
  metabolic a.
  respiratory a.
aciduria
  orotic a.
Acinetobacter
  A. anitratus
  A. calcoaceticus

  A. calcoaceticus-baumannii
   complex
  A. lwoffi
Acintomadura
ACIP
  Advisory Committee on
  Immunization Practice
acitretin
ACLAb
  anticardiolipin antibody
ACLE
  acute cutaneous lupus erythematosus
Aclovate
  A. topical
acne
  a. albida
  a. artificialis
  a. atrophica
  a. bacillus
  bromide a.
  a. cachecticorum
  a. cheloidalis
  chlorine a.
  a. ciliaris
  colloid a.
  comedo a.
  common a.
  a. conglobata
  conglobate a.
  a. cosmetica
  cystic a.
  a. cystica
  a. decalvans
  a. detergicans
  a. erythematosa
  a. estivalis
  a. frontalis
  a. fulminans
  a. generalis
  halogen a.
  a. hypertrophica
  a. indurata
  a. inversa
  iodide a.
  a. keloid
  a. keloidalis
  a. keloidalis nuchae
  a. keratosa
  a. mechanica
  a. medicamentosa
  menstrual a.
  a. miliaris
  miliary a.

a. necrotica
a. necrotica miliaris
neonatal a.
a. neonatorum
nodulocystic a.
occupational a.
papular a.
a. papulosa
picker's a.
pomade a.
premenstrual a.
a. punctata
pustular a.
a. pustulosa
a. rosacea
a. scrofulosorum
a. simplex
steroid a.
summer a.
a. surgery
a. syphilitica
tar a.
a. tetrad
tropical a.
a. tropicalis
a. urticata
a. varioliformis
a. venenata
a. vulgaris
acné
a. chéloïdique
a. excoriée des jeunes filles
acneform, acneiform
a. dermatitis
a. eruption
a. lesion
a. syphilid
acneforme, acneiforme
erythema a.
acnegen
acnegenic
acneic
acneiform (*var. of* acneform)
acneiforme (*var. of* acneforme)
acne-pustulosis-hyperostosis-osteitis
acnes
Bacillus a.

Corynebacterium a.
Propionibacterium a.
acnitis
acomia
acoustic reflex threshold
acquired
a. agammaglobulinemia
a. biotin deficiency
a. cornification disorder
a. dermatosis
a. digital fibrokeratoma
a. disorder
a. generalized lipodystrophy
a. hemolytic anemia
a. hemolytic icterus
a. hemophilia
a. hypertrichosis lanuginosa
a. hypogammaglobulinemia
a. ichthyosis
a. immune deficiency
syndrome (AIDS)
a. immunity
a. immunodeficiency
a. immunodeficiency syndrome
(AIDS)
a. leukoderma
a. leukopathia
a. melanocytic nevus
a. nevus
a. partial face-sparing
lipodystrophy
a. pellicle
a. sensitivity
a. trichoepithelioma
a. tufted angioma
a. vascular disorder
acquisita
epidermolysis bullosa a. (EBA)
acquisitum
ACR
American College of Rheumatology
**Acradinium-ester-labeled nucleic
acid probe**
acral
a. erythema
a. lentiginous melanoma
a. vitiligo

NOTES

5

Acremonium
acrivastine/pseudoephedrine
acroangiodermatitis
acroasphyxia
acrocephalosyndactyly
acrochordon
acrocyanosis
acrodermatitis
  a. chronica atrophicans
  a. continua
  a. continua of Hallopeau
  a. enteropathica
  a. hiemalis
  papular a.
  a. papulosa infantum
  a. perstans
  pustular a.
  a. pustulosa
  a. vesiculosa tropica
acrodermatosis
acrodynia
acrodynic erythema
acrofacial vitiligo
acrogeria
acrohyperhidrosis
acrokeratoelastoidosis
acrokeratosis
  a. neoplastica
  paraneoplastic a.
  a. paraneoplastica
  a. verruciformis
  a. verruciformis of Hopf
acroleukopathy
acromegalic
  a. arthropathy
acromegaly
acromioclavicular
acromiodeltoideus
  nevus fuscoceruleus a.
acro-osteolysis
acropachy
  thyroid a.
acropachyderma
acropigmentation
acropustulosis
  a. of infancy
  infantile a.
acroscleroderma
acrosclerosis
acrospiroma
  eccrine a.
  giant eccrine a.
acrosyringium

acroterica
  morphea a.
Acrotheca aquaspersa
acrotrophodynia
acrylic acid allergy
Acsorex
act
  Coinage A.
  throwing a.
Actagen
  A. Syrup
  A. Tablet
ACTH
  adrenocorticotropic hormone
  ACTH therapy
Acthar
ActHBI
ActHIB vaccine
Acticel wound dressing
Actifed
  A. Allergy Tablet
  A. Tablet
Actimmune
Actin
  A. FSL
  A. monomers
actin-binding protein
Actinex
  A. topical
actinic
  a. burn
  a. cheilitis
  a. dermatitis
  a. elastosis
  a. granuloma
  a. keratosis
  a. porokeratosis
  a. prurigo
  a. purpura
  a. reticuloid
  a. reticuloid syndrome
actinica
  dermatitis a.
actinism
Actinobacillus
  A. *actinomycetemcomitans*
  A. *equuli*
  A. *hominis*
  A. *lignieresii*
  A. *suis*
  A. *ureae*
actinodermatitis
actinodermatosis

A

Actinomadura
   A. madurae
   A. pelletieri
Actinomyces
   A. bovis
   A. hominis
   A. israelii
   A. naeslundii
actinomycetemcomitans
   Actinobacillus a.
actinomycetoma
actinomycin
actinomycoma
actinomycosis
   cervical a.
actinomycotic
actinophage
actinotherapy
   ultraviolet a.
action
   mechanism of a.
activated
   a. macrophage
   a. partial thromboplastin time
   (APTT)
   a. vitamin K-dependent factor
activation
   complement a.
activator
   plasminogen a.
   polyclonal a.
active
   a. anaphylaxis
   a. immunity
   a. immunization
   a. joint
   a. pinocytosis
   a. prophylaxis
   a. range of motion
   a. sensitization
   a. transport
activin
activity
   ATPase a.
   complement a.
   increased sympathoadrenal a.
actomyosin

Actron
Acular
   A. Ophthalmic
acuminate
   a. papular syphilid
   a. wart
acuminatum, pl. acuminata
   condyloma a.
   condylomata a.
   papilloma a.
   verruca acuminata
acuminatus
   lichen ruber a.
acupuncture
acuta
   parapsoriasis lichenoides et
   varioliformis a.
   pityriasis lichenoides et
   varioliformis a. (PLEVA)
   pustulosis vacciniformis a.
   urticaria a.
acute
   a. allergic urticaria
   a. anaphylactic reaction
   a. anterior poliomyelitis
   a. asthma attack
   a. atrophic oral candidiasis
   a. atrophic paralysis
   a. attack
   a. bacterial endocarditis (ABE)
   a. bulbar poliomyelitis
   a. cellular rejection
   a. contagious conjunctivitis
   a. cutaneous leishmaniasis
   a. cutaneous lupus
   erythematosus (ACLE)
   a. decubitus ulcer
   a. disseminated histiocytosis
   a. disseminated myositis
   a. epidemic conjunctivitis
   a. epidemic leukoencephalitis
   a. epiglottitis
   a. febrile neutrophilic
   dermatosis
   a. flaccid paralysis (AFP)
   a. follicular conjunctivitis
   a. hemorrhagic edema

NOTES

7

acute *(continued)*
a. hemorrhagic
glomerulonephritis
a. herpes zoster
a. herpetic gingivostomatitis
a. hypersensitivity pneumonitis
a. idiopathic polyneuritis
a. idiopathic thrombocytopenic
purpura
a. infectious nonbacterial
gastroenteritis
a. inflammation (AI)
a. intermittent porphyria
a. interstitial nephritis
a. intravascular hemolysis
a. laryngotracheobronchitis
a. lupus erythematosus
a. lupus pneumonitis
a. meningococcemia
a. necrotizing encephalitis
a. necrotizing ulcerative
gingivitis
a. nephritis
a. otitis media (AOM)
a. paranasal sinusitis
a. paronychia
a. peritonitis
a. phase protein
a. phase reactants
a. phase reaction
a. physiology and chronic
health evaluation (APACHE)
a. primary hemorrhagic
meningoencephalitis
a. pulmonary reaction
a. radiation pneumonitis
a. respiratory failure (ARF)
a. retinal necrosis (ARN)
a. retroviral syndrome
a. rheumatic arthritis
a. rheumatic fever (ARF)
a. rheumatoid arthritis
a. rhinitis
a. scalp cellulitis
a. transfusion reaction
a. urticaria
a. vascular purpura
acutum
ulcus vulvae a.
acutus
pemphigus a.
acyclovir
ADA deficiency

Adagen
adamantinoma
adapalene gel
ADCC
antibody-dependent cell-mediated
cytotoxicity
Addison disease
addition-deletion mutation
additive
a. arthritis
food a.
addressin
addressing ligand
adductor digiti quinti
Aden
A. fever
A. ulcer
adenine
adenitis
adeno-associated virus (AAV)
adenocarcinoma
aggressive digital papillary a.
(ADPA)
colonic a.
eccrine a.
Lucké a.
adenoepithelioma
adenoid
adenoidal facies
adenoidal-pharyngeal-conjunctival
(A-P-C)
a.-p.-c. virus
adenoidectomy
adeno-like
gallus a.-l. (GAL)
adenoma
aggressive digital papillary a.
(ADPA)
apocrine a.
sebaceous a.
a. sebaceum
adenomatoid
adenopathy
hilar a.
adenosatellite virus
adenosine
a. deaminase
a. deaminase deficiency
a. diphosphate (ADP)
a. monophosphate (AMP)
a. triphosphate (ATP)
Adenoviridae
adenovirus

A

adenovirus-mediated
  a.-m. gene transfer
  a.-m. transfer
adenylate cyclase toxin
adenylic acid
adenylosuccinic acid synthetase
adequate
  a. hydration
  a. urine output
adermal
adermia
  a. congenita
adermic
adermogenesis
adherence
  a. assay
  immune a.
adhesin-receptor interaction
adhesins
adhesion
  a. aid
  corneocyte a.
  keratinocytic a.
  a. molecule
  a. phenomenon
  a. protein
  a. test
adhesive
  a. capsulitis
  Scanpor acrylate a.
adiaphoresis
adiaphoretic
adipometer
adiponecrosis subcutanea
  neonatorum
adiposa
  blepharoptosis a.
  seborrhea a.
adiposis dolorosa
adiposity
  painful a.
adiposum
  sclerema a.
adjuvant
  Freund complete a.
  Freund incomplete a.
  a. vaccine

Adlone injection
adnata
  alopecia a.
adnexa
  ocular a.
adnexal
  a. carcinoma
  a. tumor
adolescent eczema
adoptive
  a. immunity
  a. immunotherapy
ADP
  adenosine diphosphate
  ALA dehydratase deficiency
  porphyria
ADPA
  aggressive digital papillary
  adenocarcinoma
  aggressive digital papillary adenoma
adrenal
  a. cortex disorder
  a. insufficiency
Adrenalin
α-adrenergic
  -a. agonist
  -a. blocking agent
β-adrenergic agonist
adrenergic drug
adrenocortical
  a. failure
  a. insufficiency
adrenocorticosteroid
  a. therapy
adrenocorticotropic
  a. hormone (ACTH)
  a. hormone therapy
Adriamycin
adrostenedione
Adrucil injection
Adson
  A. test
  A. toothed forceps
adsorbed
  tetanus toxoid, a.
adsorbent

NOTES

9

Adsorbotear
   A. Ophthalmic solution
adsorption
   immune a.
adult
   a. bullous dermatosis
   a. eczema
   a. respiratory distress syndrome
   (ARDS)
   a. T-cell leukemia (ATL)
   a. T-cell lymphoma
   a. T-cell lymphoma-leukemia
   a. tuberculosis
adultorum
   scleredema a.
adult-type rheumatoid arthritis
adventitia
adventitious cyst
adverse drug reaction
Advil
   Children's A.
   A. Cold & Sinus Caplets
Advisory Committee on
   Immunization Practice (ACIP)
Aedes
   A. aegypti
aegleria invadens
Aeroaid
aeroallergen
   mold a.
Aerobacter
aerobe
   obligate a.
aerobic
AeroBid
AeroBid-M
   A.-M. Oral Aerosol Inhaler
aerobiology
Aerochamber
   A. nebulizer
aerodigestive
aerogen
aerogenes
   Pasteurella a.
aerogenesis
aerogenic
aeroirritant
Aerolate III
Aerolate JR
Aerolate SR S
aerometric study
Aeromonas
   A. caviae

A. hydrophila
A. septicemia
A. shigelloides
A. sobria
A. veronii
aerophil
aerophilic
aeroplankton
Aeroseb-Dex
aerosol
   Brethaire Inhalation A.
   A. Cloud Enhancer (ACE)
   DEY albuterol inhalation a.
   Duo-Medihaler A.
   Fluro-Ethyl A.
   ipratropium bromide a.
   monodisperse a.
   Nasalide Nasal A.
   a. spray
   Tilade Inhalation A.
   Virazole A.
aerosolization
aerosolized pollutant exposure
AeroSonic personal ultrasonic
   nebulizer
AeroTech II nebulizer
AeroZoin
aeruginosa
   Pseudomonas a.
aestival (*var. of* estival)
aestivale (*var. of* estivale)
aestivalis (*var. of* estivalis)
AF-1 antigen
AF-2 antigen
AFB
   acid-fast bacillus
affective disorder
afferent nerve fiber
affinity
   a. antibody
   a. maturation
Afipia felis
AFP
   acute flaccid paralysis
African
   A. Burkitt lymphoma
   A. hemorrhagic fever
   A. histoplasmosis
   A. honeybee
   A. horse sickness
   A. horse sickness virus
   A. swine fever
   A. swine fever virus

A. tick typhus
A. tick virus
A. trypanosomiasis
Africanized honeybee sting
African-variety Kaposi sarcoma
Afrin
A. Nasal solution
A. Tablet
Aftate
after
before and a. (B&A)
aftosa
afzelii
Borrelia a.
Ag
antigen
agalactiae
Streptococcus a.
agammaglobulinemia
acquired a.
secondary a.
Swiss type a.
transient a.
X-linked a.
agar
BCYE a.
a. diffusion assay
a. gel diffusion
Kirby-Bauer a.
Löwenstein-Jensen a.
Sabouraud a.
agenesia
agenesis
pilorum a.
pulmonary a.
agent
α-adrenergic blocking a.
alkylating a.
antifibrinolytic a.
antihypertensive a.
antihyperuricemic a.
antimalarial a.
antipruritic a.
antirheumatic a.
Bittner a.
chelating a.
chemical a.

chemotherapy a.
chimpanzee coryza a. (CCA)
cholinergic a.
coloring a.
cooling a.
cytotoxic a.
delta a.
denaturing a.
Eaton a.
epsilon-aminocaproic a.
F a.
fertility a.
foamy a.
hemostatic a.
immunosuppressive a.
keratolytic a.
LDH a.
LeukoScan diagnostic a.
macrolide antimicrobial a.
MS-1 a.
MS-2 a.
noncorticosteroid anti-
inflammatory a.
Norwalk a.
Norwalk-like a.
prophylaxis a.
psychotropic a.
reovirus-like a.
sclerosing a.
topical hemostatic a.
transforming a.
Wor Ditchling a.
age-related osteoporosis
agglutinate
agglutinating antibody
agglutination
acid a.
bacteriogenic a.
cold a.
cross a.
false a.
group a.
immune a.
indirect a.
latex a.
latex particle a.
mixed a.

NOTES

11

agglutination *(continued)*
  nonimmune a.
  passive a.
  reversed passive latex a.
  spontaneous a.
agglutinative
agglutinin
  blood group a.
  chief a.
  cold a.
  cross-reacting a.
  febrile a.
  flagellar a.
  group a.
  H a.
  immune a.
  incomplete a.
  major a.
  minor a.
  O a.
  partial a.
  plant a.
  saline a.
  serum a.
  somatic a.
  warm a.
  Yersinia pseudotuberculosis a.
agglutinogen
  blood group a.
  T a.
agglutinogenic
agglutinophilic
agglutinoscope
agglutogen
agglutogenic
aggrecan
  a. CS/KS
aggregate
  a. anaphylaxis
  IgG-RF-complement a.
aggregometry
aggressin
aggressive
  a. cell cluster
  a. digital papillary
    adenocarcinoma (ADPA)
  a. digital papillary adenoma
    (ADPA)
  a. infantile fibromatosis
aging
  photo a.
  premature a.

AGM
  absorbent gelling material
agminata
agminated
agonist
  α-adrenergic a.
  β-adrenergic a.
  bronchoactive a.
agranulocytosis
  feline a.
agretope
agria
  prurigo a.
agrius
  lichen a.
Agrobacterium
  A. radiobacter
  A. tumefaciens
A-hydroCort
AI
  acute inflammation
aid
  adhesion a.
AIDS
  acquired immune deficiency
    syndrome
  acquired immunodeficiency
    syndrome
  AIDS vaccine
AIDS-related
  A.-r. complex (ARC)
  A.-r. virus (ARV)
AIHA
  autoimmune hemolytic anemia
AIL
  angioimmunoblastic
    lymphadenopathy
ainhum
air
  a. bronchogram
  a. cleaner
  a. coil
  high-efficiency particulate a.
    (HEPA)
  a. pollution
  a. pollution control
  a. spora
  a. trapping
air conditioning
airborne
  a. spore
  a. transmission
Airet

air-fluidized bed
airspace
    a. consolidation
    peripheral a.
    a. process
airway
    a. bacterial colonization
    a. pressure release ventilation
    (APRV)
    a. resistance
    a. responsiveness
airways disease
AITP
    autoimmune thrombocytopenia
Ajellomyces dermatitidis
Akabane virus
akamushi
    a. disease
    Leptotrombidium a.
    Trombicula a.
akari
    Rickettsia a.
AK-Chlor Ophthalmic
AK-Cide Ophthalmic
AKD
    atypical Kawasaki disease
AK-Dex Ophthalmic
AK-Dilate Ophthalmic solution
akeratosis
AK-Homatropine Ophthalmic
AK-Nefrin Ophthalmic solution
Akne-Mycin
    A.-M. topical
AK-Neo-Dex Ophthalmic
AK-Poly-Bac Ophthalmic
AK-Pred Ophthalmic
AkroTech mattress
AK-Spore
    A.-S. H.C. Ophthalmic
    Ointment
    A.-S. H.C. Ophthalmic
    suspension
    A.-S. H.C. Otic
    A.-S. Ophthalmic Ointment
AK-Sulf Ophthalmic
AKTob Ophthalmic
AK-Tracin Ophthalmic

AK-Trol Ophthalmic
Akwa Tears solution
AL
    A. amyloidosis
    A. protein
ALA
    δ-aminolevulinic acid
    ALA dehydratase deficiency
    porphyria (ADP)
Ala-Cort
Aladdin infant flow system
alae nasi
alanine aminotransferase
alanyl-tRNA synthetase
Ala-Quin topical
Ala-Scalp
alastrim
alba
    linea a.
    miliaria a.
    morphea a.
    phlegmasia a.
    pityriasis a.
    stria a.
albae
Albendazole
albendazole
    a. sulfoxide
albicans
    Candida a.
    linea a.
    Monilia a.
    stria a.
albicantes
    lineae a.
albida
    acne a.
albidum
    atrophoderma a.
albimanus
    Anopheles a.
albinism
    brown a.
    brown oculocutaneous a.
    circumscribed a.
    cutaneous a.
    localized a.

NOTES

albinism *(continued)*
  minimal-pigment
    oculocutaneous a.
  Nettleship-Falls ocular a.
  ocular a.
  oculocutaneous a.
  red a.
  rufous a.
  rufous oculocutaneous a.
  temperature-sensitive
    oculocutaneous a.
  type IA oculocutaneous a.
  type IB oculocutaneous a.
  type II ocular a.
  type II oculocutaneous a.
  type I-MP oculocutaneous a.
  type I ocular a.
  type I oculocutaneous a.
  type I-TS oculocutaneous a.
  tyrosinase-negative
    oculocutaneous a.
  tyrosinase-positive
    oculocutaneous a.
  tyrosinase-related
    oculocutaneous a.
  yellow a.
  yellow oculocutaneous a.
albino
albinotic
alboatrum
  Verticillium a.
Albright
  A. disease
  A. hereditary osteodystrophy
  A. syndrome
albumin
  amoxicilloyl-human serum a.
    (AX-HSA)
  ampicillin-human serum a.
    (AMP-HSA)
  Bence Jones a.
  low plasma a.
  penicillin-penicilloyl human
    serum a. (PPO-HSA)
albus
  lichen a.
  Staphylococcus a.
albuterol
  a. sulfate syrup
Alcaligenes
  A. denitrificans
  A. faecalis
  A. odorans

  A. piechaudii
  A. xylosoxidans
alclometasone dipropionate
alcohol
  benzyl a.
  isopropyl a.
  wool wax a.
Alcyonidrium
alder
  red a.
  a. tree
aldesleukin
Aldrich syndrome
alendronate
  a. sodium
Aleppo boil
aleukemic leukemia
Aleutian
  A. mink disease
  A. mink disease virus
Aleve
alexandrite laser
alexin
  a. unit
Alezzandrini syndrome
alfa
  epoetin a.
alfa-2a
  interferon a.
alfa-2b
  interferon a.
alfalfa
  a. grass
Alferon N
algid stage
alginate dressing
Algisorb wound dressing
alglucerase
algorithm
  Dermatologic Diagnostic A.
  diagnostic a.
  problem-oriented a.
Alibert disease
aliquant
aliquot
alizarin red S stain
Alkaban-AQ
alkaline phosphatase and
  pyrophosphate
alkalinization
alkali patch test
alkaloid
  Vinca a.

alkaptonuria
Alka-Seltzer Plus Cold Liqui-Gels
  Capsule
alkylating
  a. agent
  a. therapy
Allegra
allele
  HLA a.
Aller-Chlor Oral
Allercon Tablet
Allerest
  A. 12 Hour Nasal solution
  A. Maximum Strength
Allerfrin
  A. Syrup
  A. Tablet
Allergan Ear Drops
allergen
  a. contact
  environmental a.
  epidermal a.
  a. exposure
  flux a.
  inhalant a.
  a. inhalation challenge test
  Lolium perenne a.
  occupational a.
allergenic
  a. extract
allergen-induced
  a.-i. asthma
  a.-i. mediator release
allergic
  a. angiitis
  a. angioedema
  a. bronchopulmonary
   aspergillosis (ABPA)
  a. conjunctivitis
  a. contact dermatitis
  a. coryza
  a. crease
  a. diathesis
  a. eczema
  a. eczematous contact-type
   dermatitis
  a. extract

  a. facies
  a. granulomatosis
  a. granulomatous arteritis
  a. importance
  a. inflammation
  a. manifestation
  a. nonthrombocytopenic purpura
  a. purpura
  a. reaction
  a. rhinitis
  a. rhinoconjunctivitis
  a. salute
  a. sensitivity
  a. shiner
  a. stomatitis
  a. urticaria
  a. vasculitis
allergin
allergist
allergization
allergized
allergoid
allergologic
allergosis
allergy
  acrylic acid a.
  atopic a.
  bacterial a.
  car a.
  cold a.
  contact a.
  delayed a.
  drug a.
  food a.
  IgE-mediated food a.
  immediate a.
  insulin a.
  latent a.
  nickel a.
  ocular a.
  physical a.
  polyvalent a.
  seasonal a.
  a. unit (AU)
AllerMax Oral
Allerphed Syrup
Allerprick needle

NOTES

A

15

Allescheria boydii
alligator skin
alloantibody
alloantigen
allochromasia
Allodermanyssus
    A. sanguineus
AlloDerm universal dermal tissue graft
allogenic, allogeneic
allograft
    a. rejection
allogroup
allophenic
alloplast
allopurinol
allosensitization
allotope
allotransplantation
allotrichia circumscripta
allotype
    Gm a.'s
    InV a.'s
    Km a.
allotypic
    a. determinants
    a. marker
Allpyral
allscale
all-*trans*-retinoic acid
allylamine
almond
aloe
    Cortaid with a.
    Dermtex HC with a.
Alomide
    A. Ophthalmic
alopecia
    a. adnata
    androgenic a.
    a. areata
    a. capitis totalis
    Celsus a.
    cicatricial a.
    a. cicatrisata
    a. circumscripta
    a. congenitalis
    a. disseminata
    drug-induced a.
    female pattern a.
    a. follicularis
    a. furfuracea
    a. generalisata

    a. hereditaria
    hot comb a.
    Jonston a.
    a. leprotica
    a. liminaris
    a. liminaris frontalis
    lipedematous a.
    male pattern a.
    a. marginalis
    a. marginata
    a. medicamentosa
    moth-eaten a.
    a. mucinosa
    a. neoplastica
    a. neurotica
    nonscarring a.
    patterned a.
    a. pityrodes
    postpartum a.
    a. prematura
    premature a.
    a. presenilis
    pressure a.
    scarring a.
    a. senilis
    a. symptomatica
    syphilitic a.
    a. syphilitica
    tick bite a.
    a. totalis
    toxic a.
    a. toxica
    traction a.
    traumatic a.
    a. triangularis
    a. triangularis congenitalis
    a. universalis
alopecic
alpha
    a. adrenergic stimulation
    a. chain
    a., delta
    a., delta sleep anomaly
    a. fetoprotein
    a. heavy-chain disease
    interferon a. (IFN-α)
    a. lactalbumin
    a. nonrapid eye movement (alpha-NREM)
    5 a. reductase
    a. wave intrusion
alpha-2 globulin

alpha-antitrypsin
    serum a.-a.
alpha-interferon 3
alpha-lactalbumin
alpha-latrotoxin
alpha-NREM
    alpha nonrapid eye movement
    alpha-NREM sleep
Alphatrex
Alphavirus
alphos
alprazolam
ALS
    amyotrophic lateral sclerosis
    antilymphocyte serum
alteration
    ecologic a.
    metabolic a.
    red cell membrane a.
Alternaria
    A. mold
    A. *tenuis*
alternate-day therapy
aluminum
    a. acetate
    a. acetate and acetic acid
    a. chloride
    a. chloride hexahydrate
    a. Finn chamber
alum-precipitated
    a.-p. preparation
    a.-p. pyridine-extracted pollen
      extract
Alupent
alvei
    Bacillus a.
    Hafnia a.
alveolar
    a. capillary
    a. infiltration by histiocyte
    a. macrophage
    a. ventilation
    a. ventilation per minute
alveolar-arterial oxygen gradient
alveolar-septal amyloidosis
alveoli (*pl. of* alveolus)

alveolitis
    cryptogenic fibrosing a. (CFA)
    diffuse fibrosing a.
    extrinsic allergic a.
    occupational allergic a.
alveolointerstitial
alveolus, pl. **alveoli**
    ventilated a.
ALW
    arch-loop-whorl system
alymphoplasia
    Nezelof type of thymic a.
    thymic a.
amalgam
    dental a.
    a. tattoo
amantadine
    a. hydrochloride
Am antigen
Amapari virus
amaranth
    green a.
amaranth-chenopod
Ambi 10
AmBisome
Amblyomma
    A. *americanum*
    A. *cajennense*
    A. *hebraeum*
amboceptor
    a. unit
Amboyna button
ambulans
    ulcus a.
ambulant erysipelas
ambustion
ambustionis
    dermatitis a.
amcinonide
Amcort
amdinocillin
Ameba histolytica
amebiasis
    a. cutis
amebic
    a. ulcer
ameboma

NOTES

amelanotic
  a. melanoma
amelioration
Americaine
American
  A. Academy of Pediatrics (AAP)
  A. cockroach
  A. College of Rheumatology (ACR)
  A. elm
  A. elm tree
  A. leishmaniasis
  A. Rheumatism Association (ARA)
  A. Rheumatism Association index
  A. trypanosomiasis
americanum
  Amblyomma a.
americanus
  Necator a.
amerospore
Amesec
A-methaPred injection
amiantacea
  pityriasis a.
  tinea a.
amiantaceous
  a. crust
amicrobic
amidophosphoribosyltransferase
amifloxacin
amikacin
  a. sulfate
Amikin injection
amine
amino
  a. acid
  a. acid metabolism
  a. ethyl ethanolamine
aminoacyl-tRNA synthetase
aminobenzoic acid
aminoglycoside
δ-aminolevulinic acid (ALA)
Amino-Opti-E Oral
aminopenicillin
aminophylline
  a., amobarbital, and ephedrine
aminopterin syndrome
aminosalicylate sodium
aminosidine
  a. sulfate

aminotransferase
  alanine a.
amiodarone pigmentation
Ami-Tex LA
Amitril
amitriptyline
  a. hydrochloride
ammonia rash
ammonium
  quaternary a.
amnioma
A-mode ultrasound
amorolfine
amorphous
  a. parenchymal opacification
  a. substance
amoxicillin
  a. and clavulanic acid
amoxicillin/clavulanate (AMX/CL)
  a. suspension
amoxicilloyl-human serum albumin (AX-HSA)
Amoxil
AMP
  adenosine monophosphate
amphimicrobe
Amphocil
amphophilous
amphotericin
  a. B colloidal dispersion
  a. B lipid complex injection
  a. B liposomal formulation
amphotericin B
amphotropic virus
AMP-HSA
  ampicillin-human serum albumin
ampicillin
  a. and probenecid
  a. and sulbactam
ampicillin-human serum albumin (AMP-HSA)
amplification
  a. assay
  HBV bDNA signal a.
  human immunodeficiency virus DNA a.
Amplified Mycobacterium Tuberculosis Direct Test
amplifier host
amputating ulcer
α-MSH
amstelodami
  Aspergillus a

AMX/CL
amoxicillin/clavulanate
AMX/CL suspension
amyctic
amyloid
a. A protein
cutaneous a.
a. degeneration
a. disease
primary a.
a. Q
secondary a.
systemic a.
a. tumor
amyloidosis
AA a.
AL a.
alveolar-septal a.
bullous a.
a. cutis
focal a.
hemodialysis-associated a.
hereditary cardiopathic a.
immune-derived a.
immunocyte-derived a.
lichen a.
lichenoid a.
localized cutaneous a.
macular a.
mediastinal a.
neuropathic a.
nodular a.
nodular pulmonary a.
parenchymal a.
pleural a.
polyneuropathic a.
primary systemic a.
pseudotumoral mediastinal a.
pulmonary a.
secondary systemic a.
tracheobronchial a.
amyloidotic nephropathy
amyopathic
amyotrophic lateral sclerosis (ALS)
AN
acanthosis nigricans

ANA
antinuclear antibody
speckled-pattern ANA
anabolic steroid
anabrosis
anabrotic
Anacin
anaemicus (*var. of* anemicus)
anaerobe
anaerobic
a. bacterial arthritis
a. *Bifidobacterium*
a. cellulitis
Anaerobiospirillum
anaerobius
Peptostreptococcus a.
Anafranil
anagen
a. effluvium
a. phase
Ana-Guard
Anahelp
Ana-Kit
anallergic
analog
semisynthetic a.
analogous
analogue
purine a.
Analpram
analysis
displacement a.
dual-fluorescence a.
gait a.
immunofluorescence a.
post hoc a.
quantitative immunoglobulin a.
saturation a.
spectral a.
ultrastructural a.
analyte
analyzer
Electra 1000C coagulation a.
Malvern a.
MiniOX 1A oxygen a.

NOTES

19

analyzer *(continued)*
   Opti 1 portable pH/blood
     gas a.
   SPART a.
Anamine Syrup
anamnestic
   a. reaction
   a. response
ananaphylaxis
ANAP
   anionic neutrophil activating peptide
anaphylactic
   a. antibody
   a. crisis
   a. hypersensitivity reaction
   a. intoxication
   a. reaction
   a. shock
   a. state
anaphylactica
   enteritis a.
anaphylactogen
anaphylactogenesis
anaphylactogenic
anaphylactoid
   a. crisis
   a. purpura
   a. reaction
   a. shock
anaphylatoxin
   C3 a. (C3a)
   a. inactivator
   a. peptide
anaphylaxis
   active a.
   aggregate a.
   antiserum a.
   chronic a.
   controlled a.
   drug a.
   eosinophil chemotactic factor
    of a. (ECF-A)
   fire ant a.
   generalized a.
   Hymenoptera venom a.
   inflammatory factor of a. (IF-
    A)
   inverse a.
   local a.
   passive a.
   passive cutaneous a. (PCA)
   penicillin-induced a.
   pharmacologic mediators of a.

   reversed a.
   reversed passive a.
   slow-reacting factor of a.
    (SRF-A)
   slow-reacting substance of a.
    (SRS-A)
   systemic a.
anaphylotoxin
anaplasia
Anaplex Liquid
Anaprox
anatomical
   a. tubercle
   a. wart
anatoxic
anatoxin
anatripsis
anatriptic
Anatuss
Anavar
ANCA
   antineutrophilic cytoplasmic
    antibody
Ancef
Ancobon
ancylostoma
   A. braziliense
   A. caninum
   a. dermatitis
   A. duodenale
ancylostomiasis
   cutaneous a.
   a. cutis
andersoni
   Dermacentor a.
androgen
androgenic alopecia
anemia
   acquired hemolytic a.
   aregenerative a.
   autoimmune hemolytic a.
    (AIHA)
   chronic hemolytic a.
   congenital a.
   dermatopathic a.
   drug-related
    immunohemolytic a.
   equine infectious a.
   Fanconi a.
   hypochromic normocytic a.
   iron deficiency a.
   microangiopathic hemolytic a.
   neonatal a.

a. neonatorum
pernicious a.
severe a.
sickle cell a.
anemic halo
anemicus, anaemicus
nevus a.
anemone
sea a.
anemophilous
anergic
a. leishmaniasis
anergy
native a.
natural a.
negative a.
nonspecific a.
peripheral a.
positive a.
specific a.
in vitro a.
Anestacon
anesthesia
Madajet XL local a.
anesthetic
intradermal a.
a. leprosy
preoperative a.
topical a.
anetoderma
a. of Jadassohn
Jadassohn-Pellizzari a.
Schweninger-Buzzi a.
a. of Schweninger-Buzzi
a. scleroatrophy
aneuploidy
DNA a.
ANF
antinuclear factor
Angelman syndrome
angel wing deformity
angiectodes
nevus a.
angiitis
allergic a.
choroidal a.
Churg-Strauss a.

granulomatous a.
hypersensitivity a.
a. livedo reticularis
necrotizing a.
non-necrotizing a.
systemic hypersensitivity a.
angina
herpetic a.
Ludwig a.
Vincent a.
anginose scarlatina
angioblastic lymphadenopathy
angiocentric lymphoma
angiodestructive lymphoma
angioedema
allergic a.
episodic a.
hereditary a. (HAE)
hereditary vibratory a.
a. profile
vibratory a.
angioedema-urticaria-eosinophilia
syndrome
angioendotheliomatosis
malignant a.
proliferating systematized a.
reactive a.
angiogenesis
a. inhibitor
angiography
angioid streak
angioimmunoblastic
lymphadenopathy (AIL)
angioinvasive lesion
angiokeratoma
circumscriptum a.
a. corporis diffusum
a. corporis diffusum universale
a. of Fordyce
localized a.
a. of Mibelli
verrucous a.
angiokeratosis, pl. angiokeratoses
angioleiomyoma
angiolipoma
angiolupoid
angiolymphatic invasion

NOTES

angiolymphoid
  a. hyperplasia
  a. hyperplasia with eosinophilia
angioma
  acquired tufted a.
  capillary a.
  a. cavernosum
  cavernous a.
  cherry a.
  keratotic a.
  senile a.
  serpiginosum a.
  a. simplex
  spider a.
  strawberry a.
  superficial a.
angiomatosis
  bacillary a.
  cutaneomeningospinal a.
  meningo-oculofacial a.
angiomyoneuroma
angioneuromyoma
angioneurotica
  purpura a.
angioneurotic edema
angioproliferative lesion
angiosarcoma
Angiostrongylus costaricensis
angiotensin-converting enzyme (ACE)
angle
  Lovibond a.
angry
  a. back reaction
  a. back syndrome
angstrom, Angström (A)
Angström unit (A unit)
angular
  a. cheilitis
  a. conjunctivitis
  a. stomatitis
anhidrosis
  thermal a.
  thermogenic a.
anhidrotic
  a. ectodermal dysplasia
anhydride
  phthalic a.
  terpine a.
  trimellitic a.
anhydrous
  a. facial foundation
  a. theophylline

ani
  pruritus a.
anicteric virus hepatitis
animal
  control a.
  conventional a.
  a. dander
  a. dander sensitivity
  a. hair
  Houssay a.
  normal a.
  a. scabies
  sentinel a.
  a. toxin
  a. virus
anionic
  a. detergents
  a. neutrophil activating peptide (ANAP)
anisa
  Legionella a.
anisakiasis
Anisakis
anitratus
  Acinetobacter a.
Anitschkow myocyte
ankle
  retinacula of a.
ankylosing spondylitis (AS)
ankylosis
anlage
annual bluegrass
annular
  a. erythema
  a. erythematous plaque
  a. lesion
  a. lichen planus
  a. lipoatrophy
  a. syphilid
annulare
  erythema a.
  generalized granuloma a.
  granuloma a.
  localized granuloma a.
  perforating granuloma a.
  subcutaneous granuloma a.
annularis
  leukotrichia a.
  lichen a.
  lichen planus a.
  lipoatrophia a.
  psoriasis a.

annulata
thrix a.
annulatus, pl. annulati
pili a.
pseudopilus a.
annulus
a. migrans
ano
fistula in a.
anogenital
a. disorder
a. epidermal cyst
a. pilar cyst
a. sebaceous cyst
a. vestibular cyst
a. vestibular papilla
anomaly
alpha, delta sleep a.
nevoid a.
reticulate pigmented a.
sleep a.
anonychia
Anopheles
A. *albimanus*
A. *freeborni*
A. *funestus*
A. *gambiae*
anorexia
anoxia
focal a.
anserina
cutis a.
anserine
a. bursitis
ant
a. bite
black a.
fire a.
red a.
red imported fire a.
a. sting
antagonism
bacterial a.
antagonist
calmodulin a.
insulin a.
leukotriene a.

recombinant human interleukin-1 receptor a.
antecubital fossa
antemortem
antenna, pl. antennae
Antense anti-tension device
anterior
a. synechia formation
a. uveitis
anteriores
limbi palpebrales a.
anthelotic
anthema
anthesis
Anthopsis deltoidea
anthracis
Bacillus a.
anthracoid
Anthra-Derm
anthralin
anthramucin
anthrax
cutaneous a.
a. toxin
anthropi
Ochrobacterium a.
anthroponotic cutaneous leishmaniasis
anthropophaga
Cordylobia a.
anti-A antibody
antiadhesin antibody
antiagglutinin
antialexin
antiallergic
antianaphylaxis
antiandrogen
antiantibody
antiantitoxin
antiarachnolysin
antiautolysin
anti-B4 blocked ricin
antibacterial
a. therapy
anti-B antibody
anti-basement
a.-b. membrane antibody

NOTES

anti-basement *(continued)*
   a.-b. membrane antibody-
     induced glomerulonephritis
   a.-b. membrane
     glomerulonephritis
   a.-b. membrane nephritis
antibiogram
antibiont
antibiosis
AntibiOtic
   A. Otic
antibiotic
   a. enterocolitis
   a. protein
   a. sensitivity
   a. sensitivity test
antibiotic-associated colitis
antibiotic-resistant
antibodies
   HIV neutralizing a.
antibody (Ab)
   affinity a.
   agglutinating a.
   anaphylactic a.
   anti-A a.
   antiadhesin a.
   anti-B a.
   anti-basement membrane a.
   anticardiolipin a. (ACA,
     ACLAb)
   anti-CD4 a.
   anti-CD54 a.
   anti-centromere a.
   anti-CMV a.
   anti-D anti-Rh a.
   anti-DNA a.
   anti-DNA-topoisomerase I a.
   anti-EBV a.
   anti-HB$_c$ a.
   anti-HB$_e$ a.
   anti-HB$_s$ a.
   antihistone a.
   antihistone-(H2A-
     H2B)/deoxyribonucleic acid
     complex a.
   anti-idiotype a.
   anti-Jo-1 a.
   anti-Jp-1 a.
   anti-70K a.
   anti-Ku a.
   anti-La a.
   antilymphocyte a.
   anti-melanocyte a.

anti-Mi-2 nuclear a.
antineuronal a.
antineutrophilic cytoplasmic a.
   (ANCA)
antinuclear a. (ANA)
anti-nuclear matrix a.
antiparvovirus 19 a.
antiphospholipid a. (APLA)
anti-PM-Scl a.
antipneumococcal a.
anti-ribosome a.
anti-RNA pol I a.
anti-RNP a.
anti-Ro a.
antirubella a.
anti-S a.
anti-Scl-70 a.
antiscleroderma 70 a. (anti-Scl-
   70)
anti-Sm a.
anti-Smith a.
anti-smooth muscle a.
anti-SRP a.
anti-SS-A a.
anti-SS-B a.
anti-Th a.
antithyroid microsomal a.
anti-topoisomerase I a.
anti-U1 RNP a.
anti-U3 RNP a.
avidity a.
bivalent a.
blocking a.
blood group a.
BMZ a.
cell-bound a.
CF a.
chimeric a.'s
cold a.
cold-reactive a.
a. combining site
complement-fixing a.
complete a.
cross-reacting a.
cytophilic a.
cytotropic a.
a. deficiency
a. deficiency disease
a. deficiency syndrome
direct fluorescent a.
Donath-Landsteiner a.
a. dysfunction

Epstein-Barr virus-induced
early a.
Escherichia coli
polysaccharide a.
a. excess
fluorescent a.
fluorescent antimembrane a.
(FAMA)
Forssman a.
group A carbohydrate a.
hemagglutinating a.
a. to hepatitis B core antigen
(HB$_c$Ab, HBcAb)
a. to hepatitis B e antigen
(HB$_e$Ab, HBeAb)
a. to hepatitis B surface
antigen (HB$_s$Ab, HBsAb)
heterocytotropic a.
heterogenetic a.
heterophil a., heterophile a.
histone-DNA a.
homocytotropic a.
human anti-CMV a.
idiotype a.
IgA a.
IgE a.
IgG a.
IgM a.
IgM anticardiolipin a.
immobilizing a.
incomplete a.
indirect fluorescent a.
inhibiting a.
inhibition fluorescent a.
lymphocytotoxic a.
monoclonal a. (MAB, MoAb)
native type anti-DNA a.
natural a.
neutralizing a.
nonprecipitable a.
nonprecipitating a.
normal a.
P-K a.'s
polyclonal a.
polynucleotide a.
Prausnitz-Küstner a.
precipitating a.

pre-existing a.
prophylactic a.
r24 a.
reaginic a.
serum anti-glomerular-basement-
membrane a.
single-stranded anti-DNA a.
thyroid-stimulating a.
treponema-immobilizing a.
treponemal a.
univalent a.
U1 RNP a.
Vi a.
Wassermann a.
antibody-dependent cell-mediated
cytotoxicity (ADCC)
anti-C3 assay
anticardiolipin
a. antibody (ACA, ACLAb)
a. antibody syndrome
anti-CD4 antibody
anti-CD54 antibody
anti-centromere antibody
anti-Centruroides antivenin
anticholinergic drug
α_1**-antichymotrypsin**
anti-CMV
anticytomegalovirus
anti-CMV antibody
anticoagulant
circulating a.
lupus a. (LA)
anticomplement
anticomplementary
a. factor
a. serum
anticontagious
anticonvulsant
hydantoin a.
anticytokine
anticytomegalovirus (anti-CMV)
anticytotoxin
anti-D
a.-D. anti-Rh antibody
a.-D. enzyme-linked
immunosorbent assay
a.-D. immunoglobulin

NOTES

25

antideoxyribonculeic acidase
antidepressant
    heterocyclic a.
    tricyclic a.
anti-DNA antibody
anti-DNase B
anti-DNA-topoisomerase I antibody
antidouble-stranded DNA
anti-EBV
    anti-Epstein-Barr virus
    anti-EBV antibody
antiendotoxin
    XXMEN-OE5 a.
antienzyme
antiepithelial serum
anti-Epstein-Barr virus (anti-EBV)
antifibrinolytic agent
antifungal
    Absorbine Jr. A.
    Breezee Mist A.
    a. therapy
antigen (Ag)
    ABO a.'s
    acetone-insoluble a.
    AF-1 a.
    AF-2 a.
    allogeneic a.
    Am a.
    antibody to hepatitis B core a.
    (HB$_c$Ab, HBcAb)
    antibody to hepatitis B e a.
    (HB$_e$Ab, HBeAb)
    antibody to hepatitis B
    surface a. (HB$_s$Ab, HBsAb)
    Au a.
    Aus a.
    Australia a.
    Be^a a.
    Becker a.
    Bi a.
    Bile a.
    bivalent a.
    blood group a.
    bullous pemphigoid a. (BPA)
    By a.
    capsular a.
    carcinoembryonic a. (CEA)
    C carbohydrate a.
    CDE a.
    cholesterinized a.
    Chr^a a.
    cicatricial pemphigoid a.
    class I a.

class II a.
class III a.
commercial a.
common a.
complete a.
conjugated a.
D a.
delta a.
Dharmendra a.
Di a.
Duffy a.
epidermolysis bullosa
    acquisita a.
Epstein-Barr nuclear a.
    (EBNA)
a. excess
flagellar a.
food a.
Forssman a.
Frei a.
Fy a.
G a.
Ge a.
Gm a.
Good a.
Gr a.
group a.'s
H a.
H-2 a.
He a.
heart a.
hepatitis A a. (HAA)
hepatitis-associated a. (HAA)
hepatitis B core a. (HB$_c$Ag,
    HBcAg)
hepatitis Be a.
hepatitis B surface a. (HB$_s$Ag,
    HBsAg)
heterogenetic a.
heterogenic a.
heterogenic enterobacterial a.
heterophil a.
heterophile a.
hexon a.
histocompatibility a.
HL-A a.'s
Ho a.
homologous a.
Hu a.
human leukemia-associated a.'s
human leukocyte a. (HLA)
human lymphocyte a. (HLA)
I a.

Ia a.
incomplete a.
a. interferon
InV group a.
Jk a.
Jobbins a.
Js a.
K a.
KF-1 a.
KI a.
Km a.
Kveim a.
Kveim-Stilzbach a.
La a.
Lan a.
LDA-1 a.
Le a.
leukocyte common a.
Levay a.
LH 7:2 a.
Lu a.
lymphocyte function-
    associated a. (LFA)
lymphogranuloma venereum a.
Lyt a.'s
M a.
M_1 a.
Mitsuda a.
MNSs a.
Mu a.
mumps skin test a.
O a.
oncofetal a.
organ-specific a.
Ot a.
P a.
p24 a.
partial a.
P blood group a.
penton a.
peptide a.
PM-Scl a.
pollen a.
polymerized a.
polysaccharide a.
private a.

proliferating cell nuclear a.
    (PCNA)
protein a.
public a.
R a.
red cell a.
Rh a.
Rhus toxicodendron a.
Rhus venenata a.
RNP a.
Ro a.
S a.
"self" a.
sensitized a.
shock a.
Sm a.
soluble a.
somatic a.
species-specific a.
specific a.
Stobo a.
streptococcal M a.
Streptococcus M a.
streptococcus M a.
surface a.
Sw^a a.
Swann a.
T a.
Tac a.
T-dependent a.
theta a.
thymus-independent a.
tissue-specific a.
Tj a.
Tr^a a.
transplantation a.
tumor a.
tumor-associated a.
tumor-specific
    transplantation a.'s (TSTA)
a. unit
V a.
Vel a.
Ven a.
very late activation a. (VLA-1
    antigen)
Vi a.

NOTES

27

antigen *(continued)*
   VLA-1 a.
     very late activation antigen
   Vw a.
   Webb a.
   Wr^a a.
   Wright a. (Wr^a)
   Xg a.
   Yt^a a.
antigen-1
   leukocyte factor a. (LFA-1)
   lymphocyte function a. (LFA-
    1)
antigen-antibody
   complement-activating a.-a.
   a.-a. complex
   a.-a. reaction
antigen-binding
   a.-b. diversity
   a.-b. site
antigen-combining site
antigenemia
antigenemically cross-reacting food
antigenic
   a. competition
   a. complex
   a. determinant
   a. drift
   a. shift
antigenicity
antigen-nonspecific immune complex
   assay
antigen-presenting cell
antigen-recognition
antigen-sensitive cell
antigen-specific immune response
antigenuria
   pneumococcal a.
antiglobulin test
antiglomerular basement membrane
   (anti-GMB)
anti-GMB
   antiglomerular basement membrane
anti-HAV
anti-HB$_c$ antibody
anti-HB$_e$ antibody
anti-HB$_s$ antibody
anti-*Helicobacter*
antihemagglutinin
antihemolysin
antihemolytic
antihidrotic
Antihist-1

antihistamine
   H$_1$ a.
   H$_2$ a.
   nonsedating a.
   oral a.
antihistaminic
antihistone antibody
antihistone-(H2A-
   H2B)/deoxyribonucleic acid
   complex antibody
anti-hnRNP
antihormone
antihuman
   a. globulin
   a. globulin test
antihuman parvovirus
   immunoglobulin G
anti-hyaluronidase
antihydriotic
antihypertensive agent
antihyperuricemic agent
anti-idiotype
   a.-i. antibody
   a.-i. autoantibody
anti-IIb-IIIA mAB therapy
anti-inflammatory
   nonsteroidal a.-i.
   a.-i. therapy
anti-Jo-1 antibody
anti-Jp-1 antibody
anti-70K antibody
anti-kidney serum nephritis
anti-Ku antibody
anti-La antibody
antileukocidin
antileukotoxin
antiluetic
antilymphocyte
   a. antibody
   a. serum (ALS)
antilysin
antimalarial
   a. agent
   a. drug
anti-melanocyte antibody
antimetabolite
anti-Mi-2 nuclear antibody
antimicrobial
   a. spectrum
antimicrobiology susceptibility
   testing
Antiminth

A

antimonial drug therapy for
   leishmaniasis
antimycobacterials
antimycotic
antinative DNA
antineoplastic
antineuronal antibody
antineurotoxin
antineutrophilic cytoplasmic
   antibody (ANCA)
antinuclear
   a. antibody (ANA)
   a. antibody immunodiffusion
   a. antibody immunofluorescence
   a. antibody screening by
      enzyme immunoassay
   a. antibody screening test
   a. factor (ANF)
anti-nuclear matrix antibody
antioxidant
   a. vitamin
antiparasitic
antiparvovirus 19 antibody
antiperspirant
antiphagocytic
antiphospholipid
   a. antibody (APLA)
   a. antibody syndrome (APS)
α2-antiplasmin
anti-PM-Scl antibody
antipneumococcal antibody
antipneumococcic
anti-Pr cold autoagglutinin
antiprecipitin
antipruritic
   a. agent
   a. therapy
   topical a.
antipsoriatic
antipsoric
antipyretic
antipyrine and benzocaine
antipyrotic
antirabies
   a. serum
   a. serum, equine origin
antireticular cytotoxic serum

antiretroviral
antirheumatic
   a. agent
   a. drug
anti-ribosome antibody
antiricin
anti-RNA pol I antibody
anti-RNP antibody
anti-Ro antibody
anti-rotavirus IgA titer
antirubella antibody
anti-S antibody
antiscabetic
antiscabietic
anti-Scl-70
   antiscleroderma 70 antibody
   anti-Scl-70 antibody
antiscleroderma 70 antibody (anti-
   Scl-70)
antiseborrheic
antisense drug
antisepsis
antiseptic
antiserum, pl. antisera
   a. anaphylaxis
   blood group a.
   heterologous a.
   homologous a.
   monovalent a.
   nerve growth factor a.
   NGF a.
   polyvalent a.
   specific a.
anti-Sm antibody
anti-Smith antibody
anti-smooth muscle antibody
anti-SRP antibody
anti-SS-A antibody
anti-SS-B antibody
antistaphylococcic
antistaphylolysin
antisteapsin
antistreptococcic
antistreptokinase
antistreptolysin
   a.-O (ASLO)
   a. O titer

NOTES

antisubstance
antisudorific
antisynthetase syndrome
anti-tac
anti-Th antibody
antithrombin
  a. III
antithymocyte globulin
antithyroid microsomal antibody
anti-topoisomerase I antibody
antitoxic
  a. serum
antitoxigen
antitoxin
  bivalent gas gangrene a.
  bothropic a.
  Bothrops a.
  botulinum a.
  botulism a.
  bovine a.
  Crotalus a.
  despeciated a.
  diphtheria a.
  dysentery a.
  gas gangrene a.
  normal a.
  pentavalent gas gangrene a.
  plant a.
  a. rash
  scarlet fever a.
  staphylococcus a.
  tetanus a.
  tetanus-perfringens a.
  a. unit
antitoxinogen
antitrypsin
  α-1 a. deficiency panniculitis
antituberculosis
antituberculous therapy
antitumorigenesis
antitussive
antityphoid
anti-U1 RNP antibody
anti-U3 RNP antibody
antivenene
  a. unit
antivenin
  anti-Centruroides a.
  a., black widow spider
  a. (crotalidae) polyvalent
antivenom
  Latrodectus mactans a.
  tiger snake a.

Antivert
antiviral
  a. drug
  a. immunity
  a. protein (AVP)
  a. therapy
Antrizine
antrostomy
Anturane
Anucort-HC Suppository
Anuprep HC Suppository
Anusol
  A. HC-1
  A. HC-2.5%
  A.-HC Suppository
Anxanil
AOM
  acute otitis media
aortitis
Apacet
APACHE
  acute physiology and chronic health
    evaluation
  APACHE II score
  APACHE II system
apatite
A-P-C
  adenoidal-pharyngeal-conjunctival
  A-P-C virus
Apert
  A. hirsutism
  A. syndrome
apheresis
aphtha, pl. aphthae
  Bednar a.
  herpetiform a.
  Mikulicz a.
aphthoid
aphthosis
aphthous
  a. genital ulcer
  a. oral ulcer
  a. stomatitis
Aphthovirus
aphylactic
aphylaxis
apical lobe fibrosis
apicoposterior segment
apiculus
apiospermum
  Monosporium a.
  Scedosporium a.

apis
    A. mellifera
    A. mellifera sting
    Spiroplasma a.
APLA
    antiphospholipid antibody
aplasia
    a. cutis congenita
    gold-induced a.
    pure red cell a. (PRCA)
Apley maneuver
Aplisol
apnea
    obstructive sleep a. (OSA)
    sleep a.
apneustic breathing
apocrine
    a. adenoma
    a. bromhidrosis
    a. carcinoma
    a. chromhidrosis
    a. cystadenoma
    a. gland
    a. malaria
    a. miliaria
    a. retention cyst
    a. sweat gland
aponeurosis
    palmar a.
aponeurotic fibroma
apophylaxis
apophyseal joint
apoplexy
    cutaneous a.
apoptosis
apostematosa
    cheilitis glandularis a.
apparatus
    Golgi a.
    internal hair a.
    pilosebaceous a.
apparent
    a. leukonychia
AP-PCR
    arbitrary primed PCR
appearance
    cluster-of-grapes a.

enamel paint spot a.
    finger-in-glove a.
    ground-glass a.
    "slapped cheek" a.
    "slapped face" a.
appendage
    epidermal a.
appendicular tuberculosis
apple
    a. jelly nodule
    a. jelly papule of lupus
        vulgaris
appliance
    TheraSnore oral a.
appropriate culture
Aprodine
    A. Syrup
    A. Tablet
APRV
    airway pressure release ventilation
APS
    antiphospholipid antibody syndrome
APTT
    activated partial thromboplastin time
apurpuric
Aqua Care moisturizer
Aquacare topical
aquagenic
    a. pruritus
    a. urticaria
AquaMEPHYTON injection
Aquanil
Aquaphor
    A. Antibiotic topical
Aquaphyllin
AquaSite Ophthalmic solution
Aquasol E Oral
aquaspersa
    Acrotheca a.
    Rhinocladiella a.
AquaTar
aqueous
    a. epinephrine
    a. extract
    penicillin a.
    a. solution
    a. vaccine

NOTES

ARA
American Rheumatism Association
arabic
arabinoside
cytosine a.
ara-C
arachidonic
a. acid (AA)
a. acid cascade
a. acid metabolites
arachnidism
necrotic a.
arachnodactylia
arachnodactyly
congenital contractural a.
arachnoideus
nevus a.
Aralen
A. Phosphate
A. Phosphate With Primaquine Phosphate
Aramine
araneidism
araneus
nevus a.
A-range
psoralen ultraviolet A.-r. (PUVA)
aranodactylia
arbitrary primed PCR (AP-PCR)
arbor
a. vitae
a. vitae tree
arborescens
lipoma a.
arborize
arbovirus, arborvirus
ARC
AIDS-related complex
arc
mercury a.
arcade
fibrous a.
arcanobacterial pharyngitis
arch-loop-whorl system (ALW)
arciform
arcuate
arcuatus
Chortoglyphus a.
ARDS
adult respiratory distress syndrome
area
butterfly a.

Celsus a.
dermatomic a.
flush a.
intertriginous a.
Jonston a.
periocular a.
perioral a.
periorbital a.
areata
alopecia a.
pseudo-alopecia a.
areate
areatus
aregenerative anemia
arenaceous
Arenaviridae
A. virus
Arenavirus
areola
Chaussier a.
nevoid hyperkeratosis of nipple and a.
areolar
ARF
acute respiratory failure
acute rheumatic fever
Argasidae
Argentinean hemorrhagic fever
Argentine hemorrhagic fever virus
Argesic-SA
arginine codon
argininosuccinicaciduria
argon
a. laser
a. pumped tunable-dye laser
Argyll Robertson pupil
argyria
argyriasis
argyric
argyrism
Argyrol S.S. 20%
argyrosis
Aria CPAP system
ARI Group I–IV filter
Aristocort
A. Forte
A. Intralesional suspension
Syrup of A.
A. Tablet
Aristospan
Arizona
A. ash
A. ash tree

A. coral snake
A. cypress
A. cypress tree
arizonae
    Salmonella a.
Arizona/Fremont
    A. cottonwood
    A. cottonwood tree
Arm-a-Med
    A.-a.-M. Isoetharine
    A.-a.-M. Isoproterenol
    A.-a.-M. Metaproterenol
armed macrophage
ARN
    acute retinal necrosis
Arndt-Gottron syndrome
around-the-clock oral maintenance
  bronchodilator therapy
arrangement
    chromosome a.
    lesion a.
    V-D-J gene a.
array
    reticulate a.
arrector, pl. arrectores
    a. pili muscle
    a. pilus
arrest
    cardiorespiratory a.
arresting
    high efficiency particulate a.
    (HEPA)
Arrhenius-Madsen theory
arrhythmia
Arrow pneumothorax kit
arrowroot
arsenic
    a. pigmentation
    a. trioxide
arsenical keratosis
artefact (*var. of* artifact)
artefacta
    dermatitis a.
Artemisia
    A. salina
Arteparon

arterial
    a. blood gas (ABG)
    a. hypoxemia
    a. spider
    a. ulcer
arteriosclerosis
    fibrotic a.
    a. obliterans
arteriosclerotic gangrene
arteriovenous
    a. fistula
    a. malformation (AVM)
    a. shunt
arteritis
    allergic granulomatous a.
    cranial a.
    equine viral a.
    giant cell a.
    granulomatous a.
    Takayasu a.
    temporal a.
    temporal giant cell a.
Arterivirus
artery
    nutrient a.
Artha-G
arthralgia
arthritic tuberculosis
arthritide
arthritis, pl. arthritides
    acute rheumatic a.
    acute rheumatoid a.
    additive a.
    adult-type rheumatoid a.
    anaerobic bacterial a.
    axial psoriatic a.
    bacterial a.
    brucella a.
    burnt out rheumatoid a.
    Candida a.
    candidal a.
    chronic postrheumatic fever a.
    crystal-induced a.
    degenerative a.
    enteropathic a.
    erosive a.
    A. Foundation Ibuprofen

NOTES

arthritis *(continued)*
   A. Foundation Nighttime
   A. Foundation Pain Reliever
   fungal a.
   gonococcal a.
   granulomatous idiopathic a.
   hepatitis A a.
   hepatitis B a.
   herpes simplex virus a.
   idiopathic destructive a. (IDA)
   infectious a.
   juvenile a.
   juvenile chronic a.
   juvenile rheumatoid a. (JRA)
   large-joint inflammatory a.
   Lyme a.
   meningococcal a.
   a. mutilans
   nongonococcal bacterial a.
   oligoarticular seronegative
    rheumatoid a.
   pauciarticular a.
   pauciarticular juvenile
    rheumatoid a.
   peripheral a.
   phase I rheumatoid a.
   phase II rheumatoid a.
   polyarticular a.
   polyarticular gonococcal a.
   polyarticular juvenile
    rheumatoid a.
   polymicrobial a.
   post-traumatic a.
   postvenereal reactive a.
   pseudocystic rheumatoid a.
   psoriatic a.
   pyogenic a.
   reactive a.
   rheumatoid a. (RA)
   a. robustus
   Salmonella a.
   sarcoid a.
   septic a.
   seropositive rheumatoid a.
   suppurative a.
   systemic juvenile rheumatoid a.
   traumatic a.
   venereal-associated a.
   viral a.
   a. without deformity
   Yersinia a.
arthritogenicity
arthrocentesis

arthrochalasis multiplex congenita
arthrodesis
arthrography
   double-contrast a.
arthro-ophthalmopathy
   hereditary a.-o.
Arthropan
arthropathia psoriatica
arthropathy
   acromegalic a.
   cuff tear a.
   enteropathic a.
   facet joint a.
   hemophilic a.
   Jaccoud a.
   myxedematous a.
   neuropathic a.
   primary amyloidotic a.
   psoriatic a.
   pyrophosphate a.
   resorptive a.
   seronegativity, enthesopathy, a.
    (SEA)
arthropica
   psoriasis a.
arthropism
arthroplasty
   Mayo modified total elbow a.
arthropod
   a. bite
   a. sting
arthropod-borne virus
arthroscope
   Citoscope-16 a.
   30-degree oblique a.
   Medical Dynamics 5990
    needle a.
   Stryker a.
arthroscopy
   needle a.
arthrosia
   exanthesis a.
arthrosis
   uncovertebral a.
arthrospore
arthrotomy
Arthus
   A. phenomenon
   A. reaction
arthus-type reaction
articular
   a. disease
   a. leprosy

Articulose-50 injection
artifact, artefact
artificial
    a. active immunity
    a. passive immunity
    a. tears
artificialis
    acne a.
arum plant
ARV
    AIDS-related virus
aryepiglottic
AS
    ankylosing spondylitis
ASA
    acetylsalicylic acid
asaccharolyticus
    Peptostreptococcus a.
Asacol Oral
asbestos
    a. corn
    a. wart
ascariasis
ascaris
Ascaris lumbricoides
asci (*pl. of* ascus)
Ascoli reaction
Ascomycetes
ascospore
Ascriptin
ascus, pl. **asci**
asepsis
aseptic
    a. necrosis
    a. technique
ash
    Arizona a.
    green a.
    Oregon a.
    a. tree
    white a.
ashgray
    a. blister beetle
    a. blister beetle sting
ash-leaf spot
ashsphere
ashy dermatosis

Asiatic cholera
ASLO
    antistreptolysin-O
    ASLO titer
Asmalix
ASO
    A. test
    A. titer
asparagus
aspartic proteinase
aspen
    a. tree
aspergilloma
aspergillosis
    allergic bronchopulmonary a.
    (ABPA)
    disseminated a.
    invasive a.
Aspergillus
    A. amstelodami
    A. avenaceus
    A. caesiellus
    A. candidus
    A. carneus
    A. clavatus
    A. deltoidea
    A. flavus
    A. fumigatus
    A. nidulans
    A. niger
    A. oryzae
    A. osteomyelitis
    A. restrictus
    A. sydowi
    A. terreus
    A. ustus
    A. versicolor
aspirate
    nasopharyngeal a.
    (NPA)
aspiration
    a. biopsy
    fine needle a. (FNA)
    myringotomy with a.
    recurrent a.
aspirin
    Bayer A.

A

NOTES

aspirin *(continued)*
    Bayer Buffered A.
    enteric-coated a.
    Extra Strength Bayer Enteric
      500 A.
    A. Free Anacin Maximum
      Strength
    a. sensitivity
    St. Joseph Adult Chewable A.
    a. triad
Aspirin-Free Bayer Select Allergy
  Sinus Caplets
aspirin-induced papillary necrosis
aspirin-sensitive asthma
Asprimox
assassin
    a. bug
    a. bug bite
assay
    adherence a.
    agar diffusion a.
    amplification a.
    anti-C3 a.
    anti-D enzyme-linked
      immunosorbent a.
    antigen-nonspecific immune
      complex a.
    Borrelia burgdorferi DNA a.
    CH50 a.
    chemiluminescence a.
    Colorimeti A.
    competitive binding a.
    complement binding a.
    conglutinin a.
    Cotinine a.
    Crithidia luciliae
      immunofluorescence a.
    21-Day Cumulative
      Irritancy A.
    double antibody sandwich a.
    EAC rosette a.
    enzyme-linked
      immunosorbent a. (ELISA)
    Farr a.
    fluid-phase C1q-binding a.
    food immune complex a.
      (FICA)
    α-glutathione S-transferase a.
    glycoprotein-based enzyme-
      linked immunosorbent a.
      (ggELISA)
    hemolytic a.
    hepatitis B viral DNA a.

    HIV DNA amplification a.
    immune adherence
      immunosorbent a. (IAHIA)
    immune complex a.
    immunochemical a.
    immunoprecipitation a.
    immunoradiometric a.
    indirect a.
    leukocyte attachment a.
    Limulus lysate a.
    lymphocyte function a.
    PCR a.
    precipitin a.
    Premier H. pylori a.
    quantitative complement a.
    radioreceptor a.
    Raji cell radioimmune a.
    RCR a.
    recombinant immunoblot a.
      (RIBA)
    replication-competent
      retrovirus a.
    solid-phase C1q-binding a.
    staphylococcal-binding a.
    two-site immunoradiometric a.
Assess peak flow meter
associated macrophage
associates
    microbial a.
Association
    American Rheumatism A.
      (ARA)
association constant
associative reaction
astacoid rash
asteatode
asteatosis
    a. cutis
asteatotic
    a. eczema
Astech peak flow meter
Astelin
astemizole
asteroid body
asteroides
    Nocardia a.
asthenia
    neurocirculatory a.
    tropical anhidrotic a.
asthma
    allergen-induced a.
    aspirin-sensitive a.
    atopic a.

baker's a.
bronchial a.
chronic a.
cough-variant a.
exercise-induced a. (EIA)
extrinsic a.
food a.
functional abnormality in a.
hay a.
intrinsic a.
miller's a.
mixed a.
nocturnal a.
occupationally induced a. (OA)
poorly reversible a.
steroid-dependent a.
subclinical a.
summer a.
AsthmaHaler
AsthmaNefrin
asthmatic
  a. bronchitis
  tight a.
asthmaticus
  status a.
asthmogenic
astringent
astrocyte
astronyxis
  Acanthamoeba a.
Astroviridae virus
asymmetric
  a. distribution
  a. oligoarthritis
  a. oligoarthropathy
  a. peripheral sensory
    neuropathy
  a. polyarthritis
asymptomatic cricoarytenoid
  synovitis
α_1-**AT**
Atabrine
Atarax
atavism
  phylogenetic a.
ataxia
  cerebellar a.

locomotor a.
  a. telangiectasia
  a. telangiectasia syndrome
ataxia-telangiectasia
atheroma
atheromatous embolus
athlete's
  a. foot
  a. nodule
athrepsia
ATL
  adult T-cell leukemia
atlantoaxial joint
atonic ulcer
atopen
atopic
  a. allergy
  a. asthma
  a. dermatitis
  a. dermatitis rash
  a. diathesis
  a. eczema
  a. reagin
  a. sensitivity
atopy
atovaquone
Atozine
ATP
  adenosine triphosphate
ATPase activity
atra
  Stachybotrys a.
Atra-Tain
atrepsy
atretic meningocele
atrichia
atrichosis
atrichous
atrioventricular (AV)
Atrohist
Atropair Ophthalmic
atrophedema
atrophia
  a. cutis
  a. maculosa varioliformis cutis
  a. pilorum propria

NOTES

atrophic
a. candidiasis
a. glossitis
a. lichen planus
a. macule
a. papulosis
a. plaque
a. rhinitis of swine
a. white scar
atrophica
acne a.
hyperkeratosis figurata
centrifuga a.
macula a.
stria a.
atrophicae
lineae a.
lineae striae a.
atrophicans
acrodermatitis chronica a.
dermatitis a.
epidermolysis bullosa a.
keratosis pilaris a.
lichen planus et acuminatus a.
lichen sclerosus et a.
pityriasis alba a.
poikiloderma vasculare a.
poikiloderma vascularis a.
atrophicus
lichen sclerosis et a. (LS&A)
atrophie blanche
atrophoderma
a. albidum
a. biotripticum
a. diffusum
follicular a.
idiopathic a.
a. maculatum
a. neuriticum
a. of Pasini and Pierini
Pasini-Pierini idiopathic a.
progressive idiopathic a.
a. reticulatum symmetricum faciei
a. scleroatrophy
senile a.
a. striatum
a. ulerythematosa
a. vermicularis
a. vermiculatum
atrophodermatosis
atrophy
blue a.
Buchwald a.
central papillary a.
diffuse a.
a. of fat
fat-replacement a.
intrinsic muscle a.
linear a.
macular a.
optic a.
papillary a.
primary a.
primary idiopathic macular a.
skin a.
traction a.
wucher a.
Atropine-Care Ophthalmic
atropine sulfate
Atropisol Ophthalmic
Atrovent
A. Aerosol Inhalation
A. Inhalation solution
A/T/S
A. lotion
A. topical
attachment plaque
attack
acute a.
acute asthma a.
drop a.
syncopal a.
attenuant
attenuate
a. vaccinia virus
attenuated
mumps virus vaccine, live, a.
rickettsia vaccine, a.
a. tuberculosis
a. vaccine
a. virus
attenuation
attenuator
Attenuvax
atypical
a. erythema multiforme
a. fibroxanthoma
a. histiocytosis
a. ichthyosiform erythroderma
a. Kawasaki disease (AKD)
a. lipoma
a. measles
a. mole
a. mole syndrome
a. mycobacterial colonization

A

a. mycobacterial infection
a. pityriasis rosea
a. pneumonia
AU
allergy unit
Au antigen
Auchmeromyia
audiometry
screening a.
threshold a.
audouinii
Microsporum a.
augmentation therapy
Augmentin
Aujeszky
A. disease
A. disease virus
aura
Auralate
aural fistula
Auralgan
auranofin
aurantiasis
a. cutis
Aureobasidium pullulans
aureotherapy
aureus
Staphylococcus a.
auriasis
auricle
accessory a.
auriculotemporal syndrome
aurid
aurochromoderma
aurothioglucose
aurothiomalate
Auroto
Aus antigen
Auspitz sign
Australia antigen
Australian
A. parrot droppings
A. parrot feather
A. parrot protein
A. pine
A. pine tree
A. X disease

A. X disease virus
A. X encephalitis
australis
Rickettsia a.
autacoid
autoagglutination
autoagglutinin
anti-Pr cold a.
cold a.
autoallergic
autoallergization
autoallergy
autoamputate
autoanaphylaxis
autoantibody
anti-idiotype a.
brain-reactive a.
cold a.
Donath-Landsteiner cold a.
hemagglutinating cold a.
idiotype a.
monoclonal a.
myositis-associated a.
plasma protein a.
warm a.
autoanticomplement
autoantigen
autoclasis
autocrine
autocytolysin
autocytolysis
autocytotoxin
autodermic
autodigestion
a. of connective tissue
auto-eczematization
autoerythrocyte
a. sensitivity
a. sensitization
a. sensitization syndrome
autogeneic graft
autogenous
a. vaccine
autograft
autografting
autogram
autographism

NOTES

39

Autohaler
Maxair A.
autohemagglutination
autohemolysin
autohemolysis
autoimmune
a. chronic hepatitis
a. disease
a. disorder
a. hemolysis
a. hemolytic anemia (AIHA)
a. neonatal thrombocytopenia
a. neutropenia
a. panhypopituitarism
a. phenomenon
a. purpura
a. thrombocytopenia (AITP)
a. type of reaction
autoimmunity
autoimmunization
autoimmunocytopenia
autoinfection
auto-injector
autoinoculable
autoinoculation
autoisolysin
autologous
a. graft
a. mixed leukocyte reaction
autolyse
autolysin
autolysis
autolytic
autolyze
Automeris
A. io
automobile exhaust
autonomic
a. imbalance syndrome
a. nervous system
autonomous
autophagia
autophagic
autophagy
autophytica
dermatitis a.
autoplast
autoplastic
a. graft
autoplasty
autoradiography
autoreinfection
autoreproduction

autosensitivity
DNA a.
autosensitization
a. dermatitis
autosensitize
autosepticemia
autoserotherapy
autoserum
a. therapy
autosomal
a. dominant
a. dominant lamellar ichthyosis
a. recessive
a. recessive ichthyosis
a.-recessive severe combined
immunodeficiency disorder
a. recessive trait
autotherapy
autotoxicus
horror a.
autotransplant
autotransplantation
autovaccination
auxilytic
AV
atrioventricular
AV block
avascular
a. necrosis (AVN)
avascularity
Aveeno
A. Cleansing Bar
avenaceus
Aspergillus a.
Aviadenovirus
avian
a. diphtheria
a. encephalomyelitis virus
a. erythroblastosis virus
a. infectious encephalomyelitis
a. infectious laryngotracheitis
a. infectious laryngotracheitis
virus
a. influenza
a. influenza virus
a. leukosis
a. leukosis-sarcoma complex
a. leukosis-sarcoma virus
a. lymphomatosis
a. lymphomatosis virus
a. monocytosis
a. myeloblastosis
a. myeloblastosis virus

a. neurolymphomatosis virus
a. pneumoencephalitis virus
a. reticuloendotheliosis
a. sarcoma
a. sarcoma virus
a. viral arthritis virus
avidin-biotin-peroxidase staining
avidity antibody
Avipoxvirus
avirulent
avitaminosis
avium
    Mycobacterium a.
avium-intracellulare
    Mycobacterium a.-i. (MAC,
    MAI)
Avlosulfon
AVM
    arteriovenous malformation
AVN
    avascular necrosis
avoidance
Avon Skin-So-Soft
AVP
    antiviral protein
axenic
AX-HSA
    amoxicilloyl-human serum albumin
axial
    a. psoriatic arthritis
    a. type
axillaris
    trichomycosis a.
    trichonocardiosis a.
axillary
    a. freckling
    a. hair
    a. venom gland

axis
    psycho-neuro-immuno-
    endocrine a.
    a. of symmetry
Ayndet moisturizing soap
AZA
    azathioprine
Azactam
azalide
azapropazone
azar
    kala a.
azatadine maleate
azathioprine (AZA)
azelaic acid
azelastine
Azelex
azidothymidine (AZT)
azithromycin
Azlocillin
Azmacort
azo itch
azoprotein
azotemia
    progressive a.
AZT
    azidothymidine
aztreonam
azul
Azulfidine
    A. EN-tabs
azure lunula of nail
azurocidin
azurophil
    a. granule
    a. granule protein

NOTES

β (*var. of* beta)
  β corynebacteriophage
  β hemolysin
  β hemolysis
  β-MSH
  β phage
  transforming growth factor β
    (TGFβ)
B
  B cell
  B lymphocyte
  B virus
B1
  B1 cell
  Coxsackievirus B1
B2
  Coxsackievirus B2
B3
  Coxsackievirus B3
B4
  B4 blocked ricin
  Coxsackievirus B4
  leukotriene B4 (LTB4)
B5
  Coxsackievirus B5
B$_6$
  vitamin B$_6$
B19 virus
B&A
  before and after
Babesia
  B. bigemina
  B. bovis
  B. canis
  B. divergens
  B. equi
  B. felis
  B. major
  B. microti
  B. rodhaini
babesiosis
baby
  blueberry muffin b.
  collodion b.
BABYbird respirator
Baby Magic soap
bacampicillin hydrochloride
Baccharus
Baciguent topical

bacillary angiomatosis
bacillary-barren tuberculids
Bacille bilié de Calmette-Guérin
  (BCG)
bacilli (*pl. of* bacillus)
bacilliformis
  Bartonella b.
bacillosis
Bacillus
  B. abortus
  B. acnes
  B. alvei
  B. anthracis
  B. anthracis toxin
  B. Calmette-Guérin Live
  B. cereus
  B. circulans
  B. laterosporus
  B. licheniformis
  B. megaterium
  B. polymyxa
  B. pseudodiphtheriticum
  B. pumilus
  B. sphaericus
  B. stearothermophilus
  B. subtilis
bacillus, pl. bacilli
  acid-fast b. (AFB)
  acne b.
  b. Calmette-Guérin (BCG)
  Calmette-Guérin b.
  b. Calmette-Guérin vaccine
  cholera b.
  comma b.
  fusiform b.
  Gram-negative b. (GNB)
  Gram-positive b.
  Hansen b.
  Koch b.
  lepra b.
  Park-Williams b.
  vole b.
  Warthin-Starry-staining b.
  Whipple b.
bacitracin
  b., neomycin, and polymyxin
    b
  b., neomycin, polymyxin b,
    and hydrocortisone

B

bacitracin *(continued)*
  b., neomycin, polymyxin B, and lidocaine
  b. and polymyxin b
baclofen
bacoti
  Liponyssus b.
BACTEC
  B. radiometry
  B. system
bacteremia
  Gram-negative b.
  Gram-positive b.
  MAI b.
  polymicrobial b.
  Pseudomonas aeruginosa b.
bacteria (*pl. of* bacterium)
bacteria-free stage of bacterial endocarditis
bacterial
  b. allergy
  b. antagonism
  b. arthritis
  b. conjunctivitis
  b. contamination
  b. disease
  b. endocarditis
  b. exotoxin
  b. hemolysin
  b. infection
  b. interference
  b. macromolecule
  b. meningitis (BM)
  b. phagocytosis test
  b. plaque
  b. pneumococcal pneumonia
  b. septicemia
  b. synergistic gangrene
  b. toxin
  b. vaccine
  b. virus
bacterial-induced vascular damage
bacterially induced hemostatic disorder
bactericidal/permeability-increasing protein
bactericide
  specific b.
bacterid
  pustular b.
bacterioagglutinin
bacteriocide
bacteriocidin

bacteriocin factor
bacteriocinogenic plasmid
bacteriocinogens
bacteriocins
bacteriogenic agglutination
bacteriolysin
bacteriolysis
bacteriolytic
  b. serum
bacteriolyze
bacteriopexy
bacteriophage
  defective b.
  filamentous b.
  b. immunity
  mature b.
  b. resistance
  temperate b.
  typhoid b.
  b. typing
  vegetative b.
  virulent b.
bacteriophagia
bacteriophagology
bacteriopsonin
bacteriosis
bacteriostasis
bacteriostat
bacteriostatic
bacteriotoxic
bacteriotropic
  b. substance
bacteriotropin
bacterium, pl. bacteria
  Bordetella pertussis b.
  coryneform b.
  facultative b.
  lysogenic b.
  pyogenic b.
bacteriuria
Bacteroides
  B. fragilis
Bacticort Otic
Bactine
Bactocill
  B. injection
  B. Oral
BactoShield topical
Bactrim
  B. DS
Bactroban
  B. topical
Baculoviridae

B

Baelz disease
Bäfverstedt syndrome
bagassosis
Bag Balm lubricant/emollient
Bagdad
    bouton de B.
Baghdad boil
Bahia grass
Baker cyst
baker's
    b. asthma
    b. eczema
    b. itch
baking soda paste
BAL
    bronchoalveolar lavage
balanitis, pl. balanitides
    Candida b.
    b. circinata
    circinate b.
    b. circumscripta plasma
      cellularis
    erosive *Candida* b.
    Follmann b.
    plasma cell b.
    b. xerotica obliterans
    b. of Zoon
balanoposthitis
    streptococcal b.
Balantidium coli
balatus
    Acarus b.
bald
    b. cypress
    b. cypress tree
Baldex
baldness
    common b.
    congenital b.
    male pattern b.
    moth-eaten b.
    pubic b.
ball
    fungus b.
ballistospore

balloon
    b. cell
    b. cell nevus
ballooning degeneration
balm
balnea
    pruritus b.
balnei
    Mycobacterium b.
balneotherapy
Balnetar
balsam
    b. of Peru
    b. of tolu
balsamic
bamboo hair
banana
bancrofti
    Filaria b.
    Wuchereria b.
Bancroftian filariasis
band
    b. keratopathy
    marginal b.
    Muerhrcke b.
bandage
    Ace b.
    Hollister medial adhesive b.
    b. sign
    TubiFast b.
Band-Aid
    B.-A. dressing
banding
Bang disease
Bannister disease
Bannwarth syndrome
Banophen Oral
Banti syndrome
bar
    Aveeno Cleansing B.
    HI-CAL VM b.
    ZNP B.
barba, pl. barbae
    folliculitis barbae
    pseudofolliculitis barbae
    sycosis barbae

NOTES

45

barba *(continued)*
   tinea barbae
   trichophytosis barbae
Barbados leg
barbed
   b. hypostome
   b. stinger
barber's
   b. itch
   b. pilonidal sinus
barbula hirci
Barcoo
   B. disease
   B. rot
Bard-Parker blade
bare lymphocyte syndrome
bark
   b. scorpion
   b. scorpion sting
barking cough
barley
barn
   b. dust
   b. itch
barrier
   b. layer
   physical b.
   b. zone
bartholinitis
Bartonella
   B. bacilliformis
   B. henselae
   B. henselae detection
   B. quintana
bartonellosis
Bart-Pumphrey syndrome
Bart syndrome
basal
   b. cell
   b. cell carcinoma (BCC)
   b. cell epithelioma (BCE)
   b. cell layer
   b. cell membrane
   b. cell nevus
   b. cell nevus syndrome
   b. cell papilloma
   b. lamina
basaloid
   b. cell
Basan syndrome

basement
   b. membrane
   b. membrane zone (BMZ)
basic calcium phosphate (BCP)
basidiobolae
   entomophthoramycosis b.
Basidiomycetes
basidiospore
basiloma terebrans
basis
   nonimmunologic b.
basket-weave vacuolization
basophil
   b. degranulation test
   b. kallikrein
basophilic degeneration
basosquamous carcinoma
bass
Bateman disease
bath
   colloid b.
   b. itch
   b. pruritus
bathing-trunk nevus
battery
   b. acid
   b. patch testing
bayberry
   b. tree
Bayer
   B. Aspirin
   B. Buffered Aspirin
   B. Low Adult Strength
   B. Select Pain Relief Formula
bayonet hair
bay sore
Bazex syndrome
Bazin disease
Bb
   Borrelia burgdorferi
BCC
   basal cell carcinoma
BCE
   basal cell epithelioma
B-cell
   B.-c. antigen receptor
   B.-c. differentiation/growth
     factor
   B.-c. growth factor-1
   B.-c. growth factor-2
   B.-c. leukemia
   B.-c. lymphocytic leukemia
   B.-c. lymphocytoma cutis

B

B.-c. lymphoma
B.-c. memory
B.-c. pseudolymphoma
BCG
   Bacille bilié de Calmette-Guérin
   bacillus Calmette-Guérin
   TICE BCG
      TICE Bacillus Calmette-
       Guérin Live
   BCG vaccine
BCP
   basic calcium phosphate
BCYE agar
Bdellovibrio
beaded hair
beading
beads
   Sephadex b.
bean
   broad b.
   castor b.
   coffee b.
   green b.
   green coffee b.
   kidney b.
   lava b.
   lima b.
   navy b.
   string b.
Be^a antigen
beard
   ringworm of b.
Beau line
beauty mark
becaplermin
Becker
   B. antigen
   B. hairy hamartoma
   B. nevus
beclomethasone
   b. dipropionate
Beclovent
   B. Oral Inhaler
Beconase
   B. AQ Nasal Inhaler
   B. Nasal Inhaler

bed
   air-fluidized b.
   Biologics Airlift b.
   low-air-loss b.
   b. sore
   tanning b.
bedbug
   b. bite
   b. disease transmission
Bednar aphtha
bedsore
bee
   bumble b., bumblebee
   b. glue
   honey b., honeybee
   b. sting
   sweat b.
   b. venom
beech
   b. tree
beefwood
Beepen-VK Oral
beet
   sugar b.
beetle
   ashgray blister b.
   blister b.
   striped blister b.
before and after (B&A)
Behçet
   B. disease
   B. syndrome
Behring law
bejel
Belix Oral
**belladonna, phenobarbital, and
   ergotamine tartrate**
Bellergal-S
belli
   Isospora b.
Bell palsy
Bel-Phen-Ergot S
Bena-D injection
Benadryl
   B. injection
   B. Oral
   B. topical

NOTES

Benahist injection
Ben-Aqua
Bence
  B. Jones albumin
  B. Jones protein
Benemid
benign
  b. cephalic histiocytosis
  b. dry pleurisy
  b. dyskeratosis
  b. familial chronic pemphigus
  b. giant cell synovioma
  b. hemangiopericytoma
  b. hyperplasia
  b. inoculation lymphoreticulosis
  b. inoculation reticulosis
  b. intracranial hypertension
  b. juvenile melanoma
  b. lymphadenosis
  b. lymphocytoma cutis
  b. migratory glossitis
  b. monoclonal gammopathy
  b. mucosal pemphigoid
  b. papular acantholytic
    dermatosis
  b. paroxysmal peritonitis
  b. symmetric lipomatosis
  b. systemic mastocytosis
  b. tumor
benigna
  lymphadenosis cutis b.
  lymphogranulomatosis b.
  variola b.
Benoject injection
Benoquin
benoxaprofen
Benoxyl
bentonite flocculation test
Benzac
  B. AC Gel
  B. AC Wash
  B. W
benzalkonium chloride
Benzamycin
Benzashave
benzathine
  penicillin g b.
benzbromarone
benziodarone
benznidazole
benzocaine
  antipyrine and b.
  b., butyl aminobenzoate,

    tetracaine, and benzalkonium
    chloride
  b., gelatin, pectin, and sodium
    carboxymethylcellulose
  orabase with b.
benzodiazepine
  b. midazolam
benzoic acid and salicylic acid
benzoin
benzoyl
  b. peroxide
  b. peroxide and hydrocortisone
benzphetamine hydrochloride
benzyl alcohol
benzylpenicilloyl-polylysine
bergamot
  oil of b.
Berger IgA nephropathy
beriberi
Berkeley scarifier
berlock, berloque
  b. dermatitis
Bermuda
  B. grass
  B. smut
Bernard-Soulier syndrome
Berotec
berylliosis
beryllium
  b. disease
  b. granuloma
Besnier
  B. disease
  prurigo of B.
  B. prurigo
beta, β
  B.-2
  b. adrenergic stimulation
  b. carotene
  b. hemolytic streptococci
    infection
  interferon b. (IFN-β)
  b. lactoglobulin
Betachron E-R
Betadine
  B. First Aid Antibiotics +
    moisturizer
betae
  Phoma b.
betaglycan
beta-lactoglobulin
betamethasone
  b. and clotrimazole

b. dipropionate
b. sodium phosphate and
acetate suspension
b. valerate
Betapen-VK Oral
Betaseron
Betatrex
Beta-Val
Bethesda unit (BU)
Betimol Ophthalmic
Betulaceae
BHR
bronchial hyperresponsiveness
Bi antigen
Biavax II
Biaxin
B. Filmtabs
bicarbonate (HCO₃)
sodium b.
Bicillin
B. C-R 900/300 injection
B. C-R injection
B. L-A injection
bicipital tendinitis
Bicitra
biclonal
b. gammopathy
b. peak
BIDS
brittle hair, intellectual impairment,
decreased fertility, short stature
ichthyosis plus BIDS (IBIDS)
BIDS syndrome
bieneusi
Enterocytozoon b.
Biet
collarette of B.
bifida
occult spina b.
Bifidobacterium
anaerobic *B.*
bifurcatus
pilus b.
bigemina
Babesia b.
biglycan
Biken CAM vaccine

bilateral sensorineural deafness
Bile antigen
bi-level positive airway pressure
(BiPAP)
bilharzial granuloma
bilharzioma
biliaire
masque b.
Bili light
bilirubinemia
Biltricide
bimodal immunofluorescent pattern
binary nomenclature
binding
b. constant
DNA b.
bioassay
bioavailability
Biocef
biochemical
b. abnormality
b. metastasis
biocidal
Bioclot test
Biohist-LA
biologic
b. hemolysis
b. unit (BU)
biological
b. immunotherapy
b. standard unit
b. vector
Biologics Airlift bed
biomagnetic therapy
Biomox
Bion Tears solution
Biopatch antimicrobial dressing
biophylactic
biophylaxis
biopsy
aspiration b.
elliptical b.
excisional b.
incisional b.
intestinal b.
lymph node b.
muscle b.

NOTES

biopsy *(continued)*
   nasopharyngeal b.
   needle b.
   open lung b.
   peroral intestinal b.
   punch b.
   renal b.
   shave b.
   synovial b.
   temporal artery b.
   transjugular hepatic b.
Bio-Tab Oral
biotin
biotinidase
   b. deficiency
   b. enzyme
biotripticum
   atrophoderma b.
Biotropine
biotropism
Biozyme-C
BiPAP
   bi-level positive airway pressure
biphasic response
bipolar electrosurgery
Birbeck granule
birch
   red b.
   river b.
   b. tree
bird-breeder's
   b.-b. disease
   b.-b. lung
birefringent
birminghamensis
   Legionella b.
Birnaviridae
Birnavirus
Birtcher hyfrecator
birthmark
   hemangioma b.
   strawberry b.
   vascular malformation b.
Birt-Hoff-Dubé syndrome
Biskra
   bouton de B.
   B. button
Bismatrol
bismuth
   b. granule
   b. subgallate
   b. subsalicylate
Bisolvon

bisphosphonate
bitartrate
   hydrocodone b.
   levarterenol b.
   metaraminol b.
   norepinephrine b.
bite
   ant b.
   arthropod b.
   assassin bug b.
   bedbug b.
   black fly b.
   black widow spider b.
   brown recluse spider b.
   cat flea b.
   centipede b.
   chigger b.
   conenose bug b.
   Congo floor maggot b.
   copperhead snake b.
   coral snake b.
   cottonmouth snake b.
   Ctenocephalides canis b.
   Ctenocephalides felis b.
   deer fly b.
   dog flea b.
   Eastern coral snake b.
   fiddle-back spider b.
   fly b.
   giant desert centipede b.
   Gila monster b.
   Glossina b.
   gnat b.
   harvest mite b.
   Heloderma suspectum b.
   horsefly b.
   insect b.
   kissing bug b.
   Latrodectus mactans b.
   Loxosceles reclusa b.
   midge b.
   mite b.
   moccasin snake b.
   mosquito b.
   northern rat flea b.
   Nosopsyllus fasciatus b.
   oriental rat flea b.
   b. pathology
   pit viper b.
   rat flea b.
   rattlesnake b.
   red bug b.
   sand flea b.

sandfly b.
Scolopendra heres b.
sea snake b.
snake b.
spider b.
stable fly b.
Stomoxys b.
Texas coral snake b.
tick b.
Triatoma gerstaeckeri b.
Triatoma sanguisuga b.
tsetse fly b.
Tunga penetrans b.
violin-back spider b.
Xenopsylla cheopis b.
Yersinia pestis b.
biting
   b. insect
   nail b.
   b. reef worm
bitolterol mesylate
bitter dock
Bittner
   B. agent
   B. milk factor
   B. virus
biundulant meningoencephalitis
bivalent
   b. antibody
   b. antigen
   b. gas gangrene antitoxin
Bizzozero node
Bjornstad syndrome
BK virus
black
   b. ant
   b. currant rash
   b. dermatographia
   b. dot tinea capitis
   b. eschar
   b. eye
   b. fly
   b. fly bite
   b. hairy tongue
   b. heel
   b. light lamp
   b. locust

b. locust tree
b. mulberry
b. pepper
b. piedra
Sudan b.
b. toe
b. walnut
b. widow spider
b. widow spider bite
blackberry
black-dot ringworm
blackhead
black-legged tick
blade
   Bard-Parker b.
   CLM articulating
     laryngoscope b.
   Gillette Blue B.
blain
blanch
blanchable red lesion
blanche
   atrophie b.
blanched cutaneous elevation
blanching
   delayed b.
bland aerosolized liquid
blanket
   cooling b.
Blaschko line
blastema
blastoconidia
   Candida b.
blastogenesis
blastogenetic
Blastomyces
   B. brasiliensis
   B. dermatitidis
blastomycetes
   pathogenic b.
blastomycetica
   erosio interdigitalis b.
blastomycetic dermatitis
blastomycosis
   European b.
   North American b.
   South American b.

B

NOTES

blastomycosis-like pyoderma
blastomycotica
    dermatitis b.
blastomycotic osteomyelitis
blasts
    refractory anemia with
      excess b. (RAEB)
bleb
    b. stapling
blemish
Blenderm patch technique
blennorrhagia
blennorrhagic
blennorrhagica
    keratoderma b.
    keratosis b.
blennorrhagicum
    keratoderma b.
blennorrhea
    b. neonatorum
blennorrheal conjunctivitis
Blenoxane
bleomycin
    b. sulfate
Bleph-10 Ophthalmic
Blephamide
    B. Ophthalmic
blepharitis
    mixed seborrheic-
      staphylococcal b.
    staphylococcal b.
blepharochalasia
blepharochalasis
blepharochromidrosis
blepharoconjunctivitis
blepharoptosis adiposa
bleuâtre
    tache b.
blind
    b. boil
    b. loop syndrome
    b. passage
blinding disease
blindness
    river b.
blister
    b. beetle
    b. beetle sting
    blood b.
    central b.
    diabetic b.
    fever b.
    fly b.

    friction b.
    pressure b.
    subcorneal b.
blistering
    b. collodion
    b. dermatitis
    b. distal dactylitis
    b. skin
Blis-To-Sol
Blocadren Oral
Bloch-Sulzberger
    B.-S. disease
    B.-S. syndrome
block
    AV b.
    stellate ganglion b.
blockade
    stellate ganglion b.
    virus b.
blockage
    mechanical vessel b.
    vessel b.
blocker
    H2 b.
blocking
    b. antibody
    b. vagal afferent fiber
    b. vagal efferent fiber
Blomia tropicalis
blood
    b. blister
    b. chemistry
    b. coagulation
    b. coagulation test
    b. eosinophilia
    b. fluke
    b. gas
    b. group
    b. group agglutinin
    b. group agglutinogen
    b. group antibody
    b. group antigen
    b. group antiserum
    b. grouping
    b. group substance
    b. group system
    occult b.
    b. pH
    b. pressure
    b. serum
    b. transfusion
    b. transfusion therapy
    b. type

whole b.
b. worm
bloodborne
blood group-specific substances A
and B
bloodsucking
Bloom syndrome
blossom
orange b.
blot
Southern b.
Western b.
blotch
blubber finger
blue
b. atrophy
b. bottle sting
b. grass (*See* bluegrass)
b. mussel
b. nevus
b. rubber-bleb nevi
b. rubber-bleb nevus syndrome
Selsun B.
b. spot
blueberry
b. muffin baby
b. muffin child
bluecomb
b. disease of turkey
b. virus
bluegrass
annual b.
Kentucky b.
blue-gray lesion
bluetongue virus
blunt dissection
blush
blushing
BLV
bovine leukemia virus
BM
bacterial meningitis
BMD
bone mineral density
BMZ
basement membrane zone
BMZ antibody

BNLF-1 oncogene
Bockhart
B. folliculitis
B. impetigo
body
asteroid b.
Borrel b.'s
ciliary b.
Civatte b.'s
colloid b.'s
Cowdry type A inclusion b.'s
Cowdry type B inclusion b.'s
Creola b.
cytoid b.
cytoplasmic inclusion b.'s
Donovan b.
elementary b.'s (EB)
foreign b. (FB)
glomus · b.
Guarnieri b.'s
Halberstaedter-Prowazek b.'s
inclusion b.
Joest b.'s
b. lice
Lindner b.'s
loose b.
b. louse
Medlar b.'s
Miyagawa b.'s
b. moisturizer
molluscum b.
Negri b.'s
nuclear inclusion b.'s
Odland b.
Paschen b.'s
polyhedral b.
Prowazek b.'s
Prowazek-Greeff b.'s
psittacosis inclusion b.'s
rice b.'s
ringworm of b.
round b.
Russell b.'s
Schaumann b.
trachoma b.'s
vitreous b.

B

NOTES

53

Boeck
   B. sarcoid
   B. scabies
boggy swelling
Bohn nodule
boil
   Aleppo b.
   Baghdad b.
   blind b.
   botfly b.
   date b.
   Madura b.
   Oriental b.
   salt water b.
   tropical b.
bois
   pian b.
Bolivian hemorrhagic fever
bolster finger
Bombus **sting**
bone
   b. culture
   b. decay
   b. erosion
   b. marrow-derived cell
   b. marrow examination
   b. marrow transplantation
   b. mineral density (BMD)
Bonine
bony erosion
Böök syndrome
BOOP
   bronchiolitis obliterans with
      organizing pneumonia
booster
   b. dose
   b. response
boot
   Unna b.
borax
border
   coast of Maine b.
   indurated b.
   irregular b.
   raised b.
   vermilion b.
   volcanic b.
borderline
   b. leprosy
   b. malignant
      hemangiopericytoma
Bordetella
   B. parapertussis

   B. pertussis
   B. pertussis bacterium
Bordet-Gengou phenomenon
Borg scale
boric acid
Borna
   B. disease
   B. disease virus
Bornholm
   B. disease
   B. disease virus
Borrel bodies
Borrelia
   B. afzelii
   B. burgdorferi (Bb)
   B. burgdorferi DNA assay
   B. garinii
   B. lymphocytoma
   B. recurrentis
borreliosis, pl. borrelioses
   Lyme b.
BORSA strain
Borst-Jadassohn type intraepidermal
   epithelioma
bosch yaws
bossing
   frontal b.
Boston exanthema
botfly
   b. boil
   b. facultative myiasis
   b. obligate myiasis
bothropic antitoxin
Bothrops **antitoxin**
botryomycosis
botryosum
   Stemphylium b.
Botrytis cinerea
botulin
botulinum antitoxin
botulinus toxin
botulism
   b. antitoxin
   wound b.
botulismotoxin
boubas
Bouchard node
Bouffardi
   B. black mycetoma
   B. white mycetoma
bougie
bougienage
bouquet fever

Bourneville-Pringle disease
bouton
   b. de Bagdad
   b. de Biskra
boutonneuse fever
boutonnière deformity
bovine
   b. antitoxin
   b. collagen dermal implant
   b. colloid
   b. colostrum
   b. ephemeral fever
   b. herpes mammillitis
   b. leukemia virus (BLV)
   b. leukosis virus
   b. mastitis
   b. papular stomatitis
   b. papular stomatitis virus
   pegademase b.
   b. rhinoviruses
   b. rotavirus stain
   b. spongiform encephalopathy
   b. superoxide dismutase
   b. ulcerative mammillitis
   b. vaccinia mammillitis
   b. virus diarrhea
   b. virus diarrhea virus
   b. whey protein concentrate
bovis
   Actinomyces b.
   Babesia b.
Bowen
   B. disease
   B. disease of the glans penis
   B. precancerous dermatosis
bowenoid
   b. cell
   b. papulosis
Bowins suction
Bowman layer
box
   b. elder maple
   b. elder maple tree
   b. jellyfish
   b. jellyfish sting
boydii
   Allescheria b.

   Petriellidium b.
   Pseudallescheria b.
bozemanii
   Legionella b.
BP
   bullous pemphigoid
BPA
   bullous pemphigoid antigen
BQ Tablet
BR
   breathing reserve
brace
   Knight-Taylor b.
bracelet
   identification b.
brachial neuritis of Lyme disease
brachyonychia
brachytherapy
   endobronchial b.
bracket fungus
bradykinin
brain abscess
Brainerd diarrhea
brain-reactive autoantibody
branched DNA signal amplification
   assay for hepatitis B
branchial
   b. cleft
   b. cyst
B-range
   ultraviolet B.-r. (UVB)
Branhamella catarrhalis
branny
   b. desquamation
   b. scale
   b. tetter
Brasfield
   B. chest radiograph score
   B. scoring system
brasiliensis
   Blastomyces b.
   Nocardia b.
   Paracoccidioides b.
brawny
   b. edema
   b. induration

NOTES

Brazilian
B. pemphigus
B. rubber
B. rubber tree
braziliense
  Ancylostoma b.
Brazil nut
breakbone fever
Breathe
B. Right
B. Right nasal strip
breathing
apneustic b.
intermittent positive pressure b.
  (IPPB)
Ondine curse, periodic b.
pursed lips b.
b. reserve (BR)
sleep-disordered b.
breathlessness
bredeney
  Salmonella b.
breed
short-haired b.
Breezee Mist Antifungal
Brethaire
B. Inhalation Aerosol
Brethine
B. injection
B. Oral
Brett syndrome
Brevibacterium
brevicaulis
  Scopulariopsis b.
brevis
  Demodex b.
Brevoxyl
Bricanyl
B. injection
B. Oral
bridge
intercellular b.
bright erythema
Brill disease
Brill-Zinsser disease
brittle
b. hair, intellectual impairment,
  decreased fertility, short
  stature (BIDS)
b. nail
b. nail syndrome

broad
b. bean
b. spectrum
broad-spectrum
broccoli
Brocq
B. disease
pseudopelade of B.
Brodie abscess
Brofed Elixir
broken vein
Bromaline Elixir
Bromanate Elixir
Bromarest
Bromatapp
Bromavir
brome grass, bromegrass
bromelain
Bromfed
B.-PD
B. Syrup
B. Tablet
bromhexine
bromhidrosiphobia
bromhidrosis, bromidrosis
apocrine b.
eccrine b.
bromide
b. acne
ethidium b.
b. intoxication
ipratropium b.
pancuronium b.
bromidrosis
bromine
bromism
bromoderma
bromohyperhidrosis
Bromphen
B. Elixir
B. Tablet
brompheniramine
b. maleate
b. and phenylephrine
b. and phenylpropanolamine
b. and pseudoephedrine
bronchi (*pl. of* bronchus)
bronchial
b. artery embolization
b. asthma
b. epithelial cell
b. hygiene
b. hyperresponsiveness (BHR)

B

b. inhalation challenge test
b. mucous membrane
b. provocation
b. provocation test
b. smooth muscle
b. smooth muscle tone
b. stenosis
b. toilet
bronchiectasis
proximal b.
bronchiolitis
b. obliterans with organizing pneumonia (BOOP)
bronchitis
asthmatic b.
chronic b.
infectious avian b.
wheezy b.
bronchoactive agonist
bronchoalveolar
b. cell carcinoma
b. lavage (BAL)
bronchoconstriction
bronchodilatation
bronchodilator
Inhal-Aid b.
Maxi-Myst b.
nebulized b.
bronchogenic
b. carcinoma
b. cyst
bronchogram
air b.
bronchopleural fistula
bronchopneumonia
eosinophilic b.
bronchorrhea
Broncho Saline
bronchoscope
Dumon-Harrell b.
fiberoptic b.
bronchoscopy
fiberoptic b.
ultrasound-guided b.
bronchospasm
exercise-induced b.

bronchovascular markings
bronchus, pl. bronchi
lobar b.
subsegmental b.
Bronitin
Bronkaid Mist
Bronkephrine
B. injection
Bronkodyl
Bronkometer
Bronkosol
Brontex
bronzed skin
bronzinum
chloasma b.
Brooke
B. disease
B. tumor
Brooke-Spiegler syndrome
bropirimine
broth
Quant b.
b. test
Todd-Hewitt b.
brown
b. albinism
b. moth larvae sting
b. oculocutaneous albinism
b. recluse spider
b. recluse spider bite
b. tumor
brown-black lesion
brown-spot syndrome
brown-tail
b.-t. moth larva
b.-t. moth sting
b.-t. rash
brucei
Trypanosoma b.
Brucella
B. canis
B. card test
brucella
b. arthritis
b. strain 19 vaccine
brucellergin
brucellin

NOTES

brucellosis
    chronic b.
brucellum
    erythema b.
Bruch membrane
Brugia
    B. malayi
    B. timori
Brugsch syndrome
bruise
Brumpt white mycetoma
Brunsting-Perry
    localized pemphigoid of B.-P.
brush
    b. border receptor
    b. burn
    b. burn abrasion
brussel sprout
Bruton disease
bruxism
BU
    Bethesda unit
    biologic unit
buaki
buba madre
bubas
bubble
    b. gum dermatitis
    b. hair
bubo, pl. **buboes**
    malignant b.
    primary b.
    venereal b.
bubonic plague
bubonulus
Bucast
buccarum
    morsicatio b.
Buchwald atrophy
Buckley syndrome
buckwheat
Budd-Chiari syndrome
budesonide
buffalo
    b. fly
    b. hump
Bufferin
bug
    assassin b.
    conenose b.
    kissing b.
Buhler test

bulb
    hair b.
bulbar
bulbosa
    myringitis b.
bulla, pl. **bullae**
    friction b.
    hemorrhagic b.
    intraepidermal b.
    pressure b.
bullectomy
    transaxillary apical b.
bullosa
    Cockayne-Touraine
    epidermolysis b.
    Dowling-Meara
    epidermolysis b.
    dystrophic epidermolysis b.
    epidermolysis b. (EB)
    Hallopeau-Siemens
    epidermolysis b.
    Herlitz epidermolysis b.
    impetigo b.
    impetigo contagiosa b.
    inherited epidermolysis b.
    junctional epidermolysis b.
    (JEB)
    Köbner epidermolysis b.
    Pasini epidermolysis b.
    urticaria b.
bullosis
    b. diabeticorum
bullosum
    erythema b.
    erythema multiforme b.
bullosus
    herpes circinatus b.
bullous
    b. amyloidosis
    b. congenital ichthyosiform
    erythroderma
    b. disease
    b. edema
    b. erythema multiforme
    b. fever
    b. hemorrhagic pyoderma
    gangrenosum
    b. impetigo
    b. impetigo of newborn
    b. lesion
    b. lichen planus
    b. myringitis
    b. pemphigoid (BP)

b. pemphigoid antigen (BPA)
b. pemphigoid-like eruption
b. skin lesion
b. syphilid
bumble bee
bumblebee sting
bump
    goose b.
Bunnell sign
Bunyamwera
    B. fever
    B. virus
Bunyaviridae
Bunyavirus
bunyavirus encephalitis
bupivacaine
    b. hydrochloride
burgdorferi
    Borrelia b. (Bb)
Burkard
    B. spore trap
    B. trap
Burkholderia cepacia
Burkitt lymphoma
burn
    actinic b.
    brush b.
    chemical b.
    first degree b.
    flash b.
    full-thickness b.
    mat b.
    partial-thickness b.
    radiation b.
    road b.
    rope b.
    second degree b.
    superficial b.
    thermal b.
    third degree b.
burnetii
    Coxiella b.
burning
    b. mouth
    b. tongue
burnt out rheumatoid arthritis
Burow solution

burr
burrobrush
    white b.
burrow
burrowing hair
bursa, pl. **bursae**
    diarthrodial joint bursae
    distended b.
    pes anserinus b.
bursectomy
bursitis
    anserine b.
    fungal b.
    iliopectineal b.
    infrapatellar b.
    ischiogluteal b.
    olecranon b.
    prepatellar b.
    tendinitis b.
bursography
burst
    oxidative b.
    phagocyte oxidative b.
    prednisone b.
    respiratory b.
    steroid b.
Buruli ulcer
burweed
Bury disease
Buschke
    B. disease
    B. scleredema
Buschke-Löwenstein
    B.-L. giant condyloma
    B.-L. tumor
Buschke-Ollendorf
    B.-O. disease
    B.-O. sign
    B.-O. syndrome
bush
    iodine b.
    rabbit b.
    b. yaws
buspirone
Busse-Buschke disease
busulfan
butcher's tubercle

B

NOTES

butoconazole
butorphanol
butoxide
    piperonal b.
butterfly
    b. area
    b. eruption
    b. lung
    b. patch
    b. rash
    b. sign
button
    Amboyna b.
    Biskra b.
    Oriental b.

butyrate
    hydrocortisone b.
BV-ara-U
BvgAS regulon
BvgS protein
Bwamba
    B. fever
    B. virus
By antigen
bypass arthritis-dermatitis syndrome
byssinosis
Bywaters lesion

C
    C carbohydrate antigen
    C group virus
C1
    C. esterase
    C. esterase inhibitor
    C. inhibitor
C3
    C. anaphylatoxin (C3a)
    complement C.
    C. proactivator
    C. proactivator convertase
    serum C.
    C. test
C4
    complement C.
    serum C.
    C. test
C1q immune complex detection
C3/C4 receptor
C5b-C8 complex
C5b-C9 complex
CA
    croup-associated
    CA virus
C3a
    C3 anaphylatoxin
cabbage
cable rash
cachecticorum
    acne c.
    melanoderma c.
Cachexon
C5a complex
CAD
    chronic airways disease
    coronary artery disease
cadaverous
cadherin
CAE
    cefuroxime axetil suspension
caecutiens
    Onchocerca c.
caerulea (*var. of* cerulea)
caesiellus
    Aspergillus c.
Cafatine
café
    c. au lait spot
    c. coronary syndrome

Cafergot
Cafetrate
CAH
    chronic active hepatitis
cajennense
    Amblyomma c.
Cajuput oil
Calabar swelling
calamine
    c. lotion
calcaneal
    c. petechia
    c. spur
calcar
Calciferol
    C. injection
    C. Oral
calcific
    c. periarthritis
    c. tendinitis
calcification
    soft tissue c.
    subcutaneous c.
calcifying
    c. epithelioma
    c. epithelioma of Malherbe
Calcijex
calcineurin
calcinosis
    c. circumscripta
    c. cutis, osteoma cutis,
      poikiloderma, and skeletal
      abnormalities (COPS)
    c. cutis, Raynaud phenomenon,
      esophageal motility disorder,
      sclerodactyly, telangiectasia
      (CREST)
    c. cutis, Raynaud phenomenon,
      esophageal motility disorder,
      sclerodactyly, telangiectasia
      syndrome
    dystrophic c.
    tumoral c.
    c. universalis
calciphylaxis
calcipotriene
    c. therapy
calcipotriol
calcitonin
    salmon c.

calcitonin-origin amyloid deposit
calcitriol
calcium
   c. carbonate crystal
   fenoprofen c.
   c. gluconate
   c. hydroxyapatite crystal
     deposition disease
   leucovorin c.
   c. phosphate crystal deposition
     disease
   c. pyrophosphate dihydrate
     (CPPD)
   c. pyrophosphate dihydrate
     crystal deposition disease
     (CPPD)
   c. pyrophosphate dihydrate
     deposition disease (CPDD)
calcoaceticus
   Acinetobacter c.
calcofluor stain
Calcort
calculated mean organism (CMO)
Caldecort
   C. Anti-Itch spray
Caldesene topical
Caldwell-Luc procedure
Caliciviridae
   C. virus
Calicivirus
California
   C. black-legged tick
   C. encephalitis
   C. peppertree
   C. peppertree tree
   C. virus
Calliphora
Calliphoridae
callositas
callosity
callous
callus
Calmette-Guérin
   Bacille bilié de C.-G. (BCG)
   bacillus C.-G. (BCG)
   C.-G. bacillus
   C.-G. vaccine
Calmette test
calmodulin antagonist
Calm-X Oral
calor
calorica
   dermatitis c.

caloric intake
caloricum
   erythema c.
calvities
Calycophora dermatitis
Calymmatobacterium
   C. granulomatis
CAM
   cell adhesion molecule
Camcreme ECG paste
cAMP
   cyclic adenosine monophosphate
camp
   c. fever
Campbell-De Morgan spot
Campho-Phenique
camphor
   c. and phenol
camphorated menthol
camphor, menthol and phenol
camptodactyly
   congenital c.
Campylobacter
   C. jejuni
   C. pylori
Canada blue grass
canal
   external auditory c. (EAC)
canaliculitis
canary
   c. feather
   c. grass
   reed c.
canarypox virus
cancellous
cancer
   chimney sweep's c.
   c. en cuirasse
   epidermoid c.
   skin c.
cancericidal, cancerocidal
cancerophobia, cancerphobia
cancerous
cancrum
   c. oris
Candida
   C. albicans
   C. albicans IgG
   C. arthritis
   C. balanitis
   C. blastoconidia
   C. folliculitis
   C. glabrata

C. glossitis
C. glossodynia
C. granuloma
C. guillermondii
C. infection
C. intertrigo
C. krusei
C. leukoplakia
C. lusitaniae
C. onychia
C. osteomyelitis
C. parapsilosis
C. parapsilosis colonization
C. paronychia
C. septicemia
C. skin test
C. therapy
C. tropicalis

candidal
  c. angular cheilitis
  c. arthritis
  c. infection
  c. leukoplakia
  c. osteomyelitis
  c. paronychia

candidiasis
  acute atrophic oral c.
  atrophic c.
  chronic c.
  chronic atrophic c.
  chronic hyperplastic c.
  chronic mucocutaneous c.
   (CMC)
  congenital c.
  cutaneous c.
  disseminated c.
  invasive c.
  localized mucocutaneous c.
  mucocutaneous c.
  neonatal c.
  neonatal systemic c.
  oral c.
  oropharyngeal c.
  osteoarticular c.
  systemic c.
  vulvovaginal c. (VVC)

candidid

candidosis
candiduria
candidus
  Aspergillus c.
  strophulus c.
canimorsus
  Capnocytophaga c.
canine
  c. distemper virus
  c. herpesvirus
  c. herpetovirus
  c. oral papilloma
canine adenovirus 1
caninum
  Ancylostoma c.
  Dipylidium c.
canis
  Babesia c.
  Brucella c.
  Ctenocephalides c.
  Demodex c.
  Ehrlichia c.
  hepatitis contagiosa c.
  Microsporum c.
  Toxocara c.
canities
  rapid c.
  c. unguium
canium
  Neospora c.
canker
  c. sore
  water c.
Cann-Ease moisturizing nasal gel
cantaloupe
cantharic acid
cantharidal collodion
cantharidin
cantharis, pl. cantharides
canthus, pl. canthi
  inner c.
  nasal c.
  outer c.
  temporal c.
canyon ragweed
cao gio

C

NOTES

CAP
community-acquired pneumonia
cap
cradle c.
capacity
forced vital c. (FVC)
functional residual c. (FRC)
inspiratory c. (IC)
maximum breathing c. (MBC)
slow vital c. (SVC)
total lung c. (TLC)
vital c. (VC)
Capastat sulfate
CAPD
chronic ambulatory peritoneal
dialysis
capillariasis
capillaroscopy
nail fold c.
capillary, pl. capillaries
alveolar c.
c. angioma
c. fragility test
c. hemangioma
c. hemangioma of infancy
c. malformation
c. nevus
c. resistance test
synovial c.
capillitii
dermatitis papillaris c.
capillorum
defluvium c.
Capim virus
capitate
capitis
black dot tinea c.
gray patch tinea c.
inflammatory tinea c.
pediculosis c.
Pediculus c.
Pediculus humanus c.
pityriasis c.
pthiriasis c.
seborrhea c.
tinea c.
trichophytosis c.
vitiligo c.
Capitrol
Caplan syndrome
Caplets
Advil Cold & Sinus C.

Aspirin-Free Bayer Select
Allergy Sinus C.
Dimetapp Sinus C.
Dristan Sinus C.
TripTone C.
Capnocytophaga
C. canimorsus
capreomycin
c. sulfate
caprine
c. herpesvirus
c. herpetovirus
Capripoxvirus
caproate
hydroxyprogesterone c.
Caps
Drixoral Cough & Congestion
Liquid C.
capsaicin
capsid
Capsin
capsomer
capsular
c. antigen
c. precipitation reaction
capsulatum
Histoplasma c.
capsule
Alka-Seltzer Plus Cold Liqui-
Gels C.
Dapacin Cold C.
Dimetapp 4-Hour Liqui-Gel C.
Duadacin C.
Tenon c.
capsulitis
adhesive c.
Captia
C. test
C. test for syphilis
Capzasin-P
car allergy
Caraparu virus
carate
carateum
Treponema c.
carbamazepine
carbapenem
carbenicillin
Indanyl c.
carbide
cobalt in tungsten c.
carbinoxamine and pseudoephedrine
Carbiset Tablet

Carbiset-TR Tablet
Carbocaine injection
Carbodec
  C. Syrup
  C. Tablet
  C. TR Tablet
carbohydrate intolerance
carbol-fuchsin
  c. solution
carbon
  c. dioxide (CO_2)
  c. dioxide laser
  c. monoxide
carbovir
carboxamide
  imidazole c.
carboxyhemoglobin (HbCO)
carboxymethylcellulose
  benzocaine, gelatin, pectin, and
    sodium c.
  c. sodium
carboxypeptidase
carbuncle
carbuncular
carbunculoid
carbunculosis
carcinoembryonic antigen (CEA)
carcinogen
carcinogenesis
carcinoid
  c. syndrome
  c. tumor
carcinoma, pl. carcinomata
  adnexal c.
  apocrine c.
  basal cell c. (BCC)
  basosquamous c.
  bronchoalveolar cell c.
  bronchogenic c.
  cloacogenic c.
  eccrine c.
  c. en cuirasse
  epidermoid c.
  esophageal c.
  fibroepithelioma basal cell c.
  genital squamous cell c.
  infiltrative basal cell c.

  intermediate c.
  intraepidermal c.
  invasive squamous cell c.
  Lucké c.
  melanotic c.
  Merkel cell c.
  metatypical c.
  morbilliform basal cell c.
  morpheaform basal cell c.
  nasopharyngeal c.
  nevoid basal cell c.
  nodular basal cell c.
  pigmented basal cell c.
  pilomatrixoma c.
  prickle-cell c.
  sebaceous c.
  c. in situ
  in situ squamous cell c.
  spindle cell c.
  squamous cell c. (SCC)
  superficial basal cell c.
  sweat gland c.
  trabecular c.
  V-2 c.
  verrucous c.
carcinomatosis
Cardec-S Syrup
cardiac
  c. complications
  c. disease
  c. glycoside
cardiocutaneous
  c. myxoma
  c. syndrome
cardiolipin
cardiomyopathy
  restrictive c.
cardiopulmonary resuscitation
cardiorespiratory arrest
cardiovascular
  c. collapse
  c. involvement
Cardiovirus
Cardiovit AT-10 ECG/spirometry
  combination system
careless weed
Carey Coombs murmur

NOTES

carindacillin
carinii
    Pneumocystis c.
Carmol
    C.-HC topical
    C. topical
carneus
    Aspergillus c.
Carney
    C. complex
    C. syndrome
carnitine palmitoyltransferase
  deficiency
carob
carotene
    beta c.
carotenemia
carotenoderma
carotenosis
    c. cutis
carotinemia
carotinosis
    c. cutis
carpal
    c. to metacarpal ratio
    c. tunnel syndrome (CTS)
carpet-tack scale
carprofen
carrageenan
carrier
    c. cell
    convalescent c.
    incubatory c.
    c. state
    c. strain
Carrion disease
carrionii
    Cladosporium c.
carrot
Carter black mycetoma
cartilage
    hyaline articular c.
    c. matrix protein
cartilage-hair hypoplasia
cartilaginous collagen
Cartrofen
carumonam
caruncle
carunculae
    trichosis c.
Casal necklace

cascade
    arachidonic acid c.
    complementary c.
Cascade impactor
caseating
    c. granuloma
case control study
casei
    Lactobacillus c.
casein
cashew
Casoni
    C. intradermal test
    C. skin test
cassette
    susceptibility c.
cast
    erythrocyte c.
    hair c.
    spica c.
    total contact c.
Castaneda principle
Castellani
castellani
    Acanthamoeba c.
    C. Natural Formula
    C. paint
    C. point
castor bean
Castroviejo forceps
CAT
    chloramphenicol acetyltransferase
    CAT enzyme
cat
    c. dander
    c. distemper virus
    c. epithelium
    c. flea
    c. flea bite
    c. hookworm
    panleukopenia virus of c.'s
catabolism
Cataflam
    C. Oral
catagen
    c. phase
catalysis
catalyze
catamenial hemothorax
cataract
    poikiloderma atrophicans
    and c.
    secondary c.

catarrhalis
   Branhamella c.
   herpes c.
   Moraxella c.
catarrhal jaundice
catatrichy
catecholamine
caterpillar
   c. dermatitis
   puss c.
   c. rash
   saddle back c.
   c. sting
   stinging c.
catfish
   saltwater c.
   c. sting
cathepsin
   c. D
   c. G
   c. L
catholysis
Cath-Secure tape
cati
   Toxocara c.
catkins
cat-scratch disease (CSD)
cattle
   ephemeral fever of c.
   infectious papilloma of c.
   malignant catarrh of c.
   papular stomatitis virus of c.
   c. plague
   c. plague virus
   c. wart
   winter dysentery of c.
Catu virus
cauda equina syndrome
cauliflower
causalgia
causative
cauterization
cauterize
cautery
   chemical c.
   gas c.

cavernosum
   angioma c.
cavernosus
   nevus c.
cavernous
   c. angioma
   c. hemangioma
   c. lymphangioma
   c. sinusoid
caviae
   Aeromonas c.
   Nocardia c.
cavitary
cavitation
cayenne
   mal de C.
   c. pepper spot
Cazenave
   C. disease
   C. vitiligo
CAZ β-lactamase
C3b
   C. receptor
C3bBb receptor
CBH
   cutaneous basophil hypersensitivity
C4B receptor
C5b-9 receptor
C1–C9
   serum complement C1–C9
CCA
   chimpanzee coryza agent
CD2–72
   cluster of differentiation 2–72
CD4
   C. cell
   C. count
   C., human recombinant soluble rCD4
   C., human truncated-365 AA polypeptide
   C., immunoglobulin G, recombinant human
   C. T cell subset
   C. T-lymphocyte count
CD4+
   C. helper/inducer cell

C

NOTES

67

CD4+ *(continued)*
    C. measures
    C. T cell subset
CD5
    C. cell
CD8
    C. cell
    C. T cell subset
CD4/CD8 ratio
CD8+ T cell
CDC
    Centers for Disease Control
    Centers for Disease Control and
      Prevention
CDE antigen
C3dg receptor
CDM
    childhood dermatomyositis
cDNA
    complementary DNA
    cDNA probe
CEA
    carcinoembryonic antigen
Ceclor
cedar
    Japanese c.
    mountain c.
    red c.
    salt c.
    Western red c.
CeeNU Oral
cefaclor
cefadroxil monohydrate
Cefadyl
cefalexin *(var. of* cephalexin)
cefamandole
    c. nafate
Cefanex
cefazolin
    c. sodium
cefepime
cefixime
Cefizox
cefmenoxime
cefmetazole
    c. sodium
Cefobid
cefodizime
cefonicid
    c. sodium
cefoperazone
    c. sodium
ceforanide

cefotaxime
    c. sodium
cefotetan
cefoxitin sodium
cefpiramide
cefpodoxime
    c. proxetil
cefprozil
ceftazidime
ceftibuten
Ceftin
    C. Oral
ceftizoxime sodium
ceftriaxone
    c. sodium
cefuroxime
    c. axetil suspension (CAE)
Cefzil
celery
Celestone
    C. Soluspan
Celgene
celiac
    c. disease
    c. sprue
cell
    α-c.
    c. adhesion molecule (CAM)
    c. adhesion protein
    antigen-presenting c.
    antigen-sensitive c.
    B c.
    B1 c.
    balloon c.
    basal c.
    basaloid c.
    bone marrow-derived c.
    bowenoid c.
    bronchial epithelial c.
    carrier c.
    CD4 c.
    CD5 c.
    CD8 c.
    CD4+ helper/inducer c.
    CD8+ T c.
    chronic inflammatory c.
    ciliated epithelial c.
    Clara c.
    clear c.
    cleaved giant c.
    conjunctival goblet c.
    contrasuppressor c.
    cuboidal c.

cytolytic effector c.
cytomegalic c.'s
cytotoxic c.
daughter c.
dendritic c.
c. deposition
disorder of phagocytic c.
Dorothy Reed-Sternberg c.
double negative   c.
Downey c.
effector c.
end c.
endomysial mononuclear c.
endothelial c.
enterochromaffin c.
epidermal Langerhans c.
epithelioid c.
fibroblast-like c.
foam c.
foreign body giant c.
frozen-thawed red c.
germinative c.
giant c.
goblet c.
granular c.
hairy c. (HC)
HeLa c.'s
helper c.
high endothelial venule c.
hyperplastic mucus-secreting
  goblet c.
I c.
IgE-sensitized c.
immunocompetent c.
immunoglobulin-secreting c.
immunologically activated c.
immunologically competent c.
inclusion c.
inducer c.
inflammatory c.
innocent bystander c.
islet α-c.
K c.
    killer cell
killer c. (K cell, K cell)
Kulchitsky c.
c. lamina

Langerhans c.
Langhans c.
LE c.
lepra c.'s
Leu-3+ helper T c.
c. line
lupus erythematosus c.
lymph c.
lymphoid c.
lymphokine-activated killer c.
  (LAK)
c. marker
mast c.
Merkel c.
mesenchymal c.
metaplastic mucus-secreting c.
mononuclear c.
multifocal Langerhans c.
multinucleated giant c.
myeloid stem c.
naive B c.
natural killer c.
neoplastic c.
nests of nevus c.'s
nevus c., A-type
nevus c., B-type
nevus c., C-type
NK c.
non-B c.
null c.
OKT c.
    Ortho-Kung T cell
Ortho-Kung T c. (OKT cell)
Paget c.'s
pagetoid c.'s
palisade c.
pannus c.
peripheral blood
  mononuclear c. (PBMC)
plasma c.
polyclonal B c.
polymorphonuclear c.
preformed granule-associated
  mast c.
prickle c.
proliferative c.
pyknotic c.

C

NOTES

69

cell *(continued)*
    quantitation of B c.
    Raji c.
    red blood c.
    reticuloendothelial c.
    rheumatoid synovial c.
    rheumatoid synovial
      macrophage-like/dendritic c.
    rosette-forming c.
    satellite c.
    scavenger c.
    Schwann c.
    sensitized c.
    Sézary c.
    sheath c.
    sheets of nevus c.'s
    spindle c.
    squamous c.
    stem c.
    c. strain
    stromal c.
    suppressor c.
    c. surface marker
    synovial lining c. (SLC)
    T c.
    tanned red c.
    T cytotoxic c. (Tc)
    TDTH c.
    Tg c.
    T helper c. (Th)
    Tm c.
    c. transformation
    unifocal Langerhans c.
    veiled c.
    virus-transformed c.
    Warthin-Finkeldey c.
cell-bound antibody
Cellcept
cell-mediated
    c.-m. drug reaction
    c.-m. hypersensitivity
    c.-m. immunity (CMI)
    c.-m. immunologic drug
      reaction
    c.-m. reaction
Cellufresh
cellular
    c. blue nevus
    c. casts in urine
    c. immune panel
    c. immune theory
    c. immunity deficiency
      syndrome

    c. immunodeficiency with
      abnormal immunoglobulin
      synthesis
cellularis
    balanitis circumscripta
      plasma c.
    plasma c.
cellulite
cellulitis
    acute scalp c.
    anaerobic c.
    demarcated c.
    dissecting c.
    eosinophilic c.
    epizootic c.
    perianal streptococcal c.
    phlegmonous c.
cellulose
    hydroxypropyl c.
    oxidized c.
cellulosic/cuprophan
Celluvisc
CELO
    chicken embryo lethal orphan
celonychia
CELO virus
Celovirus
Celsus
    C. alopecia
    C. area
    C. kerion
    C. papule
    C. vitiligo
Cel-U-Jec
cement line
cementoma
Cenafed
    C. Plus Tablet
center
    necrotic c.
Centers for Disease Control (CDC)
Centers for Disease Control and Prevention (CDC)
centipede
    c. bite
    giant desert c.
central
    c. blister
    c. clearing
    C. European tick-borne
      encephalitis virus
    c. fibrinoid necrosis
    c. nervous system (CNS)

c. papillary atrophy
c. pruritus
c. Recklinghausen disease type II
c. stratum
c. type neurofibromatosis
centrifugum
erythema annulare c. (EAC)
leukoderma acquisitum c.
centrofacial lentiginosis
Centruroides
C. exilicauda
C. exilicauda sting
C. sculpturatus
C. sculpturatus sting
C. vittatus
C. vittatus sting
CEP
chronic eosinophilic pneumonia
cepacia
Burkholderia c.
cephalexin, cefalexin
c. monohydrate
cephalic histiocytosis
cephalo-oculocutaneous telangiectasia
cephalosporin
third-generation c.
Cephalosporium
cephalothin
c. sodium
cephapirin sodium
cephradine
Ceptaz
Ceratopogonidae
cercaria, pl. **cercariae**
cercarial
c. dermatitis
cerea
seborrhea c.
cereal
introduction of c.
cerebellar ataxia
cérébrale
tache c.
cerebral malaria
cerebri
pseudotumor c.

cerebritis
cerebrospinal
c. fever
c. meningitis
c. rhinorrhea
cerebrotendinous xanthomatosis
Ceredase injection
cereolysin
cereus
Bacillus c.
Cerezyme
Cerubidine
cerulea, caerulea
macula c.
maculae c.
ceruloplasmin
cerumen
ceruminal
ceruminous
c. gland
cervical
c. acceleration-deceleration syndrome
c. actinomycosis
c. lymph node swelling
c. patagium
cervicitis
Cetacaine
Cetamide Ophthalmic
Cetaphil
Cetapred Ophthalmic
cetirizine
CF
complement fixation
cystic fibrosis
C. antibody
Saleto C.
C. test
CFA
cryptogenic fibrosing alveolitis
CFIDS
chronic fatigue and immune dysfunction syndrome
CFU
colony-forming unit
CH50 assay
Chaetomium globosum

NOTES

C

chafe
chaffeensis
   Ehrlichia c.
Chagas disease
chagasic
chagoma
Chagres virus
chagrin
   peau de c.
chain
   alpha c.
   glycosaminoglycan c.
   heavy c.
   hemolytic c.
   homology of c.
   J c.
   kappa light c.
   lambda light c.
   light c.
   polypeptide c.
chalazion, pl. chalazia
   c. knife
chalazodermia, chalazoderma
chalk
   steroid c.
challenge
   c. diet
   dinitrochlorobenzene c.
   direct c.
   double-blind food c.
   food c.
   methacholine c.
   methacholine
     bronchoprovocation c.
   oral c.
   c. test
chamber
   aluminum Finn c.
   Finn c.
Chanarin-Dorfman syndrome
chancre
   hard c.
   hunterian c.
   mixed c.
   monorecidive c.
   c. recidive
   c. rédux
   soft c.
   sporotrichositic c.
   syphilis c.
   tuberculous c.
   tularemic c.

chancriform
   c. pyoderma
   c. syndrome
chancroid
chancroidal
chancrous
change
   clinical c.'s
   environmental c.
   fibrinoid c.
   formula c.
   histologic c.
   hormonal c.'s
   mitral valve prolapse, aortic
     anomalies, skeletal changes,
     and skin c.'s (MASS)
   nail c.
   nonspecific climatic c.
   pigment c.
   polyneuropathy, organomegaly,
     endocrinopathy, monoclonal
     gammopathy, and skin c.'s
     (POEMS)
   respiratory c.'s
   symmetric reticulonodular x-
     ray c.
   synovial fluid c.'s
   tinctorial c.
Chantemesse reaction
chappa
chapped
chapping
characteristic
   lesion surface c.
Charcot joint
Charcot-Leyden crystal
chard
   Swiss c.
Charlouis disease
Chaussier areola
Chédiak-Higashi syndrome
cheek
   c. chewing
   c. cosmetic
cheilitis, chilitis
   actinic c.
   angular c.
   candidal angular c.
   commissural c.
   contact c.
   c. exfoliativa
   c. glandularis
   c. glandularis apostematosa

c. granulomatosa
granulomatous c.
impetiginous c.
solar c.
c. venenata
Volkmann c.
cheilosis
cheiroarthropathy
diabetic c.
cheiropompholyx (*var. of*
chiropompholyx)
chelating agent
chelicera, pl. **chelicerae**
cheloid
cheloidalis
acne c.
acné chéloïdique
chelonae
Mycobacterium c.
chemes
chemexfoliation
chemical
c. agent
c. burn
c. cautery
c. depilatory
c. dermatitis
c. grouping
c. hemostasis
c. leukoderma
c. panniculitis
c. peel
c. prophylaxis
c. stimulus
c. sunscreen
chemicocautery
chemiluminescence assay
chemiluminescent
c. DNA
c. in situ hybridization for
detection of CMV DNA
chemistry
blood c.
chemoattractant
chemocautery
chemoimmunology
chemokines

chemokinetic factor
chemonucleolysis
chemonucleosis
chymopapain c.
chemoprophylaxis
chemoresistance
chemosis
chemosurgery
Mohs c.
chemotactic peptide
chemotaxis
eosinophilic c.
impaired neutrophil c.
leukocyte c.
neutrophil c.
chemotechnique
chemotherapeutic index
chemotherapy
c. agent
interleukin-2 adjunctive c.
Chenopodium
cheopis
Xenopsylla c.
cherry
c. angioma
c. spot
chest
c. cold
c. percussion and vibration
"silent" c.
chewing
cheek c.
Cheyletiella **infestation**
Cheyne-Stokes respiration
CHF
congestive heart failure
chicken
c. embryo lethal orphan
(CELO)
c. embryo lethal orphan virus
c. feather
c. pox
chickenpox
c. immune globulin (human)
c. immunoglobulin
c. vaccine
c. virus

C

NOTES

chiclero ulcer
chief agglutinin
Chiesi powder inhaler
chigga
chigger
    c. bite
    c. flea
chigoe
chikungunya virus
chilblain
    c. lupus
    c. lupus erythematosus
chilblain-like erythema
CHILD
    congenital hemidysplasia with
    ichthyosiform erythroderma and
    limb defects
        CHILD syndrome
child
    blueberry muffin c.
childbed fever
childhood
    c. bullous dermatosis
    chronic bullous dermatosis
      of c.
    c. dermatomyositis (CDM)
    c. eczema
    c. myositis
    papular acrodermatitis of c.
    polyarteritis in c.
    c. type tuberculosis
children
    chronic granulomatous disease
      of c.
Children's
    C. Advil
    C. Motrin suspension
    C. Silfedrine
    C. Vaccine Initiative (CVI)
chilitis (*var. of* cheilitis)
chimera
chimeric
    c. antibodies
chimerism
chimney sweep's cancer
chimpanzee coryza agent (CCA)
Chinese
    C. elm
    C. elm tree
    C. restaurant syndrome
Chiou equation

Chironex
    C. fleckeri
    C. fleckeri sting
chiropompholyx, cheiropompholyx
chi sequence
chitin
chive
Chlamydia
    C. disease
    C. pneumoniae
    C. psittaci
    C. trachomatis
chlamydial
    c. conjunctivitis
    c. infection
    c. urethritis
chlamydospore
Chlo-Amine Oral
chloasma
    c. bronzinum
    c. faciei
    c. gravidarum
    melanoderma c.
chloracne
Chlorafed Liquid
chlorambucil
chloramine T
chloramphenicol
    c. acetyltransferase (CAT)
    c., polymyxin b, and
      hydrocortisone
    c. and prednisolone
Chlorate Oral
chlordiazepoxide
chlorhexidine
    c. gluconate
chloride
    aluminum c.
    benzalkonium c.
    benzocaine, butyl
      aminobenzoate, tetracaine, and
      benzalkonium c.
    ethyl c.
    ferric c.
    liquid ethyl c.
    methacholine c.
    polyvinyl c. (PVC)
    sweat c.
    c. sweat test
    vinyl c.
chlorine acne
chloroguanide hydrochloride
Chloromycetin

chloroprocaine hydrochloride
Chloroptic Ophthalmic
Chloroptic-P Ophthalmic
6-chloropurine
chloroquine
    c. phosphate
    c. and primaquine
    c. therapy
chloroquine-resistant
    c.-r. *Plasmodium falciparum*
    (CRPF)
chloroxine
Chlorphed
Chlorphed-LA Nasal solution
chlorpheniramine
    c. and acetaminophen
    Efidac/24 c.
    c. maleate
    c., phenylephrine, and codeine
    c., phenylephrine, and
    phenylpropanolamine
    c., phenylephrine, and
    phenyltoloxamine
    c., phenylpropanolamine, and
    acetaminophen
        c., phenyltoloxamine,
    phenylpropanolamine and
    phenylephrine
    c. and pseudoephedrine
    c., pyrilamine, phenylephrine,
    and phenylpropanolamine
Chlor-Pro injection
chlorpromazine
    c. hydrochloride
chlortetracyline hydrochloride
Chlor-Trimeton (CTM)
    C.-T. 4 Hour Relief Tablet
    C.-T. injection
    C.-T. Oral
chocolate
cholangiolitic hepatitis
cholangitis
    sclerosing c.
Choledyl
cholera
    Asiatic c.
    c. bacillus

hog c.
    c. sicca
    c. toxin
    typhoid c.
    c. vaccine
cholerae
    Vibrio c.
choleraesuis
    Salmonella c.
choleragen
choleraic
cholera-red reaction
cholestatic hepatitis
cholesterinized antigen
cholesteroderma
cholesterol
    c. crystal
    c. embolus
cholesterolosis
    c. cutis
    extracellular c.
choline
    c. magnesium trisalicylate
    c. salicylate
cholinergic
    c. agent
    c. response
    c. urticaria
chomdromatosis
chondrification
chondritis
chondrocalcinosis
    hydroxyapatite c.
chondrocyte
chondrodermatitis
    c. helicis nodularis
    c. nodularis chronica helicis
chondrodysplasia
    lethal c.
    c. punctata
    c. punctata syndrome
    thanatophoric diastrophic c.
    twisted c.
chondrogenesis
chondroid syringoma
chondroitin
    c. sulfate

C

NOTES

chondroitin *(continued)*
   c. sulfate B
   c. sulfate/dermatan sulfate
    (CS/DS)
chondroma
chondromalacia
chondroprotective drugs
chondrosarcoma
chorda tympani syndrome
chorea
   Sydenham c.
choriomeningitis
chorioretinitis
choristoma
choroidal angiitis
choroiditis
Chortoglyphus arcuatus
Chr[a] antigen
Christmas tree pattern
chromatica
   trichomycosis c.
chromatin
chromatism
chromatogenous
chromatography
   gas c.
chromatophore
chromatophorotropic
chrome
   c. patch test
   c. ulcer
chromhidrosis, chromidrosis
   apocrine c.
   eccrine c.
chromoblastomycosis
chromomycosis
chromonychia
chromophage
chromophore
chromophototherapy
chromosomal
chromosome
   c. arrangement
   c. 6, class III MHC
   c. number
   X c.
chromotherapy
chromotrichia
chromotrichial
chronic
   c. acral dermatitis
   c. actinic dermatitis
   c. active hepatitis (CAH)

c. airways disease (CAD)
c. allograft rejection
c. ambulatory peritoneal
  dialysis (CAPD)
c. anaphylaxis
c. anterior poliomyelitis
c. asthma
c. atrophic candidiasis
c. atrophic vulvitis
c. blood loss
c. bronchitis
c. brucellosis
c. bullous dermatosis of
  childhood
c. candidiasis
c. cold agglutinin disease
c. conjunctivitis
c. cutaneous leishmaniasis
c. diarrhea
c. discoid lupus erythematosus
c. eczema
c. eosinophilic pneumonia
  (CEP)
c. Epstein-Barr virus infection
c. erythema multiforme
c. fatigue and immune
  dysfunction syndrome
  (CFIDS)
c. fatigue syndrome
c. graft-versus-host disease
c. granulomatous disease
c. granulomatous disease of
  children
c. hemolytic anemia
c. hereditary lymphedema
c. histiocytosis
c. hyperplastic candidiasis
c. hypersensitivity pneumonitis
c. idiopathic thrombocytopenic
  purpura
c. inflammation (CI)
c. inflammatory cell
c. inflammatory disease
c. interstitial lung disease
c. jejunal inflammation
c. mucocutaneous
c. mucocutaneous candidiasis
  (CMC)
c. mucocutaneous candidiasis
  syndrome
c. obstructive pulmonary
  disease (COPD)
c. otitis media

c. pain
c. pain syndrome
c. papular dermatitis
c. paranasal sinusitis
c. paronychia
c. postrheumatic fever arthritis
c. pulmonary disease
c. radiodermatitis
c. T-cell leukemia
c. thromboembolic pulmonary
   hypertension (CTEPH)
c. tophaceous gout
c. ulcer
c. undermining ulcer of
   Meleney
c. urticaria
chronica
keratosis lichenoides c.
mycosis cutis c.
c. parapsoriasis lichenoid
pityriasis lichenoides c.
urticaria c.
chronicum
erythema c.
chronicus
genital lichen simplex c.
lichen simplex c. (LSC)
chrysanthemum
chrysiasis
chrysoderma
Chrysomyia
chrysorrhoea
Euproctis c.
Chrysosporium pruinosum
chrysotherapy
Churg-Strauss
C.-S. angiitis
C.-S. granulomatosis
C.-S. syndrome (CSS)
chylidrosis
chyloderma
chylous
chymase
chymopapain
c. chemonucleosis
CI
chronic inflammation

CIC
circulating immune complex
cicatrices (*pl. of* cicatrix)
cicatricial
c. alopecia
c. horn
c. pemphigoid
c. pemphigoid antigen
c. stenosis
cicatrisata
alopecia c.
cicatrix, pl. **cicatrices**
cicatrization
exuberant c.
ciclopirox
c. olamine
CID
combined immunodeficiency disease
cidal effect
cidofovir
CIE
counterimmunoelectrophoresis
crossed immunoelectrophoresis
cigarette
c.-paper scarring
c.-paper wrinkling
c. smoke
ciguatera poisoning
cilastatin
ciliaris
acne c.
tylosis c.
ciliary
c. beat frequency
c. body
ciliated epithelial cell
Ciloxan Ophthalmic
cimetidine
Cimex lectularius
Cimicidae
cimicosis
cincinnatiensis
Legionella c.
cinerea
Botrytis c.
cinnamon
Cinobac Pulvules

C

NOTES

cinoxacin
Cipro
   C. injection
   C. Oral
ciprofloxacin
   c. hydrochloride
circinata
   balanitis c.
   impetigo c.
   pityriasis c.
   psoriasis c.
   tinea c.
circinate
   c. balanitis
circinatum
   erythema c.
circuit
   heart-lung c.
Circulaire aerosol drug delivery system
circulans
   Bacillus c.
circulating
   c. anticoagulant
   c. immune complex (CIC)
circumcised
circumflexa
   ichthyosis linearis c.
circumscribed
   c. albinism
   c. myxedema
   c. neurodermatitis
   c. precancerous melanosis of Dubreuilh
circumscripta
   allotrichia c.
   alopecia c.
   balanitis c. plasma cellularis
   calcinosis c.
   osteoporosis c.
   poliosis c.
circumscriptum
   c. angiokeratoma
   lymphangioma c.
cirrhosis
cirrhotic lacrimal gland
cisplatin
13-*cis*-retinoic acid
Citanest
   C. Forte
   C. Plain
Citoscope-16 arthroscope

citrate
   piperazine c.
   c. synthase
Citrobacter
   C. diversus
   C. freundii
citronella oil
Civatte
   C. bodies
   C. disease
   poikiloderma of C.
   C. poikiloderma
CJD
   Creutzfeldt-Jakob disease
cladiosis
cladosporioides
   Cladosporium c.
cladosporiosis
Cladosporium
   C. carrionii
   C. cladosporioides
   C. mansonii
   C. werneckii
Claforan
clamdigger's itch
Clara cell
clarithromycin
Claritin
Claritin-D
Clark level
clasmatocyte
class
   c. I antigen
   c. II antigen
   c. III antigen
   c. switch
classic
   c. allergy symptom
   c. neurofibromatosis
classification
   Gell and Coombs c.
   Lancefield c.
   Loesche c.
   Lukes-Collins c.
   morphologic c.
   Nalebuff c.
   Rappaport c.
   Runyon c.
   Steinbrocker c.
   Walter Reed c.
clastothrix
clavatus
   Aspergillus c.

clavi (*pl. of* clavus)
clavulanate
clavulanic acid
clavus, pl. clavi
clawing
    c. deformity
    rheumatoid c.
Clay-Adams stain
clean
    Dey-Wash skin wound c.
cleaner
    air c.
    unclassified air c.
cleanser
    lipid-free c.
    Saf-Clens wound c.
cleansing cream
clear
    C. Away Disc
    C. By Design
    c. cell
    c. cell acanthoma
    c. cell hidradenoma
clearance
    creatinine c.
    immune complex c.
    mucociliary c.
Clearasil
clearing
    central c.
cleavage
    lines of c.
cleaved giant cell
cleft
    branchial c.
    lucent c.
clefting
    suprabasal c.
clemastine
    c. fumarate
    c. and phenylpropanolamine
Cleocin
    C. HCl
    C. Pediatric
    C. Phosphate
Cleocin T

climacterica
    keratoderma c.
climactericum
    keratoderma c.
    keratosis c.
climatotherapy
clindamycin
clinical
    c. changes
    c. judgment
    c. manifestation
    c. myocarditis
Clinoril
clioquinol
    c. and hydrocortisone
ClipTip reusable sensor
CLM articulating laryngoscope
  blade
cloacae
    Enterobacter c.
cloacogenic carcinoma
clobetasol
    c. dipropionate
    c. propionate
Clocort Maximum Strength
clocortolone pivalate
Cloderm
    C. topical
clofazimine
    c. palmitate
clomipramine
Clomycin
clonal
    c. deletion theory
    c. expansion
    c. selection theory
clonazepam
clonidine hydrochloride
clonorchiasis
clorazepate
Clorpactin WCS-90
closed
    c. comedo
    c. patch test
"closed space" infection
clostridia

C

NOTES

clostridial
c. myonecrosis
Clostridium
Clostridium difficile
Clostridium difficile test
(CLOtest)
closure
Velcro c.
CLOtest
Clostridium difficile test
clothes louse
clotrimazole
betamethasone and c.
c. troche
Clouston syndrome
clover
sweet c.
cloxacillin
c. sodium
Cloxapen
Clr deficiency
clubbed finger
clubbing
idiopathic c.
nail c.
c. of nail
club hair
cluster
aggressive cell c.
cluster of differentiation 2–72
(CD2–72)
cluster-of-grapes appearance
Clutton joint
CMC
chronic mucocutaneous candidiasis
CMI
cell-mediated immunity
CMO
calculated mean organism
CMP-NANA
cytidine monophospho-N-acetyl
neuraminic acid
CMS AccuProbe 450 system
CMV
cytomegalovirus
cnidoblast
cnidosis
CNS
central nervous system
CO_2
carbon dioxide
CO_2 laser

coadministration
coagglutinin
coagulation
blood c.
disseminated intravascular c.
(DIC)
c. meshwork
sepsis-induced disseminated
intravascular c.
coagulopathy
consumption c.
coal
c. tar
c. tar, lanolin, and mineral oil
c. tar and salicylic acid
coalescence
coalescing
Coamatic protein C test
coarse
c. breath sound
c. rale
coast
c. of Maine border
c. sage
coated tongue
cobalamin deficiency
cobalt in tungsten carbide
cobblestoning
Cobb syndrome
cobra
c. hemotoxin
c. venom cofactor
c. venom factor
cocarde reaction
cocardiform
cocci
Gram-negative c.
Gram-positive c.
coccidioidal
c. granuloma
c. osteomyelitis
Coccidioides immitis
coccidioidin
coccidioidomycosis
cutaneous c.
coccidiosis
cockade
cockatiel feather
Cockayne syndrome
Cockayne-Touraine epidermolysis
bullosa
cocklebur

cockroach
American c.
German c.
cockscomb ulcer
cock-up deformity
cocoa
coconut
codeine
chlorpheniramine, phenylephrine,
and c.
codfish
Codiclear
coding joint
codon
arginine c.
coefficient
diffusion c.
coelenterate sting
Coe virus
cofactor
cobra venom c.
coffee bean
Coffin-Lowry syndrome
Coffin-Siris syndrome
Cogan syndrome
Cogentin
cognitive-behavioral technique
coherence therapy
Co-Hist
cohort study
coil
air c.
c. gland
secretory c.
Coinage Act
coincidental symptom
ColBENEMID
colchicine
c. and probenecid
cold
c. abscess
c. agglutination
c. agglutinin
c. allergy
C. & Allergy Elixir
c. antibody
c. autoagglutinin

c. autoantibody
chest c.
c. cream
c. exposure
c. gangrene
c. hemagglutinin disease
c. hemolysin
c. panniculitis
rose c.
c. sore
c. stage
c. ulcer
c. urticaria
c. virus
cold-dependent dermographism
Cold-Eezer Plus
cold-induced
c.-i. urticaria
c.-i. vasospasm
Coldlac-LA
Coldloc
C.-LA
cold-reactive antibody
Coleman microinfiltration system
Coleoptera
coli
Balantidium c.
Escherichia c.
c. granuloma
colic
infantile c.
colicin
colicinogeny
coliphage
colistimethate sodium
colistin, neomycin, and
hydrocortisone
colistin sulfate
colitis
antibiotic-associated c.
collagenous c.
milk-induced c.
pseudomembranous c.
colitose
collaboration
T cell-B cell c.
collacin

C

NOTES

81

collagen
cartilaginous c.
conformational kinks in c.
c. CS
c. fibril
fibrillar c.
hydroxylysine content of c.
c. implant
injectable c.
c. injection
c. polymer
short-chain type c.
short-chain type X c.
type I c.
type II c.
type III c.
type IV c.
type IX c.
type VI c.
type VII c.
type VIII c.
type XI c.
type XIV c.
c. vascular disease
c. vascular serologic test
collagenase
polymorphonuclear leukocyte c.
type IV c.
type V c.
collagenization
collagenolysis
collagenolytic enzyme
collagenoma
collagenosis
reactive perforating c.
collagenous
c. colitis
collapse
cardiovascular c.
collarette
c. of Biet
collar of Venus
collastin
collectins
collection
gravitational particle c.
isokinetic c.
collegenase
Colles fracture
colli
leukoderma c.
melanoleukoderma c.
pterygium c.

collimated bema handpiece (CBH-1)
for laser surgery
colliquativa
tuberculosis cutis c.
colliquative
c. degeneration
c. sweat
collodion
c. baby
blistering c.
cantharidal c.
hemostatic c.
iodized c.
c. membrane
salicylic acid c.
styptic c.
colloid
c. acne
c. bath
c. bodies
bovine c.
c. cyst
c. degeneration
c. milium
c. pseudomilium
colloidalis conglomerata
colloidal oatmeal
cologne
colonic adenocarcinoma
colonization
airway bacterial c.
atypical mycobacterial c.
Candida parapsilosis c.
colony-forming unit (CFU)
colony-stimulating
c.-s. factor (CSF)
c.-s. factor-developed by
Venereal Disease Research
Laboratory (CSF-VDRL)
c.-s. factor fluorescent
treponemal antibody-absorption
test (CSF-FTA-ABS)
c.-s. factor
microhemagglutination-
Treponema pallidum test
(CSF-MHA-TP)
colophony
color
constitutive skin c.
facultative skin c.
inducible skin c.
lesion c.
pale c.

Colorado
   C. microdissection needle
   C. tick fever
   C. tick fever virus
coloration
Colorimeti Assay
coloring agent
ColorZone tape
colostrum
   bovine c.
colpate
colporate
Columbia S. K. virus
columnar
   c. epithelium
Coly-Mycin
   C.-M. M Parenteral
   C.-M. S Oral
   C.-M. S Otic Drops
combination skin
combined
   c. antibody and cellular
     deficiency
   c. immunodeficiency
   c. immunodeficiency disease
     (CID)
   c. immunodeficiency syndrome
   measles, mumps and rubella
     vaccines, c.
   measles and rubella
     vaccines, c.
   penicillin g benzathine and
     procaine c.
   rubella and mumps
     vaccines, c.
combining site
combion test
combustionis
   dermatitis c.
Comby sign
comedo, pl. comedones, comedos
   c. acne
   closed c.
   comedones epidermal nevus
   c. extraction
   c. nevus
   open c.

comedocarcinoma
comedogenic
comedones (*pl. of* comedo)
comedonicus
   nevus c.
comedos (*pl. of* comedo)
Comfort Tears solution
Comhist
   C. LA
comma bacillus
commercial antigen
commissural cheilitis
Committee
   National Vaccine Advisory C.
     (NVAC)
common
   c. acne
   c. antigen
   c. baldness
   c. cold virus
   c. nevus
   c. opsonin
   c. reed
   c. reed grass
   c. striped scorpion
   c. striped scorpion sting
   c. variable immunodeficiency
     (CVI)
   c. variable unclassifiable
     immunodeficiency
   c. wart
communicable
   c. disease
community-acquired pneumonia
   (CAP)
compactum
   Fonsecaea c.
   Hormodendron c.
   stratum c.
Companion 314 nasal CPAP system
compatibility
compatible
Compeed Skinprotector dressing
competence
   immunological c.
competition
   antigenic c.

NOTES

C

83

competitive binding assay
competitor DNA
complement
   c. activation
   c. activity
   c. binding assay
   c. C3
   c. C4
   c. chemotactic factor
   component of c.
   c. deficiency
   erythrocytes, antibody, c.
     (EAC)
   c. fixation (CF)
   c. protein
   c. receptor (1–4) (CR (1–4))
   serum c. C1–C9 (C1–C9)
   c. system
   total hemolytic c.
   c. unit
complement-activating antigen-
  antibody
complementarity
   c. determining region
complementary
   c. cascade
   c. DNA (cDNA)
   c. strand
complementation
complement-fixation
   c.-f. reaction
   c.-f. test
complement-fixing antibody
complement-mediated tumor cell
  immunopurging
complete
   c. antibody
   c. antigen
   c. blood count
   c. transduction
complex
   Acinetobacter calcoaceticus-
     baumannii c.
   AIDS-related c. (ARC)
   antigen-antibody c.
   antigenic c.
   avian leukosis-sarcoma c.
   C5a c.
   Carney c.
   C5b-C8 c.
   C5b-C9 c.
   circulating immune c. (CIC)
   desmosome-tonofilament c.

   elastomeric c.
   feline leukemia-sarcoma
     virus c.
   Ghon c.
   Golgi c.
   GP ib-IX c.
   H-2 c.
   HLA c.
   IgG c.
   immune c.
   major histocompatibility c.
     (MHC)
   membrane attack c. (MAC)
   membranolytic attack c.
     (MAC)
   Mycobacterium avium c.
     (MAC)
   popliteal-arcuate c.
   primary c.
   semimembranosus c.
complexion
   T zone c.
complication
   cardiac c.'s
   delayed c.
   immunologic c.
   nonimmunologic c.
component
   absent dermal c.
   c. of complement
   matrix c.
   secretory c.
   ultrastructural c.
compound
   c. cyst
   c. nevus
   sulfhydryl c.
compress
   cool c.
   ice c.
compression
   suprascapular nerve c. (SSC)
computed tomography (CT)
Comtrex
concentrate
   bovine whey protein c.
   hyperimmune bovine colostrum
     IgC c.
   leukocyte c.
   parvum bovine
     immunoglobulin c.
   platelet c.

concentration
    geometric mean c. (GMC)
    grass pollen c.
    intradermal test c.
    minimal bactericidal c. (MBC)
    minimal inhibitory c. (MIC)
    minimum inhibitory c. (MIC)
    prick test c.
concentricum
    Trichophyton c.
concomitant
    c. immunity
concrete seborrhea
condition
    Fordyce c.
    isocapnic c.
    seborrheic dermatitis-like c.
    severe chronic allergic c.
conditional-lethal mutant
conditionally lethal mutant
conditioned hemolysis
condyloma, pl. condylomata
    c. acuminatum
    Buschke-Löwenstein giant c.
    flat c.
    giant c.
    c. latum
    c. planus
    pointed c.
condylomatous
Condylox
cone
    keratosic c.
conenose, cone-nose
    c. bug
    c. bug bite
Conex
conferta
    urticaria c.
configuration
    lesion c.
confirmation
    tissue c.
confluent
    c. and reticulate papillomatosis
conformational kinks in collagen

congelation
    c. urticaria
congelationis
    dermatitis c.
congeneric
congenita
    adermia c.
    aplasia cutis c.
    arthrochalasis multiplex c.
    cutis marmorata
      telangiectasia c.
    dyskeratosis c.
    hyperkeratosis c.
    melanosis diffusa c.
    pachyonychia c.
    type II pachyonychia c.
congenital
    c. anemia
    c. aplasia of thymus
    c. baldness
    c. camptodactyly
    c. candidiasis
    c. circumscribed hypomelanosis
    c. contractural arachnodactyly
    c. cytomegalovirus
    c. depigmentation
    c. disorder
    c. dysphagocytosis
    c. ectodermal defect
    c. ectodermal dysplasia
    c. elephantiasis
    c. erythrodermic ichthyosis
    c. erythropoietic porphyria
    c. fibromatosis
    c. generalized phlebectasia
    c. hemidysplasia
    c. hemidysplasia with
      ichthyosiform erythroderma
      and limb defects (CHILD)
    c. HIV infection
    c. ichthyosiform erythroderma
    c. ichthyosis
    c. Lyme disease
    c. nevus
    c. rubella
    c. rubella syndrome
    c. sebaceous hyperplasia

C

NOTES

congenital *(continued)*
    c. self-healing
      reticulohistiocytosis
    c. syphilis
    c. telangiectatic erythema
    c. total lipodystrophy
    c. toxoplasmosis
    c. varicella
congenitale
    poikiloderma c.
congenitalis
    alopecia c.
    alopecia triangularis c.
    erythroderma ichthyosiformis c.
Congess
    C. JR
    C. Sr
Congestac
Congestant D
congestion
    nasal c.
    Vicks 44D Cough & Head C.
congestive heart failure (CHF)
congestivum
    erythema c.
conglobata
    acne c.
conglobate
    c. abscess
    c. acne
conglomerata
    colloidalis c.
    elastosis colloidalis c.
conglutination
conglutinin
    c. assay
Congo
    C. floor maggot
    C. floor maggot bite
    C. red stain
congolensis
    Dermatophilus c.
congruence
    joint c.
conidium, pl. conidia
conjugated
    c. antigen
    c. estrogens
    c. hapten
conjugation
conjugative plasmid
conjunctiva, pl. conjunctivae
    limbi c.

conjunctival
    c. goblet cell
    c. injection
    c. testing
conjunctivitis
    acute contagious c.
    acute epidemic c.
    acute follicular c.
    allergic c.
    angular c.
    bacterial c.
    blennorrheal c.
    chlamydial c.
    chronic c.
    giant papillary c. (GPC)
    gonococcal c.
    herpes simplex c.
    infantile purulent c.
    Lymphogranuloma venereum c.
    Moraxella c.
    toxicogenic c.
    vernal c.
    viral c.
connective
    c. tissue
    c. tissue activating peptide
      (CTAP)
    c. tissue disease (CTD)
    c. tissue nevus
    c. tissue proteinase
connori
    Nosema c.
conorii
    Rickettsia c.
Conradi disease
Conradi-Hünermann syndrome
consciousness
    disturbance of c.
consistency
    lesion c.
consolidation
    airspace c.
    patchy airspace c.
    progressive acinar c.
constant
    association c.
    binding c.
    diffusion c.
    c. region
constitutional
    c. hirsutism
    c. reaction
    c. ulcer

constitutive skin color
consumption
    c. coagulopathy
    maximal oxygen c. (VO_2 max)
Contact
    C. Dermatitis Research Group
contact
    allergen c.
    c. allergy
    c. cheilitis
    c. dermatitis
    c. eczema
    c. hypersensitivity
    c. leukoderma
    c. photosensitization
    c. urticaria
contactant
contact-type dermatitis
contagion
    immediate c.
    mediate c.
contagiosa
    impetigo c.
    keratosis follicularis c.
contagiosum
    ecthyma c.
    epithelioma c.
    erythema c.
    molluscum c.
contagiosus
    pemphigus c.
contagious
    c. disease
    c. ecthyma
    c. ecthyma (pustular dermatitis)
     virus of sheep
    c. pustular dermatitis
    c. pustular stomatitis virus
contagiousness
contagium
contaminant
contaminate
contamination
    bacterial c.
content
    high liquid c.

continua
    acrodermatitis c.
continued fever
continuous
    c. low-flow oxygen
    c. passive motion (CPM)
    c. positive airway pressure
     (CPAP)
contraction
    wound c.
contracture
    Dupuytren c.
    flexion c.
contrasuppression
contrasuppressor cell
control
    air pollution c.
    c. animal
    c. of emotional factor
    mite c.
    mold c.
    odor c.
    c. proteins C1s–C3s (C1s–C3s)
controlled
    c. anaphylaxis
    c. cough
Controller
    Pepcid AC Acid C.
contusiforme
contusion
Contuss
    C. XT
convalescent
    c. carrier
    c. serum
    c. stage
conventional animal
conversion
convertase
    C3 proactivator c.
convex nail
convoluted foam mattress
convulsion
    theophylline-induced c.
cookei
    Ixodes c.
cool compress

NOTES

coolie itch
cooling
    c. agent
    c. blanket
    rapid c.
Coombs
    C. serum
    C. test
Cooperative Systematic Studies of
    the Rheumatic Disease (CSSRD)
CO-Oximeter module
COPD
    chronic obstructive pulmonary
    disease
Cophene-B injection
copious sputum
copper
    c. bromide laser
    c. deficiency
    c. deposition
    c. metabolism
    c. vapor laser
copperhead
    c. snake
    c. snake bite
copra itch
coprecipitation
coproantibodies
coproporphyria
    hereditary c. (HCP)
coproporphyrin
COPS
    calcinosis cutis, osteoma cutis,
    poikiloderma, and skeletal
    abnormalities
    COPS syndrome
Co-Pyronil 2 Pulvules
coral
    c. cut
    fire c.
    c. snake
    c. snake bite
Cordran
    C. SP topical
    C. tape
    C. topical
Cordylobia anthropophaga
Corgard
Coricidin
    C. 'D'
corii
    sclerosis c.

corium
    superficial c.
corkscrew
    c. hair
    c. spirochete
corn
    asbestos c.
    hard c.
    seed c.
    c. smut
    soft c.
cornea
    herpes c.
corneae
    ichthyosis c.
    ichthyosis sebacea c.
corneal
    c. opacification
    c. ulcer
corneocyte
    c. adhesion
    c. desquamation
corneous
corneum
    Nosema c.
    stratum c.
corneus
    c. hypertrophicus
    lichen obtusus c.
cornification
    disorder of c. (DOC)
    c. disorder
    normal c.
    type 1-24 c.
cornified
    c. cell envelope
    c. layer
cornmeal
cornoid lamella
cornu cutaneum
corona
    c. seborrheica
    c. veneris
    zona c.
coronal view
coronary
    c. artery disease
    (CAD)
    c. vasculitis
Coronaviridae
    C. virus
Coronavirus
coronavirus

corporis
  pediculosis c.
  Pediculus c.
  pthiriasis c.
  seborrhea c.
  tinea c.
  trichophytosis c.
corps ronds
cor pulmonale
corpuscle
  Meissner c.
  molluscum c.
  Negri c.'s
  Vater-Pacini c.
Corque topical
correction
  Tukey post-hoc c.
corrosive ulcer
corset
Cort
  S-T C.
CortaGel
Cortaid
  C. Maximum Strength
  C. with aloe
Cortatrigen Otic
Cort-Dome
Cortef
  C. Feminine Itch
Cortenema
cortex of hair
Corticaine cream
corticale
  Cryptostroma c.
corticosteroid
  parenteral c.
  c. rosacea
  synthetic depot c.
  systemic c.
  topical c.
corticotropin
corticotropin-releasing hormone
  (CRH)
Corticoviridae
Cortifoam
Cortin topical
cortisol

cortisone acetate
Cortisporin
  C. Ophthalmic Ointment
  C. Ophthalmic suspension
  C. Otic
  C. Topical Cream
  C. Topical Ointment
Cortizone-5
Cortizone-10
Cortone
  C. Acetate injection
  C. Acetate Oral
corymbiform
corymbose syphilid
corynebacteria
corynebacteriophage
  β c.
Corynebacterium
  C. acnes
  C. diphtheriae
  C. minutissimum
coryneform bacterium
coryza
  allergic c.
Coryzavirus
CO Sleuth
Cosmegen
cosmetic
  cheek c.
  c. dermatitis
  eyelash c.
  eyelid c.
  lip c.
  undercover c.
cosmetica
  acne c.
cosmetician
cosmetologist
cosmetology
costal fringe
costaricensis
  Angiostrongylus c.
Cotinine assay
Cotrim
  C. DS
co-trimoxazole
cotton linter

C

NOTES

cottonmouth
    c. snake
    c. snake bite
cottonseed
cottonwood
    Arizona/Fremont c.
    c. tree
cotton-wool
    c.-w. patch
    c.-w. spot
cough
    barking c.
    controlled c.
    dry c.
    huff c.
    nonproductive c.
    reflex c.
    whooping c.
coughing
    paroxysm of c.
cough-variant asthma
Coulter ICD-Prep test
coumarin
    c. necrosis
Council
    Medical Research C. (MRC)
count
    CD4 c.
    CD4 T-lymphocyte c.
    complete blood c.
    hemolysis, elevated liver
      enzymes, low platelet c.
    peripheral blood c.
    reticulocyte c.
    white blood cell c.
countenance
    Hippocratic c.
counterimmunoelectrophoresis (CIE)
counterirritant
counterirritation
coup de sabre
Covermark corrective makeup
cow dander
Cowden disease
Cowdria ruminantium
Cowdry
    C. type A inclusion bodies
    C. type B inclusion bodies
cowl
    monk's c.
cow-milk protein intolerance
cowpox
    c. virus

cow's milk
COX
    cyclooxygenase
    COX-1
      cyclooxygenase-1
    COX-2
      cyclooxygenase-2
coxarthrosis
Coxiella burnetii
Cox organism
Coxsackie
    C. B virus
    C. encephalitis
Coxsackievirus
    C. B1
    C. B2
    C. B3
    C. B4
    C. B5
CPAP
    continuous positive airway pressure
    NightBird nasal C.
CPDD
    calcium pyrophosphate dihydrate
    deposition disease
CPM
    continuous passive motion
    CPM machine
C-polysaccharide
    pneumococcal C.-p. (CPS)
CPPD
    calcium pyrophosphate dihydrate
    calcium pyrophosphate dihydrate
    crystal deposition disease
CPS
    pneumococcal C-polysaccharide
C1qR
    C. radioassay
CR (1–4)
    complement receptor (1–4)
C1r
crab
    c. grass
    c. hand
    c. louse
    c. yaws
crabro
    Vespula c.
cracked
    c. heel
    c. lips
crackle
    end-inspiratory c.

cradle cap
Crandall syndrome
cranial arteritis
craquelé
    eczema c.
    erythema c.
    onychia c.
crateriform ulcer
craw-craw, kra-kra
crazy paving dermatosis
C-reactive protein (CRP)
cream
    cleansing c.
    cold c.
    Corticaine c.
    Cortisporin Topical C.
    Elimite C.
    EMLA c.
    Eucerin c.
    facial undercover c.
    Kwell c.
    Lamisil topical c.
    Lotrimin AF C.
    masoprocol c.
    Maximum Strength Desenex Antifungal C.
    Naftin c.
    Neosporin C.
    Pramosone c.
    Psorion C.
    SSD C.
    terbinafine hydrochloride c.
    tretinoin c.
    triamcinolone c. (TAC)
    Zonalon c.
crease
    allergic c.
    earlobe c.
    palmar c.
creatinine
    c. clearance
    c. kinase
creeping
    c. eruption
    c. myiasis
    c. ulcer
    c. vesiculation

Creme
    Fungoid C.
    Fungoid HC C.
    Gormel C.
Creola body
creosote
crepitans
    peritendinitis c.
crepitant
crepitation
crepitus
crescentic glomerulonephritis
CREST
    calcinosis cutis, Raynaud phenomenon, esophageal motility disorder, sclerodactyly, telangiectasia
    CREST syndrome
Cresylate
Creutzfeldt-Jakob disease (CJD)
CRH
    corticotropin-releasing hormone
cricket
Cricket recording pulse oximeter
cricoarytenoid joint
Crimean-Congo
    C.-C. hemorrhagic fever
    C.-C. hemorrhagic fever virus
crinis, pl. crines
crinium
    fragilitas c.
    nodositas c.
crisis, pl. crises
    anaphylactic c.
    anaphylactoid c.
criteria
    Jones c.
    Steinbrocker c.
    WHO c.
Crithidia luciliae immunofluorescence assay
Crixivan
Crohn disease
Crolom
    C. Ophthalmic solution
cromoglycate
    disodium c. (DSC)
cromolyn sodium
Cronkhite-Canada syndrome

NOTES

cross
 c. agglutination
 c. infection
 Maltese c.
 c. reaction
 c. sensitization
cross-antigenicity
cross-desensitization
crossed immunoelectrophoresis (CIE)
cross-linking
cross-matching
Cross-McKusick-Breen syndrome
cross-reacting
 c.-r. agglutinin
 c.-r. antibody
 antigenemically c.-r. food
 c.-r. material
cross-reaction
cross-reactive idiotype
cross-sensitivity
cross-sensitization
cross-tachyphylaxis
Cross Top replacement oxygen
 sensor
Crotalidae
Crotalus antitoxin
crotamiton
croup
croup-associated (CA)
 c.-a. virus
croupous membrane
Crowe sign
crowned dens syndrome
crown of Venus
CRP
 C-reactive protein
CRPF
 chloroquine-resistant *Plasmodium*
 falciparum
Cruex topical
crural fold
cruris
 tinea c.
 trichophytosis c.
crust
 amiantaceous c.
 milk c.
crusta
 c. lactea
crustacean
crusted
 c. ringworm

 c. scabies
 c. tetter
cruzi
 Trypanosoma c.
crymophilic
crymophylactic
cryobiology
Cryocrit
Cryocuff
cryoglobulin
cryoglobulinemia
cryolysis
cryophilic
cryophylactic
cryoprecipitate
cryoprecipitation
cryotherapy
cryotolerant
cryptococcosis
Cryptococcus neoformans
cryptogenic
 c. fibrosing alveolitis (CFA)
 c. infection
cryptosporidiosis
Cryptosporidium **oocysts**
Cryptostroma corticale
cryptotrichotillomania
crystal
 calcium carbonate c.
 Charcot-Leyden c.
 cholesterol c.
 c. deposition disease
 lipid liquid c.
 monosodium urate c.
 oxalate c.
 plate-like c.
 c. rash
 c. violet vaccine
crystal-induced arthritis
crystallina
 miliaria c.
 uridrosis c.
Crysticillin A.S. injection
CS
 collagen C.
 invariant chain C.
C1s–C3s
 control proteins C1s–C3s
CSD
 cat-scratch disease
 CSD skin test
CS/DS
 chondroitin sulfate/dermatan sulfate

decorin C.
fibromodulin C.
seglycin C.
versican C.
CSF
colony-stimulating factor
CSF-FTA-ABS
colony-stimulating factor fluorescent
treponemal antibody-absorption
test
CSF-MHA-TP
colony-stimulating factor
microhemagglutination-*Treponema
pallidum* test
CSF-VDRL
colony-stimulating factor-developed
by Venereal Disease Research
Laboratory
Csillag disease
CS/KS
aggrecan C.
CSS
Churg-Strauss syndrome
CSSRD
Cooperative Systematic Studies of
the Rheumatic Disease
CT
computed tomography
thin-section CT
CTAP
connective tissue activating peptide
CTCL
cutaneous T-cell lymphoma
CTD
connective tissue disease
Ctenocephalides
C. canis
C. canis bite
C. felis
C. felis bite
CTEPH
chronic thromboembolic pulmonary
hypertension
CTL
cytotoxic T lymphocyte
CTM
Chlor-Trimeton

CTS
carpal tunnel syndrome
CTX
cyclophosphamide
ctx
Cytoxan
Cuban itch
cubital tunnel syndrome
cuboidal cell
cucumber
sea c.
cuff
rotator c.
c. tear arthropathy
cuirasse
cancer en c.
carcinoma en c.
culbertsoni
Acanthamoeba c.
Culex
Culicidae
culicosis
Cullen sign
cultivated
c. barley grass
c. barley smut
c. corn grass
c. corn smut
c. oat grass
c. oat smut
c. rye grass
c. rye smut
c. wheat grass
c. wheat smut
cultivation
culture
appropriate c.
bone c.
elective c.
enrichment c.
fungal c.
mixed lymphocyte c. (MLC)
organ c.
stool c.
cultured thymic epithelium
cumulative toxicity

C

NOTES

cuniculatum
epithelioma c.
cuniculus
Cupressaceae pollinosis
Cuprimine
curettage
curette, curet
currant
currens
larva c.
Curschmann spirals
Curth-Maklin cornification disorder
curve
dose-response c.
epidemic c.
Curvularia lunata
Cushing
C. disease
C. syndrome
cushingoid facies
cut
coral c.
cutanea
sclerosis c.
cutaneomeningospinal angiomatosis
cutaneous
c. abscess
c. absorption
c. albinism
c. amyloid
c. ancylostomiasis
c. anthrax
c. apoplexy
c. basophil hypersensitivity (CBH)
c. B-cell lymphocytic leukemia
c. B-cell lymphoma
c. candidiasis
c. coccidioidomycosis
c. diphtheria
c. drug eruption
c. dyschromia
c. elastosis
c. focal mucinosis
c. gangrene
c. graft versus host reaction
c. histoplasmosis
c. horn
c. hyperpigmentation
c. larva migrans
c. leishmaniasis
c. lesion
c. lupus

c. lupus erythematosus
c. manifestation
c. mastocytosis
c. meningioma
c. necrotizing venulitis
c. nodule
c. polyarteritis nodosa
c. purpura
c. reaction
c. sarcoidosis
c. sign
c. sinus
c. sporotrichosis
c. tag
c. T-cell lymphoma (CTCL)
c. test
c. toxoplasmosis
c. tuberculin test
c. tuberculosis
c. tumor
c. ulcer
c. vasculitis
cutaneous-subcutaneous nodule
cutaneum
cornu c.
sebum c.
cutaneus
nodulus c.
cutem
cuticle
c. of hair
c. of inner root sheath
cuticularization
cutireaction
c. test
cutis
amebiasis c.
amyloidosis c.
ancylostomiasis c.
c. anserina
asteatosis c.
atrophia c.
atrophia maculosa varioliformis c.
aurantiasis c.
B-cell lymphocytoma c.
benign lymphocytoma c.
carotenosis c.
carotinosis c.
cholesterolosis c.
diphtheria c.
dystrophic calcinosis c.
idiopathic calcinosis c.

c. laxa
leiomyoma c.
leukemia c.
lymphadenosis benigna c.
lymphocytoma c.
c. marmorata
c. marmorata telangiectasia
 congenita
metastatic calcinosis c.
neuroma c.
osteoma c.
osteosis c.
c. rhomboidalis nuchae
T-cell lymphocytoma c.
tuberculosis c.
c. unctuosa
c. vera
verrucosa c.
c. verticis gyrata
cutisector
Cutivate
 C. topical
cutter
 motorized c.
cutting fluid
CVI
 Children's Vaccine Initiative
 common variable immunodeficiency
Cw6
 HLA C.
cyanhidrosis
cyaniventris
 Dermatobia c.
cyanohidrosis
cyanosis
 pernio c.
cyanotic
cycle
 purine nucleotide c.
cyclic
 c. adenosine monophosphate
 (cAMP)
 c. guanosine monophosphate
 c. neutropenia
 c. nucleotides adenosine
 monophosphate
 c. urticaria

cyclizine hydrochloride
Cyclocort
 C. topical
cyclomethicone
cyclooxygenase (COX)
 c.-1 (COX-1)
 c.-2 (COX-2)
cyclophosphamide (CTX)
cycloplegic
cycloserine
cyclosporin A
cyclosporine
 c. microemulsion
cylindroma
cypress
 Arizona c.
 bald c.
 Italian c.
 Monterey c.
cyproheptadine
 c. hydrochloride
cyproterone acetate
cyst
 adventitious c.
 anogenital epidermal c.
 anogenital pilar c.
 anogenital sebaceous c.
 anogenital vestibular c.
 apocrine retention c.
 Baker c.
 branchial c.
 bronchogenic c.
 colloid c.
 compound c.
 dermoid c.
 desmoid c.
 epidermal c.
 epidermoid cyst
 epithelial c.
 false c.
 Favre-Racouchot c.
 follicular infundibular c.
 follicular isthmus c.
 implantation c.
 inclusion c.
 keratinous c.
 milia c.

NOTES

95

cyst *(continued)*
    mucinous c.
    mucous c.
    multilocular thymic c. (MTC)
    myxoid c.
    parasitic c.
    parvilocular c.
    piliferous c.
    pilonidal c.
    popliteal c.
    preauricular c.
    proliferating pilar c.
    proliferating trichilemmal c.
    renal c.
    retention c.
    sebaceous c.
    sequestration c.
    subchondral c.
    synovial c.
    thyroglossal c.
    trichilemmal c.
    unicameral c.
    unilocular c.
    vestibular c.
cystadenoma
    apocrine c.
cystatin C
cystatin C-origin amyloid deposit
cysteamine
cysteine
    c. proteinase
    c. proteinase inhibitor
cystic
    c. acne
    c. deformation
    c. fibrosis (CF)
    c. fibrosis transmembrane
      regulator
    c. hidradenoma
    c. hygroma
cystica
    acne c.
cysticercosis
cysticidal
cysticum
    acanthoma adenoides c.
    epithelioma adenoides c.
cystides
cystis
cystitis
    hemorrhagic c.
cystous
Cystoviridae

cytapheresis
cytarabine
    c. hydrochloride
cytase
cytidine monophospho-N-acetyl
    neuraminic acid (CMP-NANA)
cytoadhesion
cytochrome
    c. P450
cytocidal
cytodiagnosis
CytoGam
cytogram
cytoid body
cytokine
    IL-1β c.
    c. production
    c. synthesis inhibitory factor
    TNF mRNA c.
cytolysin
cytolysis
cytolytic
    c. effector cell
cytomegalic
    c. cells
    c. inclusion disease
cytomegalovirus (CMV)
    congenital c.
    c. disease
    c. immune globulin
    intravenous, human
    c. retinitis
cytometric indirect
    immunofluorescence
cytometry
    flow c.
cytopathic effect
cytopathogenic virus
cytophagic
    c. histiocytic panniculitis
    c. lobular panniculitis
cytophagous
cytophagy
cytophil group
cytophilic
    c. antibody
cytophylactic
cytophylaxis
cytoplasm
cytoplasmic
    c. inclusion
    c. inclusion bodies
    c. plaque

cytoryctes
Cytosar-U
cytosine
    c. arabinoside
cytoskeleton
Cytotec
cytotoxic
    c. agent
    c. cell
    c. drug
    c. immunologic drug reaction
    c. immunosuppressive therapy
    c. reaction
    c. T lymphocyte (CTL)

cytotoxicity
    antibody-dependent cell-
      mediated c. (ADCC)
    lymphocyte-mediated c. (LMC)
cytotoxin
cytotoxin-positive stain
cytotropic
    c. antibody
    c. antibody test
cytotropism
Cytovene
Cytoxan (ctx)
    C. injection
    C. Oral

NOTES

C

D2
   prostaglandin D. (PGD2)
'D'
   Coricidin 'D'
d4T, didehydrothymidine
Daae disease
dacarbazine
DaCosta syndrome
dacryoadenitis
dacryocystitis
dacryocystorhinostomy
dactinomycin
dactyledema
dactylitis
   blistering distal d.
   distal d.
   multidigit d.
   septic d.
   syphilitic d.
   tuberculous d.
dactylolysis spontanea
dactyloscopy
daisy
   oxeye d.
Dakar bat virus
Dakrina Ophthalmic solution
Dalalone
   D. D.P.
   D. L.A.
Dale reaction
Dalmane
damage
   bacterial-induced vascular d.
   immunologic organ d.
   musculotendinous d.
   sun and chemical
      combination d.
   toxic organ d.
dammini
   Ixodes d.
danazol
dandelion
dander
   animal d.
   cat d.
   cow d.
   dog d.
   inhaled d.
dandruff
dandy fever

Dane particle
Danielssen-Boeck disease
Danielssen disease
D antigen
Danysz phenomenon
Dapa
Dapacin Cold Capsule
DA pregnancy test
dapsone (DDS)
Dapsone Pharmacokinetics
dapsone/pyrimethamine
Daraprim
DAR breathing system
Darier
   D. disease
   morbus D.
   D. sign
Darier-Roussy sarcoid
Darier-White disease
dark dot disease
darkfield microscopy
dark-staining nodule
dartos
   tunica d.
date
   d. boil
   d. fever
daughter cell
daunorubicin
   d. hydrochloride
DaunoXome
Dawbarn sign
Dawson encephalitis
21-Day Cumulative irritancy assay
daylight sign
Daypro
D&C dye
ddC
   zalcitabine
ddc
   dideoxycytidine
ddi
   didanosine
DDS
   dapsone
DE
   Ru-Tuss D.
de
   d. Quervain disease
   d. Quervain tenosynovitis

dead
 d. finger
 d. space:tidal volume ratio
dead-end host
deafness
 abnormalities of genitalia,
 retardation of growth, and d.
 bilateral sensorineural d.
 keratitis d.
 lentigines, electrocardiographic
 defects, ocular hypertelorism,
 pulmonary stenosis,
 abnormalities of genitalia,
 retardation of growth, d.
 (LEOPARD)
 nerve d.
deallergize
deaminase
 adenosine d.
Debré phenomenon
debridement
debris
 phagocytosable d.
Debrisan topical
DEC
 diethylcarbamazine
Decadron
 D. and Hexadrol
 D.-LA
 D. Phosphate
 D. Phosphate Respihaler
 D. Phosphate Turbinaire
Decaject
 D.-LA
decalvans
 acne d.
 folliculitis d.
 keratosis follicularis
 spinulosa d.
 porrigo d.
decalvant
decamethonium
Decaspray
decay
 bone d.
deciduous skin
Declomycin
Decofed Syrup
decompensation
Decon
 Par D.
Deconamine
 D. SR

 D. Syrup
 D. Tablet
decongestant
 New D.
 topical d.
Deconsal
 D. II
Decontabs
decorin
 d. CS/DS
decreased
 d. fertility, short stature
 d. renal function
decubation
decubital
 d. gangrene
decubitus
 d. ulcer
deep
 d. hemangioma
 d. mycosis
deer
 d. fly
 d. fly bite
 d. fly disease
 d. hair
 d. tick
defect
 congenital ectodermal d.
 immunoregulatory d.
 neuroectodermal d.
 opsonophagocytic d.
 scleral d.
 T-cell d.
defective
 d. bacteriophage
 d. interfering (DI)
 d. interfering particle
 d. phage
 d. probacteriophage
 d. prophage
 d. virus
defects
 congenital hemidysplasia with
 ichthyosiform erythroderma
 and limb d. (CHILD)
 host d.
 humoral d.
 limb d.
Defen-LA
defense mechanism
defensin
defensins

defervesce
defervescence
defervescent stage
defibrination syndrome
deficiency
  acetylcholinesterase d.
  acquired biotin d.
  ADA d.
  adenosine deaminase d.
  antibody d.
  biotinidase d.
  carnitine palmitoyltransferase d.
  C1r d.
  cobalamin d.
  combined antibody and
    cellular d.
  complement d.
  copper d.
  essential fatty acid d.
  genetic C2 d.
  glucose-6-phosphatase d.
  HGPRT d.
  HRF d.
  hypoxanthine-guanine
    phosphoribosyltransferase d.
  IgA d.
  immune d.
  immunity d.
  immunological d.
  iron d.
  juvenile biotin d.
  leukocyte adhesion d. (LAD)
  multiple sulfatase d.
  myeloperoxidase d.
  myoadenylate deaminase d.
  myophosphorylase d.
  neonatal biotin d.
  niacin d.
  opsonic d.
  pantothenic acid d.
  phagocytic d.
  placental sulfatase d.
  primary cell-mediated d.
  prolidase d.
  α_1 proteinase d.
  protein C d.

  purine nucleoside
    phosphorylase d.
  pyridoxine d.
  pyridoxol d.
  pyruvate kinase d.
  riboflavin d.
  secondary antibody d.
  secretory component d.
  selenium d.
  steroid sulfatase d.
  thiamine d.
  tocopherol d.
  vitamin A d.
  vitamin B d.
  vitamin B_1 d.
  vitamin B_5 d.
  vitamin B_6 d.
  vitamin B_{12} d.
  vitamin C d.
  vitamin D d.
  vitamin E d.
  vitamin K d.
  zinc d.
deflazacort
deflexion
  hip d.
deflorescence
defluvium
  d. capillorum
  d. unguium
defluxion
deformans
  spondylosis d.
deformation
  cystic d.
deformity
  angel wing d.
  arthritis without d.
  boutonnière d.
  clawing d.
  cock-up d.
  opera-glass d.
  pencil and cup d.
  saddle nose d.
  swan-neck d.
defurfuration
degenerated microfilaria

D

NOTES

101

degeneration
  amyloid d.
  ballooning d.
  basophilic d.
  colliquative d.
  colloid d.
  elastoid d.
  elastotic d.
  epithelial d.
  fatty d.
  fibrinous d.
  granular d.
  hepatolenticular d.
  hyaline d.
  liquefaction d.
  malignant d.
  mucinous d.
  mucoid d.
  myxomatous d.
  reticular d.
  unilateral macular d.
degenerativa
  melanosis corii d.
degenerative
  d. arthritis
  d. collagenous plaque
Degos
  D. acanthoma
  D. disease
  malignant papillomatosis of D.
  D. syndrome
degranulation
  goblet cell d.
30-degree oblique arthroscope
dehaptenation
dehiscence
Dehist injection
dehumidification
dehumidifier
dehydration
dehydroemetine
dehydrogenase
  glucose-6-phosphate d. (G6PD)
  inosinic acid d.
  lactate d.
Dejerine-Sottas disease
delavirdine
  d. mesylate
Delaxin
delayed
  d. allergy
  d. anagen release

  d. blanching
  d. complication
  d. hypersensitivity (DH)
  d.-hypersensitivity immunologic
    drug reaction
  d. hypersensitivity reaction
  d. hypersensitivity skin testing
  d. patch test reading
  d. reaction
  d. systemic reaction
  d. tanning
  d. telogen release
  d. transfusion reaction
delayed-type hypersensitivity (DTH)
Delcort
deliensis
  Trombicula d.
delitescence
delling
Del-Mycin topical
delta
  d. agent
  alpha, d.
  d. antigen
  d. antigen hepatitis
  Galton d.
  d. sleep
  d. virus
Delta-Cortef Oral
Deltasone
  D. Dosepak
  D. Oral
Delta-Tritex
deltoidea
  Anthopsis d.
  Aspergillus d.
delusion of parasitosis
demarcated
  d. cellulitis
  d. reaction
demarcation
Dematiaceae
dematiaceous
  d. fungi
  d. fungus
d'emblée
  mycosis fungoides d.
  syphilis d.
demeclocycline hydrochloride
dementia
  transmissible d.
Demerol

demodectic
    d. acariasis
    d. mange
Demodex
    D. brevis
    D. canis
    D. equi
    D. folliculorum
demodicidosis
demodicosis
demyelinating
denaturation
denaturing agent
dendritic
    d. cell
    d. macrophage
    d. morphology
dendritiform
dengue
    d. facies
    d. fever
    hemorrhagic d.
    d. hemorrhagic fever
    d. shock syndrome
    d. virus
denitrificans
    Alcaligenes d.
Dennie
    D. infraorbital fold
    D. line
Dennie-Morgan
    D.-M. infraorbital fold
    D.-M. line
    D.-M. sign
Denorex
densa
    lamina d.
    sublamina d.
density
    bone mineral d. (BMD)
    d. gradient bone marrow
        progenitor enrichment
dental
    d. abnormality
    d. amalgam
    d. fistula
    d. plaque

d. sinus
d. sinus tract
dentifrice
dentinogenesis imperfecta
dentocariosa
    Rothia d.
denture
    d. epulis
    d. stomatitis
denudation
denude
denuded
Denys-Leclef phenomenon
deodorant
2′-deoxyadenosine
deoxycholate
deoxynucleoside
deoxyribonuclease (DNase)
    fibrinolysin and d.
    human recombinant d.
deoxyribonucleic acid (DNA)
deoxyribose
deoxyvirus
Depakene
Depakote
Depen
dependent edema
Dependovirus
dephosphorylation
depigmentation
    congenital d.
depilate
depilation
depilatory
    chemical d.
depletion
    acetylcholine d.
depMedalone injection
Depoject injection
Depo-Medrol
    D.-M. injection
Depopred injection
deposit
    calcitonin-origin amyloid d.
    cystatin C-origin amyloid d.
    immunoglobulin light chain-

D

NOTES

103

deposit *(continued)*
    origin amyloid d. (AL
      protein)
    2-microglobulin-origin
      amyloid d. (A 2M)
    prion protein-origin amyloid d.
    protein origin amyloid d.
    transthyretin-origin amyloid d.
deposition
    cell d.
    copper d.
    fibrin d.
    hemosiderin d.
    hydroxyapatite crystal d.
    nonlinear IgA d.
    silicone d.
    urate d.
depot reaction
depulization
Dercum disease
derivative
    ergotamine d.
    purified protein d.
    undecylenic acid and d.'s
    valproic acid and d.'s
Derma
    D. Smoothe Oil
    D. Soap
dermabrader
dermabrasion
Dermacentor
    D. andersoni
    D. occidentalis
    D. variabilis
Dermacomb topical
Dermacort
Dermaflex Gel
Dermagraft
dermagraphy
dermahemia
Dermaide
dermal
    d. duct tumor
    d. hypoplasia
    d. leishmanoid
    d. lesion
    d. lymphatics
    d. microvascular unit
    d. papilla
    d. system
    d. tuberculosis
dermalaxia
dermametropathism

Dermanyssus gallinae
Dermarest Dricort
Derma-Smoothe/FS topical
DermaSof sheeting
dermatalgia
dermatic
dermatica
    zona d.
dermatitic
dermatitidis
    Ajellomyces d.
    Blastomyces d.
dermatitis, pl. dermatitides
    acneform d.
    actinic d.
    d. actinica
    allergic contact d.
    allergic eczematous contact-
      type d.
    d. ambustionis
    ancylostoma d.
    d. artefacta
    atopic d.
    d. atrophicans
    d. autophytica
    autosensitization d.
    berlock d.
    blastomycetic d.
    d. blastomycotica
    blistering d.
    bubble gum d.
    d. calorica
    Calycophora d.
    caterpillar d.
    cercarial d.
    chemical d.
    chronic acral d.
    chronic actinic d.
    chronic papular d.
    d. combustionis
    d. congelationis
    contact d.
    contact-type d.
    contagious pustular d.
    cosmetic d.
    desquamative d.
    dhobie mark d.
    diaper d.
    earlobe allergic d.
    eczematoid d.
    endogenous d.
    eosinophilic d.
    erythematous macular d.

d. estivalis
ethylenediamine d.
d. exfoliativa
d. exfoliativa infantum
d. exfoliativa neonatorum
exfoliative d.
exudative discoid and
  lichenoid d.
d. factitia
factitial d.
familial rosacea-like d.
fiberglass d.
follicular nummular d.
d. gangrenosa infantum
genital atopic d.
d. herpetiformis (DH)
d. hiemalis
infectious eczematoid d.
irritant contact d.
irritant hand d.
lichenified d.
livedoid d.
mango d.
meadow grass d.
d. medicamentosa
d. multiformis
neck d.
neomycin d.
nickel d.
d. nodosa
d. nodularis necrotica
nonspecific d.
ocular atopic d.
oozing d.
d. papillaris capillitii
papulosquamous d.
paraphenylenediamine d.
d. pediculoides ventricosus
pellagra-associated d.
pellagroid d.
perfume d.
perioral d.
periorbital d.
photoallergic contact d.
photocontact d.
photoingestant d.
photosensitive nonscarring d.

photosensitivity d.
phototoxic contact d.
pigmentary atopic d.
pigmented purpuric
  lichenoid d.
plant d.
plantar d.
poison ivy d.
poison oak d.
poison sumac d.
d. pratensis striata
primary irritant d.
proliferative d.
protein contact d.
psoriasiform d.
radiation d.
ragweed d.
rat mite d.
rebound d.
d. repens
rhus d.
rosaceaform d.
rubber additive d.
sandal strap d.
Schamberg d.
schistosomal d.
seborrheic d.
d. seborrheica
d. simplex
solar d.
stasis d.
d. stasis
subcorneal pustular d.
T-cell mediated delayed type
  hypersensitivity d.
tinea d.
traumatic d.
trefoil d.
d. vegetans
d. venenata
d. verrucosa
vesicular d.
weeping d.
x-ray d.
dermatitis-arthritis-tenosynovitis
  syndrome
dermatoalloplasty

D

NOTES

dermatoarthritis
    lipoid d.
dermatoautoplasty
Dermatobia
    D. cyaniventris
    D. hominis
dermatobiasis
dermatoblepharitis
dermatocele
dermatocellulitis
dermatochalasia
dermatochalasis
dermatoconiosis
dermatocyst
dermatodynia
dermatofibroma
dermatofibrosarcoma protuberans
dermatofibrosis lenticularis
    disseminata
dermatogenic torticollis
dermatoglyph
dermatoglyphic
dermatograph
dermatographia
    black d.
    urticarial d.
    white d.
dermatographic
dermatographism
dermatography
dermatoheliosis
dermatoheteroplasty
dermatohistopathology
dermatohomoplasty
dermatoid
dermatologic
Dermatologic Diagnostic Algorithm
dermatologist
dermatology
dermatolysis
dermatoma
dermatomal
    d. distribution
    d. superficial telangiectasia
dermatome
dermatomegaly
dermatomic area
dermatomycosis
    d. pedis
dermatomyoma
dermatomyositis (DM)
    childhood d. (CDM)
    juvenile d. (JDMS)

dermatoneurosis
dermatonosology
Dermatop
dermatopathia
    d. pigmentosa reticularis
dermatopathic
    d. anemia
    d. lymphadenopathy
dermatopathology
dermatopathy
Dermatophagoides
    D. farinae
    D. microceras
    D. pteronyssinus
dermatophilosis
Dermatophilus congolensis
dermatophone
dermatophylaxis
dermatophyte
    d. fungal infection
    d. test medium (DTM)
dermatophytid, dermatophytide
    erysipelas-like d.
    d. reaction
dermatophytosis, pl. dermatophytoses
dermatoplastic
dermatoplasty
dermatopolymyositis
dermatopolyneuritis
dermatorrhagia
dermatorrhea
dermatorrhexis
dermatosclerosis
dermatoscopy
dermatosis, pl. dermatoses
    acantholytic d.
    acarine d.
    acquired d.
    acute febrile neutrophilic d.
    adult bullous d.
    ashy d.
    benign papular acantholytic d.
    Bowen precancerous d.
    childhood bullous d.
    crazy paving d.
    dermolytic bullous d.
    digitate d.
    flaky paint d.
    Gougerot-Blum d.
    ichthyosiform d.
    IgA d.
    inflammatory d.

intraepidermal neutrophilic
  IgA d.
lichenoid chronic d.
linear IgA bullous d.
d. medicamentosa
neutrophilic intraepidermal
  IgA d.
d. papulosa nigra
papulosa nigra d.
persistent acantholytic d.
pigmented purpuric
  lichenoid d.
progressive pigmentary d.
pruritic d.
pustular d.
radiation d.
Schamberg progressive
  pigmented purpuric d.
seborrheic d.
subcorneal pustular d.
temperature-dependent d.
transient acantholytic d. (TAD)
ulcerative d.
dermatotherapy
dermatothlasia
dermatothlasis
dermatotropic
dermatoxenoplasty
dermatozoiasis
dermatozoon
dermatozoonosis
dermatrophia
dermic
Dermicel tape
DermiCort
dermis
  papillary d.
  reticular d.
  upper d.
dermite
dermitis
dermoepidermal junction
dermographia
dermographism
  cold-dependent d.
  white d.

dermoid
  d. cyst
  inclusion d.
  sequestration d.
Dermolate
dermolysis
dermolytic bullous dermatosis
dermonecrotic
dermoneurosis
dermonosology
dermopathy
  diabetic d.
dermophlebitis
dermoplasty
dermostenosis
dermostosis
dermosyphilopathy
dermotoxin
dermotropic
dermotuberculin reaction
Dermoxyl
Dermtex HC with aloe
Derm-Vi Soap
DES
  diethylstilbestrol
De Sanctis-Cacchione syndrome
desaturation
Desenex
desensitization
  heterologous d.
  homologous d.
  penicillin d.
desensitize
desert
  d. ragweed
  d. sore
desetope
desiccant
desiccation
  mucous d.
Desiclovir
Design
  Clear By D.
desipramine
Desitin topical
desmoglein-1

D

NOTES

desmoid
    d. cyst
    d. tumor
desmolysis
desmon
desmoplastic
    d. malignant melanoma
    d. trichilemmoma
    d. trichoepithelioma
desmorrhexis
desmosome
desmosome-tonofilament complex
desonide
DesOwen
    ·D. topical
desoximetasone
despeciated antitoxin
despeciation
desquamans
    herpes d.
desquamate
desquamation
    branny d.
    corneocyte d.
    generalized d.
    peribronchial d.
    plantar d.
desquamative
    d. dermatitis
    d. gingivitis
    d. interstitial pneumonia (DIP)
    d. interstitial pneumonitis
desquamativum, pl. **desquamativa**
    erythema d.
    erythroderma d.
Desquam-X
destruction
    polymorphonuclear leukocyte-
    dependent tissue d.
destructor
    Lepidoglyphus d.
desynchronized sleep
detection
    Bartonella henselae d.
    C1q immune complex d.
    hepatitis B DNA d.
    hepatitis C RNA d.
    hepatitis C virus antibody d.
    Ki-67 marker d.
    Lyme disease DNA d.
    Mycobacterium tuberculosis d.
    myelin-associated glycoprotein
    antibody d.

detergens
    liquor carbonis d. (LCD)
detergent
    anionic d.'s
    superfatted synthetic d.
    synthetic d. (syndet)
detergicans
    acne d.
determinant
    allotypic d.'s
    antigenic d.
    genetic d.
    d. group
    idiotypic antigenic d.
    isoallotypic d.'s
determination
    fecal fat d.
    IgG subclass d.
detersive
detoxicate
detoxication
detoxification
detoxified toxin
detoxify
detritus
    tissue d.
Deuteromycetes
DEV
    duck embryo origin vaccine
deviation
    immune d.
    standard d. (SD)
    ulnar d.
device
    Antense anti-tension d.
    Flexi-Trak skin anchoring d.
    flutter d.
    Handisol phototherapy d.
    Orion d.
    pulse oximetry d.
    SkinTech medical tattooing d.
    SomnoStar apnea testing d.
    Venture demand oxygen
    delivery d.
    Vitrasert intraocular d.
devil
    d. grip
DeVilbiss Pulmon-Aid nebulizer
Devrom
Dewar flask
dew itch
DEXA
    dual-energy x-ray absorptiometry

Dexacidin Ophthalmic
Dexacort
    D. Turbinaire
dexamethasone (DXM)
    d. acetate
    neomycin, polymyxin b,
        and d.
    d. sodium phosphate
    tobramycin and d.
Dexasone
    D. L.A.
Dexasporin Ophthalmic
Dexchlor
dexchlorpheniramine maleate
Dexone
    D. LA
Dexotic
dextran 1
dextranomer
    d. granule
dextromethorphan
    pseudoephedrine and d.
dextrose
    tetracaine with d.
DEY albuterol inhalation aerosol
Dey-Dose
    D.-D. Isoproterenol
    D.-D. Metaproterenol
Dey-Drop Ophthalmic solution
Dey-Lute Isoetharine
Dey-Wash skin wound clean
DF2 septicemia
D/Flex
DH
    delayed hypersensitivity
    dermatitis herpetiformis
Dharmendra antigen
D.H.E. 45 injection
d'Herelle phenomenon
dhobie
    d. itch
    d. mark
    d. mark dermatitis
DHS
    D. Tar
    D. zinc

DI
    defective interfering
    DI particle
diabetes mellitus
diabetic
    d. blister
    d. cheiroarthropathy
    d. dermopathy
    d. foot ulcer
    d. gangrene
    d. hand syndrome
    d. muscle infarction (DMI)
    d. stiff-hand syndrome
    d. ulcer
diabeticorum
    bullosis d.
    eczema d.
    necrobiosis lipoidica d.
    xanthoma d.
diacetate
    diflorasone d.
diacylglycerol
diadermic
diagnosis
    differential d.
    EIA d.
    problem-oriented d.
diagnostic
    d. algorithm
    d. diphtheria toxin
    d. principle
    d. surgical therapy
    d. test
dialysis
    chronic ambulatory
        peritoneal d. (CAPD)
    equilibrium d.
diameter
    mass median aerodynamic d.
        (MMD)
Diamine T.D. Oral
diamond skin
Diamox
Di antigen
diapedesis
diaper
    d. dermatitis

NOTES

109

diaper *(continued)*
  d. granuloma
  d. rash
  d. rash intertrigo
diaphoresis
diaphoretic
diaphragmatic
  d. hernia
  d. pleurisy
diaphysis
diapnoic
diarrhea
  bovine virus d.
  Brainerd d.
  chronic d.
  prolonged d.
  wean-ling d.
diarthrodial joint bursae
diascope
diascopy
diathesis, pl. **diatheses**
  allergic d.
  atopic d.
  hemorrhagic d.
diazepam
Diazo paper
Dibenzyline
DIC
  disseminated intravascular
    coagulation
dichlorodifluoromethane and
  trichloromonofluoromethane
dichlorofluoromethane
dichlorotetrafluoroethane
  ethyl chloride and d.
Dick
  D. method
  D. test
  D. test toxin
diclazuril
diclofenac
  d. sodium
dicloxacillin
  d. sodium
Dictyocaulus viviparus
dictyospore
didanosine (ddi)
didehydrothymidine
  d4T, d.
2'-3'-dideoxyadenosine
dideoxycytidine (ddc)
  2'-3' d.
dideoxyinosine

dideoxynucleoside
Didrex
Didronel
didymospore
diet
  challenge d.
  elimination d.
  Feingold d.
  gluten-free d.
  sippy d.
Dieterle stain
diethylcarbamazine (DEC)
diethyledithiocarbamate
diethylstilbestrol (DES)
diethyltoluamide
difference
  geographic d.
differential diagnosis
differentiation
  cluster of d. 2–72 (CD2–72)
Differin gel
difficile
  Clostridium d.
Diff-Quick stain
diffusa
  leishmaniasis tegumentaria d.
  psoriasis d.
diffuse
  d. atrophy
  d. cutaneous leishmaniasis
  d. cutaneous mastocytosis
  d. erythema
  d. fibrosing alveolitis
  d. histiocytic reaction
  d. idiopathic skeletal
    hyperostosis (DISH)
  d. infiltrative lymphocytosis
  d. infiltrative lymphocytosis
    syndrome
  d. inflammation
  d. interstitial fibrosis of the
    lung
  d. interstitial lung disease
    (DILD)
  d. phlegmon
  d. plane
  d. plane xanthoma
  d. progressive systemic
    sclerosis
  d. proliferative
    glomerulonephritis
  d. pulmonary infiltrate
  d. scleritis

d. scleroderma
d. staining
diffusing capacity for carbon monoxide (DLCO)
diffusion
  agar gel d.
  d. coefficient
  d. constant
  gel d.
  d. of the lunula
diffusum
  angiokeratoma corporis d.
  atrophoderma d.
  papilloma d.
diflorasone diacetate
Diflucan
  D. injection
  D. Oral
diflunisal
DiGeorge syndrome
digestion
  intracellular d.
digit
  sausage d.
  supernumerary d.
digital
  d. fibrokeratoma
  d. whorl
digitalis
  herpes d.
digitata
  verruca d.
digitate
  d. dermatosis
  d. wart
Digitrapper MkIII sleep monitor
dihomogamm
dihydrate
  calcium pyrophosphate d. (CPPD)
dihydrocodeine
dihydroergotamine mesylate
dihydrotestosterone
3,4-dihydroxyphenylalanine (DOPA, dopa)
dihydroxypropyl theophylline
Dilantin

dilated
  d. pore
  d. pore of Winer
DILD
  diffuse interstitial lung disease
DILE
  drug-induced lupus erythematosus
Dilocaine
Dilor
diloxanide
  d. furoate
diluent
dilute Russell viper venom time
dilution
Dimaphen
  D. Elixir
  D. Tablet
dimenhydrinate
dimension
  double (gel) diffusion precipitin test in one d.
  gel diffusion precipitin tests in one d.
  single (gel) diffusion precipitin test in one d.
Dimetabs Oral
Dimetane
  D. Decongestant Elixir
  D. Oral
Dimetapp
  D. Elixir
  D. Extentabs
  D. 4-Hour Liqui-Gel Capsule
  D. Sinus Caplets
  D. Tablet
dimethicone
dimethylgloxime
  d. spot test
dimethyl sulfoxide
dimidiatum
  Scytalidium d.
diminished breath sound
dimorphic
dimorphous leprosy
dimple
  d. sign

D

NOTES

dimpling
dinitrochlorobenzene (DNCB)
   d. challenge
dinoflagellate toxin
dioecious
dioxide
   carbon d. (CO_2)
   end-tidal carbon d. ($ETCO_2$)
   partial pressure of carbon d.
      (PCO_2)
   solid carbon d.
   sulfur d. (SO_2)
DIP
   desquamative interstitial pneumon
   distal interphalangeal
Dipentum
Dipetalonema
   D. perstans
   D. streptocerca
diphasic milk fever
diphenhydramine
   acetaminophen and d.
   d. hydrochloride
   parenteral d.
diphenidol hydrochloride
Diphenylan Sodium
diphosphate
   adenosine d. (ADP)
diphosphonate
diphtheria
   d. antitoxin
   d. antitoxin unit
   avian d.
   cutaneous d.
   d. cutis
   false d.
   fowl d.
   d. and tetanus toxoid
   d., tetanus toxoids, and
      acellular pertussis vaccine
   d., tetanus toxoids, and whole-
      cell pertussis vaccine
      d., tetanus toxoids, and
      whole-cell pertussis vaccine
      and haemophilus b conjugate
      vaccine
   d. toxin
   d. toxoid, tetanus toxoid, and
      pertussis vaccine (DTP)
diphtheriae
   Corynebacterium d.
diphtheria-pertussis-tetanus (DPT)
diphtheritic ulcer

diphtheroid
diphtherotoxin
diplococcin
diplopia
Diprolene
   D. AF
dipropionate
   alclometasone d.
   beclomethasone d.
   betamethasone d.
   clobetasol d.
Diprosone
Dipylidium caninum
dipyridamole
Direct
   Mycobacterium Tuberculosis D.
      (MTD)
direct
   d. agglutination test
   d. challenge
   d. Coombs test
   d. fluorescent antibody
   d. fluorescent antibody test
   d. histamine releaser
directory
   Haines d.
dirithromycin
Dirofilaria immitis
dirofilariasis
   subcutaneous d.
disaccharide intolerance
Disalcid
Disc
   Clear Away D.
disciform
   d. thickening
discoid
   distinctive exudative d.
   exudative d.
   d. LE
   d. lupus
   d. lupus erythematosus (DLE)
discoidea
   psoriasis d.
discontinuous sterilization
discrete
   d. pit
   d. umbilicated papule
discrimination
   self-nonself d.
disease
   Addison d.

airways d.
akamushi d.
Albright d.
Aleutian mink d.
Alibert d.
alpha heavy-chain d.
amyloid d.
antibody deficiency d.
articular d.
atypical Kawasaki d. (AKD)
Aujeszky d.
Australian X d.
autoimmune d.
bacterial d.
Baelz d.
Bang d.
Bannister d.
Barcoo d.
Bateman d.
Bazin d.
Behçet d.
beryllium d.
Besnier d.
bird-breeder's d.
blinding d.
Bloch-Sulzberger d.
Borna d.
Bornholm d.
Bourneville-Pringle d.
Bowen d.
brachial neuritis of Lyme d.
Brill d.
Brill-Zinsser d.
Brocq d.
Brooke d.
Bruton d.
bullous d.
Bury d.
Buschke d.
Buschke-Ollendorf d.
Busse-Buschke d.
calcium hydroxyapatite crystal deposition d.
calcium phosphate crystal deposition d.
calcium pyrophosphate

dihydrate crystal deposition d. (CPPD)
calcium pyrophosphate dihydrate deposition d. (CPDD)
cardiac d.
Carrion d.
cat-scratch d. (CSD)
Cazenave d.
celiac d.
central Recklinghausen d. type II
Chagas d.
Charlouis d.
Chlamydia d.
chronic airways d. (CAD)
chronic cold agglutinin d.
chronic graft-versus-host d.
chronic granulomatous d.
chronic inflammatory d.
chronic interstitial lung d.
chronic obstructive pulmonary d. (COPD)
chronic pulmonary d.
Civatte d.
cold hemagglutinin d.
collagen vascular d.
combined immunodeficiency d. (CID)
communicable d.
congenital Lyme d.
connective tissue d. (CTD)
Conradi d.
contagious d.
Cooperative Systematic Studies of the Rheumatic D. (CSSRD)
coronary artery d. (CAD)
Cowden d.
Creutzfeldt-Jakob d. (CJD)
Crohn d.
crystal deposition d.
Csillag d.
Cushing d.
cytomegalic inclusion d.
cytomegalovirus d.
Daae d.

D

NOTES

disease *(continued)*
Danielssen d.
Danielssen-Boeck d.
Darier d.
Darier-White d.
dark dot d.
deer fly d.
Degos d.
Dejerine-Sottas d.
de Quervain d.
Dercum d.
diffuse interstitial lung d.
  (DILD)
DNA probe test for Lyme d.
dog d.
Dowling-Degos d.
Duhring d.
Dukes d.
Duncan d.
Dupuytren d.
Dutton d.
Epstein d.
exanthematous d.
extramammary Paget d.
exudative papulosquamous d.
Fabry d.
Fabry-Anderson d.
Farber d.
Favre-Racouchot d.
fifth d.
Filatov d.
Filatov Dukes d.
first d.
Flegel d.
fly-borne d.
food-borne d.
food-induced respiratory d.
foot-and-mouth d. (FMD)
Fordyce d.
Forestier d.
Fothergill d.
Fournier d.
fourth d.
Fox-Fordyce d.
Freiberg d.
Friend d.
fungal d.
furuncular d.
fusospirochetal d.
gamma heavy-chain d.
gasping d.
Gaucher d.
Gerhardt d.

Gerhardt-Mitchell d.
Gianotti-Crosti d.
Gibert d.
glycogen storage d.
Gougerot-Blum d.
Gougerot-Sjögren d.
graft versus host d.
granulomatous d.
Graves d.
Greenhow d.
Griesinger d.
Grover d.
Günther d.
GVH d.
Hailey-Hailey d.
Hallopeau d.
hand-foot-and-mouth d.
Hand-Schüller-Christian d.
Hansen d.
hard pad d.
Hartnup d.
Hashimoto d.
Hashimoto-Pritzker d.
heavy-chain d.
Hebra d.
helminthic parasitic d.
hemoglobin C d.
hemoglobin S d.
hemolytic sickle cell d.
hepatobiliary d.
heritable connective tissue d.
hidebound d.
HLA class 1 associated d.
Hodgkin d.
hoof-and-mouth d.
Hurler d.
Hyde d.
idiopathic cold agglutinin d.
idiopathic eczematous d.
immune complex d.
immune-mediated d.
immunobullous d.
immunodeficiency d.
immunologic inflammatory d.
inclusion body d.
infarctive inflammatory d.
infectious d. (ID)
inflammatory d.
inflammatory bowel d. (IBD)
interstitial lung d. (ILD)
iron storage d.
island d.
itchy red bump d.

Jakob-Creutzfeldt d.
Jessner-Kanof d.
Kaposi d.
Kawasaki d. (KD)
Ketron-Goodman d.
Kienböck d.
Kikuchi d.
Kimura d.
kinky-hair d.
Köbberling-Duncan d.
Köhler d.
Kyasanur Forest d.
Kyrle d.
Lane d.
Legg-Calvé-Perthes d.
Legionnaire d.
Leiner d.
Lemierre d.
Letterer-Siwe d.
linear IgA bullous d.
lipid storage d.
livedo patterned d.
liver d.
Lobo d.
Lou Gehrig d.
lumpy skin d.
lung d.
Lyell d.
Lyme d.
Lyme d. (stage 1–3)
lymphocytic d.
lymphoproliferative d.
Madelung d.
Majocchi d.
malignant neoplastic d.
mammary Paget d.
Marburg virus d.
Marek d.
margarine d.
Marie-Strümpell d.
market men d.
McArdle d.
mechanobullous d.
metabolic bone d.
Mibelli d.
Mikulicz d.
Milian d.

Milroy d.
Milton d.
Mitchell d.
mixed connective tissue d.
  (MCTD)
Mkar d.
Mondor d.
Moschcowitz d.
mosquito-borne d.
Mucha-Habermann d.
mucocutaneous d.
mucosal d.
mycoplasma d.
myeloproliferative d.
neoplastic d.
Nettleship d.
Neumann d.
neurodegenerative d.
neuropsychiatric d.
neutral lipid storage d.
Newcastle d. (ND)
Niemann-Pick d.
non-neoplastic d.
Ockelbo d.
Ofuji d.
"oid-oid" d.
orbital inflammatory d.
orphan d.
Osler d.
Osler-Weber-Rendu d.
overlap d.
Paget d.
parasitic d.
Parkinson d.
patellofemoral d.
Paxton d.
pelvic inflammatory d. (PID)
perforating d.
perna d.
Pette-Döring d.
Peyronie d.
phytanic acid storage d.
pigeon breeder's d.
pink d.
Poncet d.
porcupine d.
post-thrombotic d.

D

NOTES

disease *(continued)*
  poultry handler's d.
  Preiser d.
  primary pulmonary
    parenchymal d.
  Pringle d.
  proliferative inflammatory d.
  protozoal parasitic d.
  psychocutaneous d.
  Quincke d.
  Quinquaud d.
  Ranikhet d.
  Raynaud d.
  reactive airways d.
  Recklinghausen d.
  Recklinghausen d. type I
  Refsum d.
  Reiter d.
  Rendu-Osler-Weber d.
  restrictive lung d.
  rheumatoid d.
  Ribas-Torres d.
  Ritter d.
  Robinson d.
  Rosai-Dorfman d.
  Rosenbach d.
  Rubarth d.
  runt d.
  salivary gland virus d.
  sandworm d.
  saprophytic d.
  Schamberg d.
  Schenck d.
  Schönlein d.
  secondary d.
  Senear-Usher d.
  serum d.
  sexually transmitted d. (STD)
  shimamushi d.
  sickle cell d. (SCD)
  sinopulmonary d.
  sixth d.
  sixth venereal d.
  Sjögren d.
  skinbound d.
  slim d.
  slow virus d.
  Sneddon-Wilkinson d.
  specific d.
  SS hemoglobin d.
  stellate patterned d.
  Sticker d.
  Still d.

  Strümpell d.
  Sulzberger-Garbe d.
  Sutton d.
  Sweet d.
  Swift d.
  swine vesicular d.
  Sylvest d.
  d. syndrome
  systemic autoimmune d.
  systemic febrile d.
  Takahara d.
  Takayasu d.
  Tangier d.
  Taylor d.
  Tay-Sachs d.
  T-cell-mediated autoimmune d.
  Teschen d.
  Theiler d.
  Thiemann d.
  third d.
  tick-borne d.
  traumatically induced
    inflammatory d.
  tropical d.
  tsutsugamushi d.
  type I glycogen storage d.
  Underwood d.
  undifferentiated connective
    tissue d. (UCTD)
  Unna d.
  Unna-Thost d.
  Urbach-Wiethe d.
  vagabond's d.
  vagrant's d.
  valvular d.
  varicella d.
  vaso-occlusive d.
  venereal d.
  Vidal d.
  viral d.
  virus X d.
  Voerner d.
  von Economo d.
  von Gierke glycogen
    storage d.
  von Recklinghausen d.
  von Zumbusch d.
  Wardrop d.
  wasting d.
  Weber-Christian d.
  Weber-Cockayne d.
  Weil d.
  Well d.

Werlhof d.
Werther d.
Wesselsbron d.
Whipple d.
white spot d.
Willan d.
Wilson d.
Winkler d.
winter vomiting d.
Woringer-Kolopp d.
yellow d.
Zoon d.
Zumbusch d.
disease-modifying
   d.-m. antirheumatic drug
   (DMARD)
   d.-m. drugs
DISH
   diffuse idiopathic skeletal
   hyperostosis
disinfect
disinfectant
   phenolated d.
   Sactimed-I-Sinald d.
disinfection
disjunctum
   stratum d.
disk
   hair d.
   d. sensitivity method
Diskhaler inhaler
dismutase
   bovine superoxide d.
disodium
   d. cromoglycate (DSC)
   lobenzarit d.
   ticarcillin d.
disorder
   acquired d.
   acquired cornification d.
   acquired vascular d.
   adrenal cortex d.
   affective d.
   anogenital d.
   autoimmune d.
   autosomal-recessive severe

   combined
   immunodeficiency d.
   bacterially induced
   hemostatic d.
   congenital d.
   cornification d.
   d. of cornification (DOC)
   Curth-Maklin cornification d.
   hematologic d.
   hemostatic d.
   hereditary vascular d.
   heritable d.
   immune complex d.
   immune-mediated coagulation d.
   immunodeficiency d.
   immunologic d.
   immunoproliferative d.
   keratitis-deafness
   cornification d.
   lymphoreticular d.
   metabolic d.
   mineral-related nutritional d.
   National Institute of Arthritis,
   Musculoskeletal and
   Skin D.'s (NIAMS)
   neurologic d.
   nutritional d.
   pancreatic d.
   papulosquamous d.
   partial combined
   immunodeficiency d.
   periarticular d.
   d. of phagocytic cell
   pituitary d.
   psychophysiologic d.
   secondary psychiatric d.
   severe combined
   immunodeficiency d. (SCID)
   thyroid d.
   unilateral hemidysplasia
   cornification d.
   vascular d.
dispar
   Lymantria d.
dispersion
   amphotericin B colloidal d.

D

NOTES

displacement
  d. analysis
  odontoid process d.
Dispos-a-Med Isoproterenol
dissecans
  osteochondritis d.
dissecting
  d. cellulitis
  d. cellulitis of scalp
  d. perifolliculitis
dissection
  blunt d.
  d. cellulitis of scalp
  sharp d.
  d. tubercle
disseminata
  alopecia d.
  dermatofibrosis lenticularis d.
  osteitis fibrosa cystica d.
  tuberculosis cutis follicularis d.
disseminated
  d. aspergillosis
  d. candidiasis
  d. cutaneous gangrene
  d. cutaneous leishmaniasis
  d. gonococcal infection
  d. herpes simplex
  d. intravascular coagulation
    (DIC)
  d. lupus erythematosus
  d. neurodermatitis
  d. pagetoid reticulosis
  d. recurrent
    infundibulofolliculitis
  d. superficial actinic
    porokeratosis
  d. vaccinia
dissemination
  skin d.
  xanthoma d.
disseminatum
  keratoma d.
  xanthoma d.
disseminatus
disseminées parapsoriasis en plaques
distal
  d. dactylitis
  d. interphalangeal (DIP)
  d. intestinal obstruction
    syndrome
  d. nail matrix
distemper virus
distended bursa

distensae
  striae cutis d.
distichia
distichiasis
distinctive exudative discoid
distortum
  Microsporum canis, var d.
distress
  respiratory d.
distribution
  asymmetric d.
  dermatomal d.
  lesion d.
  linear d.
  pattern of d.
  shawl d.
districhiasis
distrix
disturbance of consciousness
ditiocarb
diuretic
  loop d.
diutinum
  erythema elevatum d.
  scleredema d.
divergens
  Babesia d.
diversiloba
  Rhus d.
diversilobum
  Toxicodendron d.
diversity
  antigen-binding d.
diversus
  Citrobacter d.
Division (I–IV) lesion
Dizac injection
Dizmiss
DLCO
  diffusing capacity for carbon
  monoxide
DLE
  discoid lupus erythematosus
DM
  dermatomyositis
  Iobid D.
  Iohist D.
  Poly-Histine D.
DMARD
  disease-modifying antirheumatic
  drug
D-Med injection

DMI
   diabetic muscle infarction
DM/PM
DMSA
   Tc-dimercaptosuccinic acid
DNA
   deoxyribonucleic acid
   D. aneuploidy
   antidouble-stranded D.
   antinative D.
   D. autosensitivity
   D. binding
   chemiluminescent D.
   chemiluminescent in situ
      hybridization for detection of
      CMV D.
   competitor D.
   complementary D. (cDNA)
   double-stranded D. (dsDNA)
   D. gyrase
   HBV D.
   D. homology
   human cloned D.
   D. hybridization
   D. hybridization test
   improper repair of D.
   PCR for HIV D.
   D. probe test
   D. probe test for Lyme
      disease
   D. repair
   single-stranded D.
   D. virus
DNA-anti-DNA system
DNA-binding test
DNase
   deoxyribonuclease
DNCB
   dinitrochlorobenzene
DOC
   disorder of cornification
dock
   bitter d.
   d.-plantain
   tall d.
   yellow d.

dog
   d. dander
   d. disease
   d. distemper virus
   d. epithelium
   d. fennel
   d. flea
   d. flea bite
   nonshedding d.
   d. tapeworm
dolens
   phlegmasia alba d.
Dolichorespula
   D. sting
Dolobid
dolor
Dolorac
dolorimeter
dolorosa
   adiposis d.
   tubercula d.
domains
   immunoglobulin d.
Domeboro
   Otic D.
domesticus
   Glycyphagus d.
dominant
   autosomal d.
   lamellar d.
Donath-Landsteiner
   D.-L. antibody
   D.-L. cold autoantibody
Donizetti potion
donor
   d. sclera
   universal d.
Donovan body
donovani
   Leishmania d.
Donovania granulomatis
donovanosis
DOPA, dopa
   3,4-dihydroxyphenylalanine
dopamine
dopa-oxidase
Doppler ultrasound

NOTES

D

d'orange
    peau d.
Dorcol
Dorfman-Chanarin syndrome
Dormin Oral
Dorothy Reed-Sternberg cell
dorsalis
    tabes d.
dorsal surface
dorsi
    elastofibroma d.
Doryx Oral
dose
    booster d.
    effective d. (ED)
    infecting d. (ID)
    L d.'s
    L+ d.
    lethal d. (LD)
    Lf d.
    Lo d.
    Lr d.
    maintenance d.
    minimal infecting d. (MID)
    minimal lethal d. (MLD)
    minimal reacting d. (MRD)
    sensitizing d.
    shocking d.
Dosepak
    Deltasone D.
    Medrol D.
dose-related effect
dose-response curve
dosimeter
    Rosenthal-French d.
dosing
    once-daily d. (ODD)
dots
    Trantas d.
double
    d. antibody immunoassay
    d. antibody method
    d. antibody precipitation
    d. antibody sandwich assay
    d. (gel) diffusion precipitin
    test in one dimension
    d. immunodiffusion
    d. negative cell
double-blind food challenge
double-contrast arthrography
double-crush syndrome
double-sandwich IgM ELISA
double-stranded DNA (dsDNA)

Douche
    Yeast-Gard Medicated D.
Douglas
    D. fir
    D. fir tree
Dovonex
dowager hump
Dowling-Degos disease
Dowling-Meara epidermolysis
    bullosa
down
    malignant d.
Downey cell
down-regulation
Down syndrome
doxepin
    d. HCl
Doxil
doxofylline
doxorubicin
    liposomal d.
Doxychel
    D. injection
    D. Oral
doxycycline
    d. pleurodesis
Doxy Oral
D.P.
    Dalalone D.
DPAP interactive airway
    management system
d-penicillamine
DPT
    diphtheria-pertussis-tetanus
Dr
    D. Scholl's Athlete's Foot
    D. Scholl's Maximum Strength
    Tritin
dracontiasis
dracunculiasis
dracunculosis
Dracunculus medinensis
drainage
    paranasal sinus d.
    percussion and postural d. (P
    and PD)
    postural d.
Draize Repeat Insult patch test
Dramamine
    D. II
    D. Oral
drawer test
Drechslera

dressing
Acticel wound d.
alginate d.
Algisorb wound d.
Band-Aid d.
Biopatch antimicrobial d.
Compeed Skinprotector d.
hydrocolloid d.
hydrogel d.
hydrophilic polymer d.
Kaltostat alginate d.
LYOfoam d.
Mesalt d.
nonocclusive d.
occlusive d.
OpSite semipermeable d.
plastic adhesive d.
polymer film d.
polymer foam d.
Royl-Derm wound hydrogel d.
semipermeable d.
Siloskin d.
Sorbsan alginate d.
Tegaderm semipermeable d.
d. therapy
Vigilon d.
water-impermeable, non-silicone-
based occlusive d.
wet d.
Dricort
Dermarest D.
dried human serum
drift
antigenic d.
drip
postnasal d. (PND)
Drisdol Oral
Dristan
D. Long Lasting Nasal
solution
D. Sinus Caplets
Drithocreme
Dritho-Scalp
Drixoral
D. Cough & Congestion
Liquid Caps
D. Non-Drowsy
D. Syrup

dronabinol
drop attack
droplet
d. infection
d. nucleus
drop-like psoriasis
droppings
Australian parrot d.
pigeon d.
Drops
Allergan Ear D.
Coly-Mycin S Otic D.
Moisture Ophthalmic D.
Myapap D.
Rondec D.
Triaminic Oral Infant D.
Drotic Otic
drowsiness
drug
adrenergic d.
d. allergy
d. anaphylaxis
anticholinergic d.
antimalarial d.
antirheumatic d.
antisense d.
antiviral d.
chondroprotective d.'s
cytotoxic d.
disease-modifying d.'s
disease-modifying
antirheumatic d. (DMARD)
d. eruption
d. hypersensitivity
immunosuppressive d.
d. interaction
d. intolerance
large-molecular-weight d.
lysosomotropic anti-malarial d.
non-cross-reactive d.
nonsteroidal anti-
inflammatory d. (NSAID)
orphan d.
d. overdose
d. rash
rauwolfia d.
d. reaction

NOTES

D

drug *(continued)*
    second-line d. (SLD)
    simple d.
    slow-acting antirheumatic d.
      (SAARD)
    sulfa d.
    uricosuric d.
drug-associated erythema multiforme
drug-fast
drug-induced
    d.-i. acanthosis nigricans
    d.-i. alopecia
    d.-i. bullous photosensitivity
    d.-i. depression of immune
      system
    d.-i. lupus
    d.-i. lupus erythematosus
      (DILE)
    d.-i. lymphadenopathy
    d.-i. progressive symptom
      sclerosis
    d.-i. purpura
    d.-i. SLE syndrome
    d.-i. systemic lupus
      erythematosus
    d.-i. thrombocytopenia
drug-related
    d.-r. immunohemolytic anemia
    d.-r. myopathy
dry
    d. cough
    d. cutaneous leishmaniasis
    D. Eyes solution
    D. Eye Therapy solution
    d. flush
    d. gangrene
    d. ice
    d. leprosy
    d. lips
    d. mouth
    d. skin
    d. tetter
Drysol
DS
    Bactrim D.
    Cotrim D.
    Septra D.
    Sulfatrim D.
    Tolectin D.
    Uroplus D.
DSC
    disodium cromoglycate

dsDNA
    double-stranded DNA
d4T
    Zerit
DTH
    delayed-type hypersensitivity
DTIC-Dome
DTM
    dermatophyte test medium
DTP
    diphtheria toxoid, tetanus toxoid,
      and pertussis vaccine
Duadacin Capsule
dual-beam photon absorptiometry
dual-energy x-ray absorptiometry
    (DEXA)
dual-fluorescence analysis
duazomycin
duboisii
    Histoplasma d.
Dubreuilh
    circumscribed precancerous
      melanosis of D.
duck
    d. embryo origin vaccine
      (DEV)
    d. feather
    d. hepatitis virus
    d. influenza virus
    d. plague
    d. plague virus
ducreyi
    Haemophilus d.
Ducrey test
duct
Duffy antigen
Duhring disease
Dukes disease
Dulbecco medium
dumas
dumoffii
    Legionella d.
Dumon-Harrell bronchoscope
Duncan
    D. disease
    D. syndrome
Dunnigan syndrome
duodenale
    Ancylostoma d.
Duofilm solution
Duo-Medihaler Aerosol
Duo-Trach
duovirus

Duplex T
Dupuytren
  D. contracture
  D. disease
Dura-Gest
Duralone injection
Duralutin injection
Duranest injection
Duration
  D. Nasal solution
duration of treatment
Duratuss
Dura-Vent
  D.-V./DA
Duricef
Durrax
durum
  fibroma d.
  heloma d.
  papilloma d.
  ulcus d.
dust
  barn d.
  grain d.
  house d.
  d. mite
  mushroom d.
dustborne
Dutton
  D. disease
  D. relapsing fever
Duvenhaga virus
Dwelle Ophthalmic solution
DXM
  dexamethasone
Dycill
dye
  D&C d.
  food d.
  injectable d.
  d. laser
Dynabac
Dyna-Care pressure pad system
Dynacin Oral
Dyna-Hex topical
Dynapen

Dyonics
  D. basket forceps
  D. Dyosite office arthroscopy
    system
  D. InteliJet fluid management
    system
  D. suction punch
dyphylline
dysarthria
dyschroia
dyschromatosis
dyschromia
  cutaneous d.
dyschromicum
dyscrasia
dysenteriae
  Shigella d.
  Shigella flexneri d.
  viral d.
dysentery
  d. antitoxin
dysesthesia
  d. pedis
dysfunction
  antibody d.
  emotional d.
  meibomian gland d.
  phagocyte d.
  small airways d.
  temporomandibular d. (TMD)
  vascular d.
dysgammaglobulinemia
dysgenesis
  gonadal d.
  reticular d.
dyshidria
dyshidrosis, dyshydrosis, dysidrosis,
  pl. dyshidroses
  lamellar d.
  sole d.
dyshidrotic
  d. eczema
dysidria
dysidrosis (var. of dyshidrosis)
dyskeratinization
dyskeratoma
  acantholytic d.

D

NOTES

dyskeratoma *(continued)*
    focal acantholytic d.
    warty d.
dyskeratosis, pl. **dyskeratoses**
    acantholytic d.
    benign d.
    d. congenita
    focal acantholytic d.
    malignant d.
    transient acantholytic d.
dyskeratotic
    d. keratinocyte
dyslipoidosis
dysmetabolism
    tryptophan d.
dyspareunia
dyspeptic
dysphagia
dysphagocytosis
    congenital d.
dyspigmentation
dysplasia
    anhidrotic ectodermal d.
    congenital ectodermal d.
    ectodermal d.
    fibrous d.
    hidrotic ectodermal d.
    hypohidrotic ectodermal d.
    late-onset spondyloepiphyseal d.
    lymphopenic thymic d.
    mesodermal d.
    multiple epiphyseal d.

    polyostotic fibrous d.
    sphenoid d.
    spondyloepiphyseal d. (SED)
dysplastic
    d. nevus
    d. nevus syndrome
dyspnea
dyspneic
dysprosium ferric hydroxide
dysproteinemia
dysraphism
dyssebacea
dyssebacia
dyssynchrony
    thoracoabdominal d.
dysthymia
dystrophia
    d. unguium
dystrophic
    d. calcinosis
    d. calcinosis cutis
    d. epidermolysis bullosa
    d. variant
dystrophica
    elastosis d.
    epidermolysis bullosa d.
dystrophin
dystrophy
    muscular d.
    reflex sympathetic d. (RSD)
    twenty-nail d.

E1
 prostaglandin E. (PGE1)
E2
 prostaglandin E. (PGE2)
EAC
 erythema annulare centrifugum
 erythrocytes, antibody, complement
 external auditory canal
 EAC rosette
 EAC rosette assay
EAE
 experimental allergic encephalitis
 experimental allergic
  encephalomyelitis
ear
 middle e.
 Otocalm E.
 e. pit
Earle L fibrosarcoma
earlobe
 e. allergic dermatitis
 e. crease
early
 e. latent syphilis
 e. reaction
early-phase response
Easprin
Eastern
 E. coral snake
 E. coral snake bite
eastern
 e. equine encephalomyelitis
  (EEE)
 e. equine encephalomyelitis
  virus
 e. tick-borne rickettsiosis
Eaton
 E. agent
 E. agent pneumonia
Eaton-Lambert syndrome
EB
 elementary bodies
 epidermolysis bullosa
 Epstein-Barr
 EB nuclear antigen test
 EB simplex
 EB viral capsid antigen test
 EB virus
EBA
 epidermolysis bullosa acquisita

ebastine
EBNA
 Epstein-Barr nuclear antigen
 EBNA IgG ELISA test
Ebola
 E. hemorrhagic fever
 E. virus
EB-specific IgM test
EBV
 Epstein-Barr virus
 EBV glycoprotein gp110
 EBV infection
ECASA
 enteric-coated acetylsalicylic acid
ECBO
 enteric cytopathogenic bovine
 orphan
 ECBO virus
eccentrica
 hyperkeratosis e.
 keratoderma e.
ecchymosed
ecchymosis, pl. ecchymoses
ecchymotic
 e. mark
 e. rash
eccrine
 e. acrospiroma
 e. adenocarcinoma
 e. bromhidrosis
 e. carcinoma
 e. chromhidrosis
 e. gland
 e. hidradenitis
 e. hidrocystoma
 e. poroma
 e. spiradenoma
 e. sweat gland
ECF-A
 eosinophil chemotactic factor of
 anaphylaxis
echidninus
 Laelaps e.
echinococcosis
Echinococcus
 E. granulosus
 E. multilocularis
echinococcus
echinoderm

E

ECHO
  enteric cytopathogenic human
    orphan
    ECHO virus
    ECHO virus 28
echoviral exanthema
eclipse
  e. period
  e. phase
ECM
  extracellular matrix
ECM-degrading proteinase
ECMO
  enteric cytopathogenic monkey
    orphan
  extracorporeal membrane
    oxygenation
    ECMO virus
EcoCheck oxygen monitor
ecologic alteration
econazole
  e. nitrate
Econopred
  E. Ophthalmic
  E. Plus Ophthalmic
ecotaxis
Ecotrin
ecotropic virus
ecphyma
ECSO
  enteric cytopathogenic swine orphan
    ECSO virus
ectasia
  papillary e.
  senile e.
Ectasule
ecthyma
  e. contagiosum
  contagious e.
  e. gangrenosum
  e. infectiosum
ecthymatiform
ecthymatous syphilid
ectoantigen
ectoderm
ectodermal dysplasia
ectodermatosis
ectodermosis
  e. erosiva pluriorificialis
ectogenous
ectoparasite
ectopic
  e. cutaneous schistosomiasis

  e. keratinization
  e. sebaceous gland
ectothrix
  e. infection
ectotoxin
ectozoon
ectromelia
  e. virus
eczema
  adolescent e.
  adult e.
  allergic e.
  asteatotic e.
  atopic e.
  baker's e.
  childhood e.
  chronic e.
  contact e.
  e. craquelé
  e. diabeticorum
  dyshidrotic e.
  e. epilans
  e. erythematosum
  flexural e.
  follicular nummular e.
  hand e.
  e. herpeticum
  e. hypertrophicum
  idiopathic late-onset e.
  infantile e.
  e. intertrigo
  lichenoid e.
  e. marginatum
  nummular e.
  e. nummulare
  orbicular e.
  e. papulosum
  e. parasiticum
  e. pustulosum
  e. rubrum
  seborrheic e.
  e. squamosum
  stasis e.
  tropical e.
  e. tyloticum
  e. vaccinatum
  varicose e.
  e. verrucosum
  e. vesiculosum
  weeping e.
  winter e.
  xerotic e.
eczematization

eczematize
eczematodes
   impetigo e.
eczematogenic
eczematogenous
eczematoid
   e. dermatitis
   e. pruritic plaques
   e. seborrhea
eczematous
   e. lesion
   e. patch
   e. PMLE
   e. polymorphous light eruption
   e. reaction
ED
   effective dose
edema
   acute hemorrhagic e.
   angioneurotic e.
   brawny e.
   bullous e.
   dependent e.
   e. of feet
   e. of hand
   hemorrhagic e.
   hereditary angioneurotic e.
    (HANE)
   indolent nonpitting e.
   inflammatory e.
   intracellular e.
   laryngeal e.
   e. neonatorum
   noninflammatory e.
   palpebral e.
   periodic e.
   persistent e.
   pitting e.
   Quincke e.
   Yangtze e.
edematous
Edmonston-Zagreb vaccine
edobacomab
Edwardsiella
EEE
   eastern equine encephalomyelitis
   EEE virus

E.E.S. Oral
Efedron
effect
   cidal e.
   cytopathic e.
   dose-related e.
   isomorphic e.
   Köbner e.
   secondary e.
   side e.
   squeeze e.
   tattooing e.
   tendonesis e.
effective dose (ED)
effector
   e. cell
   e. molecule
   e. pathway
Effersyl
efficacy
efficiency
   sleep e.
effluvium
   anagen e.
   short anagen telogen e.
   telogen e.
effort syndrome
effusion
   joint e.
   parapneumonic e.
Efidac/24
   E. chlorpheniramine
eflornithine
   e. hydrochloride
Efodine
Efudex
   E. topical
EGF
   epidermal growth factor
egg-passage
   rabies vaccine, Flury strain e.-
   p.
eggplant
egg shell nail
Ehlers-Danlos syndrome
Ehrlich
   E. phenomenon

E

NOTES

Ehrlich *(continued)*
   E. postulate
   E. side-chain theory
   E. theory
Ehrlichia
   E. canis
   E. chaffeensis
   E. sennetsu
ehrlichiosis
EI
   erythema infectiosum
EIA
   enzyme immunoassay
   enzyme-linked immunoassay
   exercise-induced asthma
   EIA diagnosis
eicosanoid
   e. inhibition
eicosapentaenoic acid
Eikenella
EI.U
   ELISA unit
ekiri
elacin
E-LAM
   endothelial-leukocyte adhesion
     molecule
ELAM-1
   endothelial leukocyte adhesion
     molecule-1
elapid
Elapidae
Elase-Chloromycetin topical
Elase topical
elastase
   neutrophil e.
   polymorphonuclear leukocyte e.
   Pseudomonas e.
elastic
   e. fiber
   e. recoil
   e. skin
   e. tissue
   e. wrap
elastic-fiber fragmentation
elasticity
   sputum viscosity and e.
elasticum
   pseudoxanthoma e.
elastin
elastofibroma dorsi
elastoid degeneration

elastolysis
   generalized e.
elastolytic giant cell granuloma
elastoma
   juvenile e.
   Miescher e.
elastomeric
   e. complex
   e. pump
elastorrhexis
elastosis
   actinic e.
   e. colloidalis conglomerata
   cutaneous e.
   e. dystrophica
   linear focal e.
   nodular e.
   e. perforans serpiginosa
   senile e.
   solar e.
elastotic
   e. degeneration
   e. stria
Elavil
elbow
   golfer e.
   Little League e.
   Mayo classification of
     rheumatoid e.
   tennis e.
Eldecort
elder
   marsh e.
   rough marsh e.
elective culture
Electra 1000C coagulation analyzer
Electro-Acuscope
electrocardiogram
   12-lead e.
electrocautery
electrocoagulated
electrocoagulation
   pinpoint e.
electrodermal testing
electrodermatome
electrodesiccation
electrofulguration
electroimmunodiffusion
electrolysis
electromagnetic
   e. field
   e. radiation

electromyographic feature
electromyography (EMG)
electron
  e. microscope (EM)
  e. microscopy
electronic filter
electro-oculogram
electrophoresis
  immunodeficiency e.
  polyacrylamide gel e. (PAGE)
  pulsed field gel e. (PFGE)
  serum protein e.
  urinary e.
electrophototherapy
electrosection
electrosurgery
  bipolar e.
element
  kappa-deleting e.
  trace e.
elementary
  e. bodies (EB)
  e. lesion
elephantiac
elephantiasic
elephantiasis
  congenital e.
  filarial e.
  e. neuromatosa
  nevoid e.
  e. nostras
  e. nostra verrucosa
  e. telangiectodes
elephant leg
elevation
  blanched cutaneous e.
  rest, ice, compresses, e.
  (RICE)
elevator grain dust mite
elevatum
ELF
  epithelial lining fluid
Elgiloy
elimination
  e. diet
  food e.

  e. procedure
  sweat chloride e.
Elimite
  E. Cream
ELISA
  enzyme-linked immunosorbent assay
  double-sandwich IgM ELISA
  ELISA test
  ELISA unit (EI.U)
ELISPOT test
Elixicon
Elixir
  Brofed E.
  Bromaline E.
  Bromanate E.
  Bromphen E.
  Cold & Allergy E.
  Dimaphen E.
  Dimetane Decongestant E.
  Dimetapp E.
  Genatap E.
Elixophyllin
Ellipse compact spacer
elliptical
  e. biopsy
  e. incision
elm
  American e.
  Chinese e.
  fall e.
  slippery e.
  e. tree
Elocon
  E. topical
eluate
  glomerular e.
EM
  electron microscope
  erythema migrans
emaculation
ematode
emboli (pl. of embolus)
embolic gangrene
embolism
  pulmonary e.

E

NOTES

embolization
    bronchial artery e.
embolus, pl. emboli
    atheromatous e.
    cholesterol e.
    septal e.
    septic e.
embryology
EMC
    encephalomyocarditis
    EMC virus
emerging virus
emetine
EMG
    electromyography
Emgel topical
EMIT
    enzyme-multiplied immunoassay
    technique
EMLA
    E. cream
    E. topical
emollient
emotional
    e. dysfunction
    e. flushing
    e. stress
emphlysis
emphractic
emphraxis
emphysema
    subcutaneous e.
empiric therapy
Empirin
empyema
empyesis
EMS
    eosinophilia-myalgia syndrome
emulsion
E-Mycin Oral
EN
    erythema nodosum
en
    e. coup de sabre
    e. passant
enamel paint spot appearance
enanthem
enanthema
enanthematous
enanthesis
encapsulated
    e. neuroma
    e. organism

encephalitide
encephalitis
    acute necrotizing e.
    Australian X e.
    bunyavirus e.
    California e.
    Coxsackie e.
    Dawson e.
    epidemic e.
    equine e.
    experimental allergic e. (EAE)
    Far East Russian e.
    fox e.
    herpes simplex e.
    hyperergic e.
    Ilhéus e.
    inclusion body e.
    Japanese B e.
    e. japonica
    e. lethargica
    Mengo e.
    Murray Valley e. (MVE)
    postvaccinal e.
    Powassan e.
    Russian autumn e.
    Russian tick-borne e.
    secondary e.
    St. Louis e.
    subacute inclusion body e.
    varicella e.
    vernal e.
    e. virus
    von Economo e.
    woodcutter's e.
encephalitogen
encephalitogenic
Encephalitozoon
encephalocele
encephalomyelitis
    avian infectious e.
    eastern equine e. (EEE)
    enzootic e.
    equine e.
    experimental allergic e. (EAE)
    herpes B e.
    infectious porcine e.
    mouse e.
    Venezuelan equine e. (VEE)
    viral e.
    virus e.

western equine e. (WEE)
zoster e.
encephalomyocarditis (EMC)
e. virus
encephalopathy
bovine spongiform e.
HIV e.
subacute spongiform e.
transmissible mink e.
end cell
endemia
endemic
e. fungal infection
e. index
e. nonbacterial infantile
gastroenteritis
e. syphilis
e. typhus
endemica
urticaria e.
endemicum
granuloma e.
endemoepidemic
Endep
endermic
endermism
end-inspiratory crackle
End Lice
endobronchial
e. brachytherapy
endocardial fibroproliferative
endocarditis
acute bacterial e. (ABE)
bacteria-free stage of
bacterial e.
bacterial e.
enterococcal e.
infectious e.
subacute bacterial e. (SBE)
endocrine
e. hormone imbalance
e. rhinitis
endocrinopathy
endocytosis
endoderm
Endodermophyton
endogenote

endogenous
e. dermatitis
e. factor
e. infection
e. ochronosis
endoluminal
endomysial mononuclear cell
endoparasitism
endophthalmitis
endoscopy
intragastral provocation
under e. (IPEC)
endosteal
endothelial
e. cell
e. cell proliferation
e. leukocyte adhesion
molecule-1 (ELAM-1)
e. lysis
e. relaxing factor
**endothelial-leukocyte adhesion
molecule (E-LAM)**
endothelioma
endothelium
endothrix
e. infection
endotoxemia
endotoxic
endotoxicosis
endotoxin
e. shock
end-tidal carbon dioxide (ETCO$_2$)
Engerix-B
English plantain
englobe
englobement
enhancement
immunological e.
Enhancer
Aerosol Cloud E. (ACE)
Enomine
Enovil
enoxacin
enrichment
e. culture
density gradient bone marrow
progenitor e.

E

NOTES

131

Enseals
Potassium Iodide E.
EN-tabs
Azulfidine E.-t.
entactin
Entamoeba histolytica
entemophilous
Entemopoxvirus
enteric
e.-coated acetylsalicylic acid (ECASA)
e. cytopathogenic bovine orphan (ECBO)
e. cytopathogenic bovine orphan virus
e. cytopathogenic human orphan (ECHO)
e. cytopathogenic human orphan virus
e. cytopathogenic monkey orphan (ECMO)
e. cytopathogenic monkey orphan virus
e. cytopathogenic swine orphan (ECSO)
e. cytopathogenic swine orphan virus
e. fever
e. orphan virus
e. virus
enteric-coated aspirin
enteritidis
Salmonella e.
enteritis
e. anaphylactica
feline infectious e.
e. of mink
transmissible e.
enteroadherent
enteroaggregative
Enterobacter cloacae
Enterobacteriaceae
Enterobius
E. vermicularis
enterochromaffin cell
enterococcal endocarditis
enterococci
vancomycin-resistant e. (VRE)
Enterococcus faecalis
enterocolitica
Yersinia e.
enterocolitis
antibiotic e.

gold-induced e.
necrotizing e. (NEC)
Enterocytozoon bieneusi
enterohemorrhagic
enteroinvasive
enteropathic
e. arthritis
e. arthropathy
enteropathica
acrodermatitis e.
enteropathy
gluten e.
gluten-sensitive e.
protein-losing e.
enterosepsis
enterotoxigenic
enterotoxin
Escherichia coli e.
staphylococcal e.
enteroviral
e. exanthema
e. infection
Enterovirus
enterovirus (EV)
myelitic e.
non-polio e.
Entex
E. LA
E. PSE
enthesitis
enthesopathy
enthetic
entomophthoramycosis basidiobolae
entrapment
genitofemoral nerve e.
nerve e.
e. neuropathy
peroneal nerve e.
saphenous nerve e.
sciatic nerve e.
suprascapular nerve e.
sural nerve e.
enucleation
envelope
cornified cell e.
viral e.
envenomation
env gene
environmental
e. allergen
e. change
e. illness
e. mite infestation

e. mycobacterial infection
e. mycobacteriosis
e. scabies
e. scleroderma
e. survey
environment progressive symptom sclerosis
enzootic
e. bovine leukosis
e. encephalomyelitis
e. encephalomyelitis virus
enzymatic saliva
enzyme
angiotensin-converting e. (ACE)
biotinidase e.
CAT e.
collagenolytic e.
epoxide hydrolase e.
e. immunoassay (EIA)
lysosomal e.
lytic e.
proteolytic e.
e. replacement
enzyme-linked
e.-l. immunoassay (EIA)
e.-l. immunosorbent assay (ELISA)
enzyme-multiplied immunoassay technique (EMIT)
EOA
erosive osteoarthritis
eosin
hematoxylin and e. (H&E)
eosinophil
e. cationic protein
e. chemotactic factor of anaphylaxis (ECF-A)
e. peroxidase
e. protein X
eosinophil-derived neurotoxin
eosinophilia
angiolymphoid hyperplasia with e.
blood e.
peripheral blood e.
prolonged pulmonary e.

pulmonary infiltrate with e. (PIE)
simple pulmonary e.
tropical e.
eosinophilia-myalgia syndrome (EMS)
eosinophilic
e. abscess
e. bronchopneumonia
e. cellulitis
e. chemotaxis
e. dermatitis
e. fasciitis
e. fasciitis syndrome
e. granuloma
e. granulomatosis
e. myalgia
e. myalgia syndrome
e. myositis
e. pneumonia
e. pulmonary syndrome
e. pustular folliculitis
e. spongiosis
EPAP
expiratory positive airway pressure
EpDRF
epithelium-derived relaxation factor
ephedrine
aminophylline, amobarbital, and e.
e. sulfate
Ephedsol
ephelides
nevi, atrial myxoma, myxoid neurofibromas, and e. (NAME)
ephelis, pl. ephelides
ephemeral
e. fever of cattle
e. fever virus
epicanthus
Epicauta
E. fabricii
E. fabricii sting
E. vitlata
E. vitlata sting
Epicel skin graft material

E

NOTES

Epicoccum purpurascens
epicondylitis
epicutaneous
  e. reaction
  e. test
epidemic
  e. benign dry pleurisy
  e. cerebrospinal meningitis
  e. curve
  e. diaphragmatic pleurisy
  e. encephalitis
  e. exanthema
  e. gastroenteritis virus
  e. hemorrhagic fever
  e. hepatitis
  e. keratoconjunctivitis
  e. keratoconjunctivitis virus
  e. myalgia
  e. myalgia virus
  e. myositis
  e. nausea
  e. nonbacterial gastroenteritis
  e. parotiditis
  e. parotitis virus
  e. pleurodynia
  e. pleurodynia virus
  e. polyarthritis
  e. roseola
  e. transient diaphragmatic
    spasm
  e. tremor
  e. typhus
  e. vomiting
epidemica
  nephropathia e.
epidemicity
epidemicum
  erythema arthriticum e.
epidemiography
epidemiologic
epidemiology
epidermal
  e. allergen
  e. appendage
  e. cyst
  e. growth factor (EGF)
  e. Langerhans cell
  e. nevus
  e. stacking
  e. testing
epidermal-melanin unit
epidermic-dermic nevus
epidermides (*pl. of* epidermis)

epidermidis
  Staphylococcus e.
epidermidosis
epidermis, pl. epidermides
  hyperkeratotic e.
  hyperplastic e.
epidermitis
epidermization
epidermodysplasia
  e. verruciformis
  e. verruciformis of
    Lewandowski-Lutz
epidermoid
  e. cancer
  e. carcinoma
  e. cyst
epidermolysis
  e. bullosa (EB)
  e. bullosa acquisita (EBA)
  e. bullosa acquisita antigen
  e. bullosa atrophicans
  e. bullosa, dermal type
  e. bullosa dystrophica
  e. bullosa, epidermal type
  e. bullosa, junctional type
  e. bullosa lethalis
  e. bullosa simplex
  e. bullosa simplex
    herpetiformis
  e. simplex
epidermolytic
  e. acanthoma
  e. hyperkeratosis
  e. keratosis palmaris et
    plantaris
  e. palmoplantar keratoderma
Epidermophyton
  E. floccosum
  E. inguinale
epidermophytosis
epidermosis
epidermotropic
  e. cutaneous toxoplasmosis
epidermotropism
EpiE-ZPen
Epifoam
epiglottiditis
epiglottitis
  acute e.
epilans
  eczema e.
epilate
epilation

epilatory
epilepticus
    status e.
epiloia
Epilyt
epimastical fever
epimerization
epinephrine
    aqueous e.
    lidocaine and e.
    self-injecting e.
    subcutaneous e.
    Xylocaine with e.
EpiPen
    E. Jr.
epiphora
epiphysiodesis
Epiquick
episclera
episcleritis
    nodular e.
    nonrheumatoid e.
    rheumatoid e.
episodic
    e. angioedema
    e. bronchial obstruction
    e. malnutrition
episome
    resistance-transferring e.
epispastic
epistaxis
epithelial
    e. cyst
    e. degeneration
    e. keratitis
    e. keratopathy
    e. lining fluid (ELF)
    e. nevus
    e. tumor
epithelialization
epithelioid
    e. cell
    e. cell nevus
    e. sarcoma
epithelioma
    e. adenoides cysticum
    basal cell e. (BCE)

Borst-Jadassohn type
    intraepidermal e.
    calcifying e.
    e. contagiosum
    e. cuniculatum
    Ferguson-Smith e.
    Jadassohn e.
    e. of Malherbe
    multiple benign cystic e.
    prickle-cell e.
    squamous cell e.
    superficial basal cell e.
epitheliomatosis
epitheliomatous
epitheliopathy
epitheliotropic
epithelite
epithelium
    cat e.
    columnar e.
    cultured thymic e.
    dog e.
    ferret e.
    goat e.
    monkey e.
    mouse e.
    rabbit e.
    sheep e.
    sloughed bronchial e.
    swine e.
epithelium-derived relaxation factor
    (EpDRF)
epithelization
epithelize
Epitol
epitope
epitoxoid
epitrichium
Epivir
    lamivudine, E. (3TC)
Epivir/3TC
epizootic cellulitis
EPO
epoetin alfa
Epogen
eponychia
eponychium

E

NOTES

135

epoprostenol
epoxide hydrolase enzyme
epoxy resin
epsilometric test
epsilon-aminocaproic agent
Epsom salts
Epstein
    E. disease
    E. pearls
Epstein-Barr (EB)
    E.-B. exanthema
    E.-B. nuclear antigen (EBNA)
    E.-B. nuclear antigen test
    E.-B. virus (EBV)
    E.-B. virus-induced early
      antibody
    E.-B. virus test
epulis
    denture e.
    e. fissuratum
equation
    Chiou e.
equi
    Babesia e.
    Demodex e.
    Rhodococcus e.
equilibrium dialysis
equine
    e. abortion virus
    e. arteritis virus
    e. coital exanthema virus
    e. encephalitis
    e. encephalomyelitis
    e. infectious anemia
    e. infectious anemia virus
    e. influenza
    e. influenza virus
    e. Morbillivirus
    e. rhinopneumonitis
    e. rhinopneumonitis virus
    e. rhinoviruses
    e. serum hepatitis
    e. viral arteritis
equinia
equivalence zone
equuli
    Actinobacillus e.
E-R
    Betachron E.-R.
eradicate
Ercaf
Ergamisol
ergocalciferol

Ergomar
Ergostat
ergosterole
Ergotamine
    Medihaler E.
ergotamine derivative
ergotism
E rosette
erosio interdigitalis blastomycetica
erosion
    bone e.
    bony e.
    subchondral e.
erosiva
erosive
    e. arthritis
    e. *Candida* balanitis
    e. lichen planus
    e. osteoarthritis (EOA)
    e. polyarthritis
erubescence
erubescent
eruption
    acneform e.
    bullous pemphigoid-like e.
    butterfly e.
    creeping e.
    cutaneous drug e.
    drug e.
    eczematous polymorphous
      light e.
    erythematous psoriasiform e.
    evanescent e.
    e. evolution
    familial polymorphous light e.
    feigned e.
    fixed drug e.
    hypopigmented macular e.
    iodine e.
    juvenile spring e.
    Kaposi varicelliform e.
    lichenoid e.
    medicinal e.
    morbilliform e.
    pemphigus-like e.
    pityriasis rosea-like e.
    polymorphous light e. (PMLE)
    post-traumatic pustular e.
    psoriasiform e.
    purpuric e.
    pustular e.
    scarlatiniform e.
    scleroderma-like e.

seabather's e.
serum e.
skin e.
summer e.
vesicopustular e.
vesicular e.
eruptione
variola sine e.
eruptive
e. fever
e. xanthoma
ERV
expiratory residual volume
Erwinia
Erycette topical
Eryc Oral
EryDerm topical
Erygel topical
Erymax topical
EryPed Oral
erysipelas
ambulant e.
e. internum
e. migrans
e. perstans faciei
phlegmonous e.
e. pustulosum
surgical e.
e. verrucosum
wandering e.
erysipelas-like
e.-l. dermatophytid
e.-l. skin lesion
erysipelatous
erysipeloid
Erysipelothrix rhusiopathiae
erysipelotoxin
Ery-Tab Oral
erythema
e. ab igne
e. acneforme
acral e.
acrodynic e.
annular e.
e. annulare
e. annulare centrifugum (EAC)

e. annulare rheumaticum
e. arthriticum epidemicum
bright e.
e. brucellum
e. bullosum
e. caloricum
chilblain-like e.
e. chronicum
e. chronicum migrans
e. circinatum
congenital telangiectatic e.
e. congestivum
e. contagiosum
e. craquelé
e. desquamativum
diffuse e.
e. dyschromicum perstans
e. elevatum diutinum
e. exfoliativa
facial e.
e. figuratum
e. figuratum perstans
e. fugax
e. gyratum
e. gyratum perstans
e. gyratum repens
hemorrhagic exudative e.
e. induratum
e. infectiosum (EI)
e. intertrigo
e. iris
Jacquet e.
e. keratodes
macular e.
malar e.
e. marginatum
e. migrans (EM)
Milian e.
e. multiforme
e. multiforme bullosum
e. multiforme exudativum
e. multiforme major
e. multiforme minor
necrolytic migratory e.
ninth-day e.
e. nodosum (EN)
e. nodosum leprosum

E

NOTES

erythema *(continued)*
  e. nodosum migrans
  e. nuchae
  palmar e.
  e. palmare
  e. palmare hereditarium
  e. papulatum
  e. paratrimma
  periungual e.
  e. pernio
  e. perstans
  e. polymorphe
  e. pudoris
  e. punctate
  e. scarlatiniform
  scarlatiniform e.
  e. simplex
  e. solare
  symptomatic e.
  telangiectatic e.
  e. threshold
  toxic e.
  e. toxicum
  e. toxicum neonatorum
  e. tuberculatum
  e. venenatum
  violet-blue e.
erythematic
erythematodes
  lupus e.
erythematosa
  acne e.
erythematosum
  eczema e.
erythematosus
  acute cutaneous lupus e.
    (ACLE)
  acute lupus e.
  chilblain lupus e.
  chronic discoid lupus e.
  cutaneous lupus e.
  discoid lupus e. (DLE)
  disseminated lupus e.
  drug-induced lupus e. (DILE)
  drug-induced systemic lupus e.
  lupus e. (LE)
  neonatal lupus e. (NLE)
  pemphigus e.
  subacute cutaneous lupus e.
    (SCLE)
  subacute lupus e.
  systemic lupus e. (SLE)
  tumid lupus e.

erythematous
  e. macular dermatitis
  e. mark
  e. plaque
  e. psoriasiform eruption
  e. syphilid
erythematovesicular
erythemogenic
erythermalgia
erythralgia
erythrasma
erythredema
erythrism
erythristic
erythroblastosis
  fetal e.
  e. fetalis
erythroblastotic
erythrocatalysis
Erythrocin Oral
erythrocyanosis
erythrocyte
  e. adherence phenomenon
  e. adherence test
  e. cast
  e. sedimentation rate (ESR)
erythrocytes, antibody, complement
  (EAC)
erythrocytolysin
erythrocytolysis
erythroderma, erythrodermia
  atypical ichthyosiform e.
  bullous congenital
    ichthyosiform e.
  congenital ichthyosiform e.
  e. desquamativum
  e. exfoliativa
  exfoliative e.
  ichthyosiform e.
  e. ichthyosiformis congenitalis
  lamellar congenital
    ichthyosiform e.
  nonbullous congenital
    ichthyosiform e.
  e. psoriaticum
  Sézary e.
erythrodermas
erythrodermatitis
erythrodermia *(var. of* erythroderma)
erythrodermic psoriasis
erythrodysesthesia syndrome
erythrogenic
  e. toxin

erythrokeratodermia
  e. figurata variabilis
  e. progressive symmetrica
  e. variabilis
erythrokeratolysis hiemalis
erythrolysin
erythrolysis
erythromelalgia
erythromelanin
erythromelia
erythromycin
  e. and benzoyl peroxide
  e. and sulfisoxazole
  e. topical
erythromycin-sulfisoxazole
erythrophagia
erythrophagocytosis
erythroplakia
erythroplasia
  e. of Queyrat
  Zoon e.
erythropoietic
  e. porphyria
  e. protoporphyria
erythropoietin
erythropolis
  Rhodococcus e.
erythroprosopalgia
erythrose pigmentaire péribuccale
Eryzole Oral
eschar
  black e.
escharotic
escharotica
  rupia e.
Escherichia
  E. coli
  E. coli enterotoxin
  E. coli polysaccharide antibody
E-selectin
E-Solve-2 topical
esophageal
  e. carcinoma
  e. hypomotility
espundia
ESR
  erythrocyte sedimentation rate

ESS
  excited skin syndrome
essential
  e. fatty acid deficiency
  e. fever
  e. pruritus
  e. telangiectasia
  e. thrombocytopenic purpura
established cell line
Estar
  E. Gel
ester
  phorbol e.
esterase
  C1 e.
  lymphocyte serine e.
  serine e.
esthiomene
estivae
estival, aestival
estivale, aestivale
  hydroa e.
estivalis, aestivalis
  acne e.
  dermatitis e.
  prurigo e.
  pruritus e.
estrogen
  conjugated e.'s
estrone
ETCO$_2$
  end-tidal carbon dioxide
E-test
ethambutol
  e. hydrochloride
ethanolamine
  amino ethyl e.
ethidium bromide
Ethilon suture
ethinylestradiol
ethionamide
ethmoidectomy
ethmoid sinusitis
ethyl
  e. chloride
  e. chloride and
    dichlorotetrafluoroethane

E

NOTES

ethyl-2,3-dihydroxybenzoate
ethylenediamine
    e. dermatitis
ethylene oxide
ethylnorepinephrine
    e. hydrochloride
ethylsuccinate
    oral erythromycin e.
etidocaine
    e. hydrochloride
etidronate
    sodium e.
etiolation
etiologic
etiology
    monoarticular arthritis of
    unknown e.
etodolac
etoposide
ETO Sleuth
etretinate
ETS-2% topical
Eubacterium
eucalyptus
    e. saligna
    e. tree
Eucerin
    E. cream
    E. moisturizer
    E. Plus moisturizer
Eudal-SR
eudiaphoresis
eumelanin
eumycetoma
eupeptic
euphoria
Euproctis
    E. *chrysorrhoea*
    E. *chrysorrhoea* sting
Eurax
    E. topical
Euroglyphus maynei
europaeus
    ulex e.
European
    E. blastomycosis
    E. blister beetle sting
eustachian tube
eutrichosis
EV
    enterovirus

evaluation
    acute physiology and chronic
    health e. (APACHE)
evanescent
    e. eruption
    e. macule
E-Vista
evolution
    eruption e.
    lesion e.
evulsion
Ewart sign
Ewing tumor
exacerbation
Exact skin product
examination
    bone marrow e.
    full-body cutaneous e.
    immunofluorescent e.
    KOH e.
    retinal e.
    Wood light e.
exanthema, pl. exanthemas,
  exanthemata
    Boston e.
    echoviral e.
    enteroviral e.
    epidemic e.
    Epstein-Barr e.
    keratoid e.
    ordinal designation of the
    exanthemata
    polymorphous e.
    e. subitum
    vesicular e.
    viral e.
exanthematicus
    ichthyismus e.
exanthematous
    e. disease
    e. fever
exanthesis
    e. arthrosia
excavatum
    pectus e.
Excedrin
    E. IB
    E. PM
EXCEL
    Simplastin E.
excess
    antibody e.
    antigen e.

excessive
    e. hairiness
    e. secretion
    e. sweating
    e. water immersion
excessive dryness
exchange
    e. plasmapheresis
    e. transfusion
exchanger
    heat/moisture e. (HME)
excision
    fusiform e.
    wide e.
excisional
    e. biopsy
    e. removal
excited
    e. skin syndrome (ESS)
    e. state
exclamation point hair
excoriate
excoriated
excoriation
    neurotic e.
excrescence
    wart-like e.
excretion
    xanthine stone e.
excursion
Exelderm
    E. topical
exercise
    isometric e.
    passive range of motion e.
exercise-induced
    e.-i. asthma (EIA)
    e.-i. bronchospasm
exertion
exfoliant
exfoliate
exfoliatio areata linguae
exfoliation
exfoliativa
    cheilitis e.
    dermatitis e.
    erythema e.

    erythroderma e.
    glossitis areata e.
    keratolysis e.
exfoliative
    e. dermatitis
    e. erythroderma
    e. psoriasis
Exgest
exhaust
    automobile e.
exhaustion
    nervous e.
    obvious physical e.
Exidine Scrub
exilicauda
    Centruroides e.
exine
Exirel
exoantigen
exocrine
exocrinopathic process
exocytosis
exogenetic
exogenote
exogenous
    e. factor
    e. ochronosis
    e. pigmentation
    e. substance
Exophiala
    E. jeanselmei
    E. werneckii
exophytic
exopolysaccharide
    mucoid e.
exoserosis
exostosis, pl. exostoses
    subungual e.
exotoxic
exotoxin
    bacterial e.
    streptococcal pyrogenic e.
    (SPE)
expansion
    clonal e.
expectorant
    Fedahist E.

E

NOTES

expectorant *(continued)*
  Genamin E.
  Myminic E.
  Silaminic E.
  Theramin E.
  Triaminic E.
  Tri-Clear E.
  Triphenyl E.
expectorate
experimental
  e. allergic encephalitis (EAE)
  e. allergic encephalomyelitis
    (EAE)
expiration
  prolongation of e.
expiratory
  e. positive airway pressure
    (EPAP)
  e. prolongation
  e. residual volume (ERV)
explant
explantation
exposure
  aerosolized pollutant e.
  allergen e.
  cold e.
  heat e.
  light e.
  limitation of e.
  occupational e.
  prior drug e.
  repeated e.
  sun e.
  vinyl chloride e.
Exsel
Extendryl
extensor
  e. surface
extensum
  hemangioma planum e.
Extentabs
  Dimetapp E.
exteriorization
externa
  otitis e.
external
  e. absorption
  e. auditory canal (EAC)
  e. otitis
extra-articular
  e.-a. tissue
extracellular
  e. cholesterolosis

  e. matrix (ECM)
  e. matrix remodeling
  e. toxin
extrachromosomal
extracorporeal
  e. membrane oxygenation
    (ECMO)
  e. photochemotherapy
  e. photophoresis
extract
  allergenic e.
  allergic e.
  alum-precipitated pyridine-
    extracted pollen e.
  aqueous e.
  glycerinated e.
  e. of henna
  inhalant allergen e.
  lyophilized e.
  phenol-preserved e.
  pollen e.
  tobacco leaf e.
  venom e.
  whole-body e.
extraction
  comedo e.
extractor
  Schamberg comedo e.
  Unna comedo e.
extralobar
extramammary Paget disease
extrapulmonary
  e. pneumocystosis
  e. sarcoidosis
  e. tuberculosis
Extra Strength Bayer Enteric 500
  Aspirin
extravascular granulomatous
  features
extrinsic
  e. allergic alveolitis
  e. asthma
  e. compression of trachea
exuberant cicatrization
exudate
  retinal e.
exudation
exudative
  e. discoid
  e. discoid and lichenoid
    dermatitis
  e. papulosquamous disease

exudativum
    erythema multiforme e.
exude
eye
    black e.
    raccoon e.'s
    red e.

eyebrow loss
eyelash
    e. cosmetic
    e. loss
eyelid cosmetic
eyeline tattoo
Eye-Lube-A solution

NOTES

E

F

F agent
F genote
F pilus
F plasmid

f

f. factor (I, II, IIa, III)

FA

fluorescent antibody stain
FA virus

Fab

F. fragment
F. piece

Faba

F. faba
F. vulgaris

fabism
fabric
fabricii

Epicauta f.

Fabry

F. disease
F. syndrome

Fabry-Anderson disease
faccinia
face

Hippocratic f.
f. peel

face-lift
facetal joint
facet joint arthropathy
facial

f. erythema
f. foundation
f. moisturizer
f. nerve palsy
f. powder
f. undercover cream
f. vitiligo

faciale

granuloma f.
pyoderma f.

facialis

herpes f.
pyodermia f.
zona f.

faciei

atrophoderma reticulatum
symmetricum f.
chloasma f.

erysipelas perstans f.
keratosis pilaris atrophicans f.
lupus miliaris disseminatus f.
seborrhea f.
tinea f.

facies

adenoidal f.
allergic f.
cushingoid f.
dengue f.
Hippocratic f.
f. Hippocratica
hound-dog f.
leonine f.
moon f.

FACS

fluorescence-activated cell sorter

factitia

dermatitis f.
urticaria f.

factitial dermatitis
factitious

f. purpura
f. urticaria

factor

f. (A, B, C, D, E, H, I)
activated vitamin K-
dependent f.
anticomplementary f.
antinuclear f. (ANF)
bacteriocin f.
B-cell differentiation/growth f.
Bittner milk f.
chemokinetic f.
cobra venom f.
colony-stimulating f. (CSF)
complement chemotactic f.
control of emotional f.
cytokine synthesis inhibitory f.
endogenous f.
endothelial relaxing f.
epidermal growth f. (EGF)
epithelium-derived relaxation f.
(EpDRF)
exogenous f.
fertility f.
fibroblast growth f. (FGF)
f f. (I, II, IIa, III)
genetic f.
f. Gm

F

factor *(continued)*
granulocyte colony-stimulating f. (G-CSF)
granulocyte-macrophage colony-stimulating f. (GM-CSF)
growth f. (GF)
Hageman f.
hemopoietic f.
heparin binding growth f. (HBGF)
histamine-releasing f. (HRF)
f. (I, II, VII, VIII, IX, X, XI, XII)
immunoglobulin G rheumatoid f. (IgG RF)
immunoglobulin M rheumatoid f. (IgM RF)
inhibition f.
f. Inv
kappa binding nuclear f.
LE f.
leukocytosis-promoting f.
leukopenic f.
lymph node permeability f. (LNPF)
macrophage-activating f. (MAF)
migration-inhibitory f. (MIF)
milk f.
monocyte chemotactic f. (MCF)
monocyte-derived neutrophil chemotactic f.
myeloma growth f.
natural killer cell stimulating f. (NKSF)
nephritic f.
nerve growth f. (NGF)
neutrophil activating f. (NAF)
neutrophil chemotactant f.
nuclear f.
osteoclast-activating f. (OAF)
platelet-activating f. (PAF)
platelet-aggregating f. (PAF)
platelet-derived growth f. (PDGF)
positive rheumatoid f.
psychogenic f.
R f.
recognition f.
releasing f. (RF)
f. replacement therapy
resistance f.
resistance-inducing f.

resistance-transfer f.
Rheumatex test for rheumatoid f.
rheumatoid f. (RF)
Rheumaton test for rheumatoid f.
secretor f.
sex f.
steel f.
stimulating f. (SF)
sun protection f. (SPF)
T-cell growth f.
T-cell replacing f.
thymic lymphopoietic f.
thyrotoxic complement-fixation f.
transfer f.
transforming f.
transforming growth f. (TGF)
transforming growth f. α (TGFα)
trigger f.
tumor lysis f.
tumor necrosis f. (TNF)
f. VIII:C inhibitor
factor-1
B-cell growth f.
heparin binding growth f. (HBGF-1)
T-cell growth f.
factor-2
B-cell growth f.
T-cell growth f.
factor-3
leukocyte antigen f. (LAF-3)
factor-4
platelet f.
factor-beta
tumor necrosis f.-b.
factor-inducing monocytopoiesis
facultative
f. bacterium
f. myiasis
f. skin color
faecalis
Alcaligenes f.
Streptococcus f.
faeni
Micropolyspora f.
Faget sign
fagopyrism
failure
acute respiratory f. (ARF)

adrenocortical f.
congestive heart f. (CHF)
impending respiratory f.
primary adrenocortical f.
renal f.
respiratory f.
secondary adrenocortical f.
severe respiratory f.
f. to thrive
ventilatory f.
Fairbanks arthritis phenotype
falciparum
    Plasmodium f.
fall
    f. elm
    f. elm tree
    hair f.
false
    f. agglutination
    f. cyst
    f. diphtheria
    f. membrane
    f. ragweed
false-negative
    f.-n. patch test
    f.-n. reaction
false-positive
    f.-p. patch test
    f.-p. reaction
    f.-p. syphilis test
FAMA
    fluorescent antimembrane antibody
famciclovir
familial
    f. amyloidotic polyneuropathy
    syndrome
    f. atypical multiple mole
    melanoma syndrome
    (FAMMM)
    f. benign chronic pemphigus
    f. cholestasis syndrome
    f. continuous skin peel
    f. hypocalciuric hypercalcemia
    f. Mediterranean fever
    f. nephropathic amyloidosis
    syndrome
    f. paroxysmal polyserositis

f. PMLE
f. polymorphous light eruption
f. pulmonary fibroproliferative
f. recurrent polyserositis
f. reticuloendotheliosis
f. rosacea-like dermatitis
f. spondyloepiphyseal dysplasia
    tarda
f. thrombocytopenia
family
    immunoglobulin supergene f.
FAMMM
    familial atypical multiple mole
    melanoma syndrome
famotidine
Famvir
Fanconi anemia
Fansidar
Fansimef
Farber disease
farcinica
    Nocardia f.
farcy
Far East Russian encephalitis
farinae
    Dermatophagoides f.
farmer's
    f. lung
    f. skin
Farr
    F. assay
    F. law
    F. test
fascia
    f. lata
    palmar f.
    plantar f.
fasciatus
    Nosopsyllus f.
fasciitis
    eosinophilic f.
    necrotizing f.
    nodular f.
    pseudosarcomatous f.
fascioliasis
Fasject
fastidious

F

NOTES

fat
  atrophy of f.
  f. malabsorption
  f. necrosis
fatigue
fat-replacement atrophy
fatty degeneration
faucium
  Mycoplasma f.
faun tail nevus
favid
favism
favosa
  porrigo f.
  tinea f.
Favre-Racouchot
  F.-R. cyst
  F.-R. disease
  F.-R. skin
  F.-R. syndrome
favus
FB
  foreign body
5-FC
  5-fluorocytosine
Fc
  F. fragment
  F. piece
  F. receptor
FCP
  florid cutaneous papillomatosis
feather
  Australian parrot f.
  canary f.
  chicken f.
  cockatiel f.
  duck f.
  goose f.
  f. hydroid
  mixed f.
  parakeet f.
  parrot f.
  pigeon f.
  turkey f.
feature
  electromyographic f.
  immunologic f.
  pathologic f.
features
  extravascular granulomatous f.
febricitans
  pes f.
febricula

febrile
  f. agglutinin
  hydroa f.
  f. urticaria
febrilis
  herpes f.
  urticaria f.
fecal fat determination
faecalis
  Enterococcus f.
Fedahist
  F. Expectorant
  F. Expectorant Pediatric
  F. Tablet
feeleii
  Legionella f.
feet (*pl. of* foot)
  edema of f.
  reddening of soles of f.
FEF
  forced expiratory flow
FEF$_{25-75\%}$
  mean forced expiratory flow during
  the middle of FVC
feigned eruption
Feingold diet
Feldene
feline
  f. agranulocytosis
  f. infectious enteritis
  f. infectious peritonitis
  f. leukemia
  f. leukemia-sarcoma virus
  complex
  f. leukemia virus (FeLV)
  f. panleukopenia virus (FPV)
  f. rhinotracheitis virus
  f. viral rhinotracheitis
felineum
  Microsporum f.
felis
  Afipia f.
  Babesia f.
  Ctenocephalides f.
felon
Felty syndrome
FeLV
  feline leukemia virus
female pattern alopecia
Femstat
fenbufen
fennel
  dog f.

fenoprofen
    f. calcium
fenoterol
fentanyl
Ferguson-Smith
    F.-S. epithelioma
    F.-S. keratoacanthoma
fermentans
    Acidaminococcus f.
fermented food
Fernandez reaction
ferox
    prurigo f.
ferret
    f. epithelium
ferric
    f. chloride
    f. subsulfate
ferrugineum
    Microsporum f.
fertility
    f. agent
    f. factor
FES
    flame emission spectroscopy
    forced expiratory spirogram
fescue
    meadow f.
fester
festooning
fetal
    f. erythroblastosis
    f. liver transplantation
    f. thymus transplantation
fetalis
    erythroblastosis f.
    ichthyosis f.
    keratosis diffusa f.
fetoprotein
    alpha f.
fetus
    harlequin f.
FEV
    forced expiratory volume
FEV$_{1\%VC}$
    forced expiratory volume in 1
    second as percent of FVC

FEV$_1$
    forced expiratory volume in 1
    second
fever
    acute rheumatic f. (ARF)
    Aden f.
    African hemorrhagic f.
    African swine f.
    Argentinean hemorrhagic f.
    f. blister
    Bolivian hemorrhagic f.
    bouquet f.
    boutonneuse f.
    bovine ephemeral f.
    breakbone f.
    bullous f.
    Bunyamwera f.
    Bwamba f.
    camp f.
    cerebrospinal f.
    childbed f.
    Colorado tick f.
    continued f.
    Crimean-Congo hemorrhagic f.
    dandy f.
    date f.
    dengue f.
    dengue hemorrhagic f.
    diphasic milk f.
    Dutton relapsing f.
    Ebola hemorrhagic f.
    enteric f.
    epidemic hemorrhagic f.
    epimastical f.
    eruptive f.
    essential f.
    exanthematous f.
    familial Mediterranean f.
    flood f.
    food f.
    Fort Bragg f.
    glandular f.
    grain f.
    Haverhill f.
    hay f.
    hemoglobinuric f.
    hemorrhagic f.

F

NOTES

fever *(continued)*
  herpetic f.
  hospital f.
  humidifier f.
  Ilhéus f.
  inundation f.
  island f.
  jail f.
  Japanese river f.
  jungle yellow f.
  Katayama f.
  kedani f.
  Korean hemorrhagic f.
  Lassa hemorrhagic f.
  laurel f.
  louse-borne relapsing f.
  low-grade f.
  malignant catarrhal f.
  Malta f.
  Manchurian hemorrhagic f.
  Marseilles f.
  Mediterranean f.
  Mediterranean exanthematous f.
  metal fume f.
  miliary f.
  mill f.
  miniature scarlet f.
  monoleptic f.
  mud f.
  nodal f.
  Omsk hemorrhagic f.
  o'nyong-nyong f.
  pappataci f.
  papular f.
  pharyngoconjunctival f.
  Phlebotomus f.
  polka f.
  polyleptic f.
  pretibial f.
  protein f.
  puerperal f.
  Pym f.
  pyogenic f.
  Q f.
  rat-bite f.
  recrudescent typhus f.
  relapsing f.
  rheumatic f.
  Rift Valley f.
  Rocky Mountain spotted f.
  rose f.
  Ross River f.
  sandfly f.

  San Joaquin f.
  scarlet f.
  ship f.
  shipping f.
  Sindbis f.
  slow f.
  solar f.
  f. sore
  spotted f.
  steroid f.
  swamp f.
  swine f.
  symptomatic f.
  syphilitic f.
  three-day f.
  tick f.
  tick-borne relapsing f.
  traumatic f.
  tsutsugamushi f.
  typhoid f.
  undifferentiated type f.'s
  f. of unknown origin (FUO)
  viral hemorrhagic f.
  viral sandfly f.
  Wesselsbron f.
  West African f.
  West Nile f.
  wound f.
  yellow f.
  Zika f.
Feverall
fexofenadine
FGF
  fibroblast growth factor
fiber
  afferent nerve f.
  blocking vagal afferent f.
  blocking vagal efferent f.
  elastic f.
  lattice f.
  parasympathetic nerve f.
  reticulin f.
  reticulum f.
fiberglass
  f. dermatitis
fiberoptic
  f. bronchoscope
  f. bronchoscopy
fibril
  collagen f.
fibrillar
  f. collagen
fibrillarin

fibrillation
fibrillin
fibrin
    f. deposition
fibrinogen level
fibrinoid
    f. change
    f. necrosis
fibrinolysin and deoxyribonuclease
fibrinolytic purpura
fibrinopeptide
fibrinous
    f. degeneration
fibroblast
    f. growth factor (FGF)
    human embryonic lung f.
    f. interferon
    f. mediation
fibroblastic tissue
fibroblast-like cell
fibrocartilage
fibroepithelial polyp
fibroepithelioma
    f. basal cell carcinoma
fibrofolliculoma
fibrogenesis imperfecta ossium
fibrokeratoma
    acquired digital f.
    digital f.
fibroma
    aponeurotic f.
    f. durum
    infantile digital f.
    irritation f.
    f. molle
    f. molle gravidarum
    f. pendulum
    peripheral ossifying f.
    periungual f.
    rabbit f.
    senile f.
    Shope f.
fibromatosis
    aggressive infantile f.
    congenital f.
    gingival f.
    juvenile hyalin f.

    juvenile palmo-plantar f.
    palmoplantar f.
    f. virus of rabbit
fibromodulin
    f. CS/DS
fibromyalgia (FM)
    f. syndrome (FMS)
    f. trigger point
fibronectin
    large, external transformation-
        sensitive f. (LETS)
    plasma f.
    f. receptor
fibroplasia
    papular f.
fibroproliferative
    endocardial f.
    familial pulmonary f.
fibrosa
    osteitis f.
fibrosarcoma
    Earle L f.
fibrosis
    apical lobe f.
    cystic f. (CF)
    glomerular f.
    idiopathic pulmonary f. (IPF)
    interstitial f.
    nodular subepidermal f.
    obliterative granulomatous f.
    parenchymal f.
    perineural f.
    peripheral f.
    progressive interstitial f.
    retroperitoneal f.
    subepidermal nodular f.
fibrositis
fibrosum
    molluscum f.
fibrosus
    nevus f.
fibrothorax
fibrotic arteriosclerosis
fibrous
    f. arcade
    f. bacterial virus
    f. dysplasia

F

NOTES

fibrous *(continued)*
    f. histiocytoma
    f. hyperplasia
    f. papule
    f. sheath
    f. synovium (FS)
    f. xanthoma
fibroxanthoma
    atypical f.
FICA
    food immune complex assay
ficosis
fiddle-back
    f.-b. spider
    f.-b. spider bite
fiddler neck
field
    electromagnetic f.
fifth disease
fig
    f. wart
    weeping f.
figurata
    keratosis rubra f.
figurate
figuratum
    erythema f.
figuratus
figure
    flame f.
filament
    intermediate f.
filamentary keratitis
filamentous
    f. bacterial virus
    f. bacteriophage
Filaria
    F. bancrofti
    F. loa
filaria, pl. **filariae**
filarial
    f. elephantiasis
    f. nematode
filariasis
    Bancroftian *f.*
    Loiasis *f.*
Filatov
    F. disease
    F. Dukes disease
    F. spot
filgrastim
filiform
    f. wart

filiformis
    verruca f.
filles
    acné excoriée des jeunes f.
Filmtab
    Biaxin F.'s
    Rondec F.
Filoviridae
    F. virus
Filovirus
filter
    ARI Group I–IV f.
    electronic f.
    HEPA f.
    membrane f.
filtrable
    f. virus
fimbriatum
    Gliocladium f.
finding
    immunofluorescence f.
    serum protein electrophoretic f.
    x-ray f.
fine needle aspiration (FNA)
finger
    blubber f.
    bolster f.
    clubbed f.
    dead f.
    Hippocratic f.
    sausage f.
    seal f.
    snapping f.
    spade f.
    speck f.
    trigger f.
    waxy f.
    whale f.
    white f.
finger-in-glove appearance
fingernail
    half-and-half f.
Finger Phantom pulse oximeter testing system
fingerprint
    Galton system of classification of f.
Finkelstein test
Finn chamber
FIO$_2$
    fraction of inspired oxygen
fir
    Douglas f.

fire
    f. ant
    f. ant anaphylaxis
    f. ant sting
    f. coral
    f. coral sting
    Saint Anthony's f.
firebush
fireweed
firm lesion
first
    F. Check rapid diagnostic test
    f. degree burn
    f. degree frostbite
    f. disease
first-set rejection
fish
    f. oil
    scorpion f.
    f. skin
    f. tank granuloma
    tuna f.
Fisher
    F. exact test
    F. two-tailed exact test
fish-mouth healing
fissuratum
    acanthoma f.
    epulis f.
    granuloma f.
fissure
    interpalpebral f.
fissured tongue
fissuring
fistula, pl. fistulae, fistulas
    f. in ano
    arteriovenous f.
    aural f.
    bronchopleural f.
    dental f.
    pilonidal f.
FITC
    fluorescein isothiocyanate
Fitz-Hugh and Curtis syndrome
fixation
    complement f. (CF)
    Ilizarov external f.

    open reduction and internal f.
    (ORIF)
    f. reaction
fixed
    f. airflow obstruction
    f. cutaneous sporotrichosis
    f. drug eruption
    f. drug reaction
    f. pulmonary infiltrate
    f. virus
flaccid
flagellar
    f. agglutinin
    f. antigen
flag sign
Flagyl
    F. Oral
flake
    sulfur f.
flaky paint dermatosis
flame
    f. emission spectroscopy (FES)
    f. figure
    f. nevus
flammeus
    nevus f.
Flantadin
flare
    wheal and f.
Flarex Ophthalmic
flash
    f. burn
flashlamp-pumped pulsed-dye laser
    (FLPD, FPDL)
Flash portable spirometer
flask
    Dewar f.
flat
    f. condyloma
    f. papular syphilid
    f. wart
flavedo
Flavimonas orzihabitans
Flaviviridae
Flavivirus
Flavobacterium meningosepticum

F

NOTES

flavus
>Aspergillus f.

flaxseed
flea
>cat f.
>chigger f.
>dog f.
>northern rat f.
>oriental rat f.
>sand f.
>f. venom

fleck
fleckeri
>Chironex f.

Flegel disease
Fleischner syndrome
flesh
>goose f.
>proud f.

flesh-colored
fleshflies
flexion contracture
Flexi-Trak skin anchoring device
flexneri
>Shigella f.

flexor
>f. surface

flexural eczema
flexure
floccosum
>Epidermophyton f.

flocculation
>f. reaction
>f. test

Flolan
Flonase
flood fever
flora
>saprophytic f.

Florey unit
florid
>f. cutaneous papillomatosis (FCP)
>f. oral papillomatosis

Florinef Acetate
floristic zone
Florone
>F. E topical
>F. topical

flour
>soybean f.
>wheat f.

flow
>f. cytometry
>forced expiratory f. (FEF)
>peak expiratory f. (PEFR)

Floxin
>F. injection
>F. Oral

FLPD
>flashlamp-pumped pulsed-dye laser vascular FLPD

flu
fluconazole
fluctuance
fluctuant
fluctuation
flucytosine
>5-f.

fludrocortisone acetate
flufenamic acid
fluffy alveolar infiltrate
fluid
>cutting f.
>epithelial lining f. (ELF)
>intravenous f.'s
>middle ear f. (MEF)
>synovial f. (SF)
>tetanus toxoid, f.
>f. therapy

fluid-phase C1q-binding assay
Flu-Imune
fluke
>blood f.
>intestinal f.
>tissue f.

Flumadine Oral
flunisolide
>f. nasal solution

fluocinolone
>f. acetonide

fluocinonide
Fluogen
Fluonex topical
Fluonid topical
fluoresce
fluorescein isothiocyanate (FITC)
fluorescence
>f. quenching

fluorescence-activated cell sorter (FACS)
fluorescent
>f. antibody
>f. antibody stain (FA)
>f. antibody technique

f. antimembrane antibody
(FAMA)
f. treponemal antibody
absorption (FTA-ABS)
f. treponemal antibody-
absorption test
Fluori-Methane Topical Spray
fluorochrome
fluorochroming
5-fluorocytosine (5-FC)
fluorometholone
sodium sulfacetamide and f.
fluorometric procedure
Fluoroplex
F. topical
Fluor-Op Ophthalmic
fluoroquinolone
fluoroscopy
fluorouracil
5-fluorouracil (5-FU)
fluoxetine
f. HCl
f. hydrochloride
flurandrenolide
flurazepam
flurbiprofen
Fluro-Ethyl
F.-E. Aerosol
Flurosyn topical
Flury
F. strain rabies virus
F. strain vaccine
flush
f. area
dry f.
histamine f.
wet f.
flushing
emotional f.
menopausal f.
neural-mediated f.
paroxysmal f.
thermal f.
fluticasone
f. propionate
Flutter
flutter device

flux
f. allergen
soldering f.
Fluzone
fly
f. bite
black f.
f. blister
buffalo f.
deer f.
horse f.
house f.
may f.
sarcophagi f.
screw-worm f.
sewer f.
Spanish f.
stable f.
tsetse f.
tumbu f.
fly-borne disease
Flynn-Aird syndrome
FM
fibromyalgia
FMD
foot-and-mouth disease
FMD virus
FML
F. Forte Ophthalmic
F. Ophthalmic
FML-S Ophthalmic suspension
FMS
fibromyalgia syndrome
FNA
fine needle aspiration
foam cell
foamy
f. agent
f. virus
focal
f. acantholytic dyskeratoma
f. acantholytic dyskeratosis
f. acral hyperkeratosis
f. amyloidosis
f. anoxia
f. dermal hypoplasia
f. embolic glomerulonephritis

F

NOTES

155

focal *(continued)*
    f. epithelial hyperplasia
    f. histiocytosis
    f. infection
    f. inflammation
    f. reaction
    f. rupture of basement
      membrane
focus, pl. **foci**
    granulomatous foci
focusing
    isoelectric f. (IEF)
fogo selvagem
FOII powder inhaler
foil bath PUVA
fold
    crural f.
    Dennie infraorbital f.
    Dennie-Morgan infraorbital f.
    lateral nail f.
    Morgan f.
    nail f.
    nasolabial f. (NLF)
    villous f.
Folex PFS
foliacée
    lame f.
foliaceous
    f. pemphigus
foliaceus
    pemphigus f.
folic acid
folinic acid
follicle
    hair f.
    hypertrophic lymphoid f.
    pilosebaceous f.
follicular
    f. abscess
    f. accentuation
    f. atrophoderma
    f. degeneration syndrome
    f. ichthyosis
    f. impetigo
    f. infundibular cyst
    f. isthmus cyst
    f. keratosis
    f. lichen planus
    f. mange
    f. melanin unit
    f. mucinosis
    f. nummular dermatitis
    f. nummular eczema

    f. occlusion triad
    f. orifice
    f. papule
    f. plug
    f. poroma
    f. pustule
    f. syphilid
    f. vulvitis
follicularis
    alopecia f.
    ichthyosis f.
    isolated dyskeratosis f.
    keratosis f.
    lichen planus f.
folliculis
folliculitis
    f. abscedens et suffodiens
    f. barbae
    Bockhart f.
    Candida f.
    f. decalvans
    eosinophilic pustular f.
    f. et perifolliculitis abscedens
      et suffodiens
    keloidal f.
    f. keloidalis
    f. nares perforans
    perforating f.
    Pityrosporum f.
    pustular f.
    f. ulerythema reticulata
    f. ulerythematosa reticulata
folliculorum
    Acarus f.
    Demodex f.
    pityriasis f.
Follmann balanitis
fomes
fomite
Fonsecaea
    F. compactum
    F. pedrosoi
food
    f. additive
    f. allergy
    f. antigen
    antigenemically cross-reacting f.
    f. asthma
    f. challenge
    f. dye
    f. elimination
    fermented f.
    f. fever

f. hypersensitivity
f. immune complex assay
(FICA)
Tetramune fish f.
food-borne disease
Food and Drug Administration
food-induced respiratory disease
foot, pl. **feet**
athlete's f.
Dr Scholl's Athlete's F.
fungous f.
Hong Kong f.
immersion f.
Madura f.
moccasin f.
mossy f.
neuropathic f.
perforating ulcer of f.
ringworm of f.
sea boot f.
shelter f.
tennis shoe f.
trench f.
f. yaws
foot-and-mouth
f.-a.-m. disease (FMD)
f.-a.-m. disease virus
f.-a.-m. disease virus vaccine
Foradil
foramen of Monro
forced
f. expiratory flow (FEF)
f. expiratory spirogram (FES)
f. expiratory volume (FEV)
f. expiratory volume in 1
second (FEV$_1$)
f. expiratory volume in 1
second as percent of FVC
(FEV$_{1\%VC}$)
f. vital capacity (FVC)
forceps
Adson toothed f.
Castroviejo f.
Dyonics basket f.
IM Jaws alligator f.
jeweler's f.
Lalonde hook f.

mosquito f.
suction loose body f.
forces
van der Waals f.
Fordyce
angiokeratoma of F.
F. condition
F. disease
F. granule
F. spot
forearm ischemic exercise test
forefoot
foreign
f. body (FB)
f. body giant cell
f. body granuloma
f. body rhinitis
f. protein
f. protein therapy
f. serum
foreign-body reaction
forelock
occipital f.
white frontal f.
Forestier disease
forest yaws
fork
tuning f.
form
hyphal f.
involution f.
pentamidine in aerosol f.
replicative f. (RF)
yeast f.
formaldehyde
f. resin
formalin
formalinize
formation
anterior synechia f.
keloid f.
posterior synechia f.
scar f.
web f.
formication
formoterol
Formo-Test test

F

NOTES

formula
  Bayer Select Pain Relief F.
  Castellani Natural F.
  f. change
  Grecian F.
  Nursoy f.
  Poisson-Pearson f.
  Triaminic AM Decongestant F.
formulary
formulation
  amphotericin B liposomal f.
fornix, pl. **fornices**
  inferior f.
Forssman
  F. antibody
  F. antigen
  F. antigen-antibody reaction
Fortaz
Fort Bragg fever
Forte
  Aristocort F.
  Citanest F.
  Robinul F.
fortuitum
  Mycobacterium f.
Fosamax
foscarnet
  f. sodium
Foscavir
  F. injection
fosfomycin tromethamine
Foshay test
Fos proto-oncogene
fossa, pl. **fossae**
  antecubital f.
  popliteal f.
Fostex
Fothergill disease
Fototar
foundation
  anhydrous facial f.
  facial f.
  oil-based facial f.
  water-based facial f.
  water-free facial f.
Fournier
  F. disease
  F. gangrene
fourth disease
foveation
fowl
  f. diphtheria
  f. erythroblastosis virus

  f. leukosis
  f. lymphomatosis
  f. lymphomatosis virus
  f. myeloblastosis virus
  f. neurolymphomatosis virus
  f. paralysis
  f. pest
  f. plague
  f. plague virus
fowleri
  Naegleria f.
fowlpox
  f. virus
fowls
  leukemia of f.
fox
  f. encephalitis
  f. encephalitis virus
Fox-Fordyce disease
foxtail
  meadow f.
FPDL
  flashlamp-pumped pulsed-dye laser
FPV
  feline panleukopenia virus
fractional sterilization
fraction of inspired oxygen (FIO$_2$)
fracture
  Colles f.
  Segond f.
  stress f.
  transchondral f.
fragilis
  Bacteroides f.
fragilitas
  f. crinium
  f. unguium
fragment
  Fab f.
  Fc f.
fragmentation
  elastic-fiber f.
frambesia
frambesiform
  f. syphilid
frambesiformis
  sycosis f.
frambesioma
framboesioides
  mycosis f.
frame-shift
  f.-s. mutagen
  f.-s. mutation

Franceschetti-Jadassohn syndrome
Francisella tularensis
Frankfort horizontal plane
FRC
    functional residual capacity
freckle
    f. of Hutchinson
    melanotic f.
freckling
    axillary f.
free
    f. radical
    f. salicylate level
freeborni
    Anopheles f.
freeze-dried protein
freezing
    surface f.
Freezone solution
Frei
    F. antigen
    F. test
Freiberg disease
Frei-Hoffmann reaction
Freon
frequency
    f. of allergy symptom
    ciliary beat f.
    f. doubled neodymium:yttrium-
        aluminum-garnet laser
fresh frozen plasma
Freund
    F. complete adjuvant
    F. complete adjuvant test
    F. incomplete adjuvant
freundii
    Citrobacter f.
Frey
    F. hair
    F. syndrome
friction
    f. blister
    f. bulla
Friedländer pneumonia
Friend
    F. disease

F. leukemia virus
F. virus
Frigiderm
fringe
    costal f.
frond
    villous f.
frontal bossing
frontalis
    acne f.
    alopecia liminaris f.
frost
    f. itch
    urea f.
frostbite
    first degree f.
frozen
    f. plasma
    f. shoulder
frozen-thawed red cell
FS
    fibrous synovium
    FS Shampoo topical
FSL
    Actin F.
FTA-ABS
    fluorescent treponemal antibody
    absorption
    FTA-ABS test
5-FU
    5-fluorouracil
fucosidosis
fugax
    erythema f.
fugitive
    f. swelling
    f. wart
fulguration
full-body cutaneous examination
full-coverage facial powder
full-thickness burn
fulminans
    acne f.
    purpura f.
fulminant
fulminating smallpox

NOTES

159

Fulvicin
    F. P/G
    F.-U/F
fulvum
    Microsporum f.
fumagillin
fumarate
    clemastine f.
fumes
    soldering f.
fumigation
fumigatus
    Aspergillus f.
function
    decreased renal f.
    phagocytic f.
    poor marrow f.
    pulmonary f. (PF)
functional
    f. abnormality in asthma
    f. C1 esterase inhibitor
    f. impairment
    f. residual capacity (FRC)
functional class II–IV
funestus
    Anopheles f.
fungal
    f. arthritis
    f. bursitis
    f. culture
    f. disease
    f. id reaction
    f. infection
    f. scraping
fungate
fungating sore
fungemia
fungi (*pl. of* fungus)
fungicidal
fungicide
fungiform
Fungi Imperfecti
fungistasis
fungistat
fungistatic
fungitoxic
Fungizone
    F. Intravenous
Fungoid
    F. Creme
    F. HC Creme
    F. tincture
    F. Topical solution

fungoid
fungoides
    granuloma f.
    microabscess of mycosis f.
    mycosis f.
fungosity
fungous
    f. foot
    f. infection
fungus, pl. fungi
    f. ball
    bracket f.
    dematiaceous fungi
    dematiaceous f.
    mosaic f.
    nonpathogenic f.
    Phoma f.
FUO
    fever of unknown origin
Furacin topical
Furadantin
Furalan
Furan
Furanite
furazolidone
furfur, pl. *furfures*
    Malassezia f.
    Microsporum f.
furfuracea
    alopecia f.
    impetigo f.
    seborrhea f.
furfuraceous
    f. impetigo
furfurans
    porrigo f.
furfures (*pl. of* *furfur*)
furoate
    diloxanide f.
    mometasone f.
Furoxone
furrow
    transverse f.
furrowed tongue
furuncle
furuncular
    f. disease
furunculoid
furunculosis
    f. orientalis
furunculous
furunculus

Fusarium
    F. moniliforme
fusca
    lamina f.
fuscoceruleus
    nevus f.-c.
    nevus f.-c. acromiodeltoideus
    nevus f.-c. ophthalmomaxillaris
fusidic acid
fusiform
    f. bacillus
    f. excision
Fusobacterium
    F. nucleatum

fusospirochetal
    f. disease
    f. stomatitis
Futcher line
FVC
    forced vital capacity
    forced expiratory volume in 1
    second as percent of FVC
    ($FEV_{1\%VC}$)
    mean forced expiratory flow
    during the middle of FVC
    ($FEF_{25\text{-}75\%}$)
Fy antigen

NOTES

F

γ
γ globulin
γ hemolysis

G
G antigen
G unit of streptomycin
G5 massage and percussion machine
GABA
gamma-aminobutyric acid
Gabbromicina
GABHS
group A beta-hemolytic streptococcus
Gaboon ulcer
gadolinium
GAG
glycosaminoglycan
gag gene
gait analysis
GAL
gallus adeno-like
galactidrosis
gallinae
Dermanyssus g.
gallinarum
neurolymphomatosis g.
osteopetrosis g.
gallium-aluminum-arsenide 904-nm laser
gallus
g. adeno-like (GAL)
g. adeno-like virus
GALT
gut-associated lymphoid tissue
Galton
G. delta
G. system of classification of fingerprint
GAL virus
Gamasidae
gamasoidosis
Gamastan
Gambel
G. oak
G. oak tree
gambiae
Anopheles g.
gametophyte
Gamimune N

gamma
g. globulin
g. heavy-chain disease
interferon g. (IFN-γ)
gamma-aminobutyric acid (GABA)
gamma-1b
interferon g.
Gammagard S/D
gamma-glutamyltranspeptidase
Gammar
gammopathy
benign monoclonal g.
biclonal g.
monoclonal g.
polyclonal g.
ganciclovir
ganglion, pl. ganglia
sensory g.
gangrene
arteriosclerotic g.
bacterial synergistic g.
cold g.
cutaneous g.
decubital g.
diabetic g.
disseminated cutaneous g.
dry g.
embolic g.
Fournier g.
gas g.
hemorrhagic g.
hospital g.
hot g.
infected vascular g.
Meleney g.
moist g.
nosocomial g.
peripheral g.
Pott g.
presenile spontaneous g.
pressure g.
progressive bacterial synergistic g.
senile g.
static g.
symmetrical g.
synergistic g.
thrombotic g.
venous g.

G

gangrene *(continued)*
    wet g.
    white g.
gangrenescens
    granuloma g.
gangrenosa
    phagedena g.
    pyodermia g.
    vaccinia g.
    varicella g.
gangrenosum
    bullous hemorrhagic
      pyoderma g.
    ecthyma g.
    hemorrhagic pyoderma g.
    pyoderma g.
gangrenosus
    pemphigus g.
gangrenous
    g. stomatitis
Gantanol
Gantrisin Oral
Garamycin
    G. injection
    G. Ophthalmic
    G. topical
Gardner-Diamond
    G.-D. purpura
    G.-D. syndrome
Gardnerella vaginitis
Gardner syndrome
gargoylism
garinii
    Borrelia g.
garlic
garment nevus
garnet
    neodymium:yttrium-aluminum-g.
    (Nd:YAG)
GAS
    group A streptococcus
gas
    arterial blood g. (ABG)
    blood g.
    g. cautery
    g. chromatography
    g. gangrene
    g. gangrene antitoxin
gasping disease
Gasterophilus
Gastrocrom Oral
gastroenteritis
    acute infectious nonbacterial g.

    endemic nonbacterial
      infantile g.
    epidemic nonbacterial g.
    infantile g.
    porcine transmissible g.
    viral g.
    g. virus type A
    g. virus type B
gastroenteropathy
gastroesophageal (GE)
    g. reflux (GER)
gastrointestinal
    g. symptom
    g. ulceration
gastropathy
    NSAID g.
gastroschisis
gastrotoxin
Gaucher disease
gauze
    nonstick g.
GBS
    group B streptococcus
GC
    glucocorticoid
G-CSF
    granulocyte colony-stimulating
      factor
GE
    gastroesophageal
Ge antigen
gel
    adapalene g.
    Benzac AC G.
    Cann-Ease moisturizing
      nasal g.
    Dermaflex G.
    Differin g.
    g. diffusion
    g. diffusion precipitin test
    g. diffusion precipitin tests in
      one dimension
    g. diffusion reaction
    Estar G.
    H.P. Acthar G.
    Keralyt G.
    precipitate in g.
    PreSun lotion and g.
    Vergogel G.
gelatin
gelatinase
    72-kD g.
    92-kD g.

Gelfoam
Gell
 G. and Coombs classification
 G. and Coombs classification
  system
 G. and Coombs reaction
gelsolin
gemellus
 Paederus g.
geminata
 Solenopsis g.
Genac Tablet
Genahist Oral
Genamin Expectorant
Genapap
Genaspor
Genatap Elixir
gene
 env g.
 gag g.
 HLA-DR3 g.
 JH g.
 recombinase activating g.
 g. transcription
 transfer g.
 transforming g.
 V g.
 vanA g.
 vanH g.
 vanS g.
 V-D-J g.
 VH g.
general
 g. immunity
 g. transduction
generalis
 acne g.
generalisata
 alopecia g.
generalisatus
 herpes g.
 herpes zoster g.
generalized
 g. anaphylaxis
 g. desquamation
 g. elastolysis
 g. epidermolytic hyperkeratosis

 g. eruptive histiocytoma
 g. granuloma annulare
 g. hyperhidrosis
 g. lentiginosis
 g. maculopapular rash
 g. melanosis
 g. morphea
 g. morphea variant
 g. myxedema
 g. pustular psoriasis
 g. pustular psoriasis of von
  Zumbusch
 g. Shwartzman phenomenon
 g. vaccinia
 g. vitiligo
 g. weakness
 g. xanthelasma
genetic
 g. C2 deficiency
 g. depression of immune
  system
 g. determinant
 g. factor
 g. marker
 microbial g.'s
 g. recombination
Gengou phenomenon
genital
 g. aphthous ulcer
 g. atopic dermatitis
 g. erosive lichen planus
 g. hair
 g. herpes
 g. herpes simplex virus
 g. hidradenitis suppurativa
 g. lentigo
 g. lichen sclerosus
 g. lichen simplex chronicus
 g. neurodermatitis
 g. papulosquamous lesion
 g. plasma cell mucositis
 g. pruritus
 g. psoriasis
 g. Reiter syndrome
 g. squamous cell carcinoma
 g. tumor
 g. wart

G

NOTES

genitalis
    herpes g.
genitalium
    Mycoplasma g.
genitofemoral nerve entrapment
genitourinary lesion
genodermatology
genodermatosis
    neurologic g.
genome
    viral g.
genomic
Genoptic
    G. Ophthalmic
    G. S.O.P. Ophthalmic
genospecies
genote
    F g.
genotype
genotyping
Genpril
Gen-Probe rapid tuberculosis test
Gensan
Gentab-LA
Gentacidin Ophthalmic
Gentak Ophthalmic
gentamicin
    prednisolone and g.
    g. sulfate
gentian violet
genu valgum
Geocillin
geode
geographic
    g. difference
    g. pattern
    g. stippling of nail
    g. tongue
geographica
    lingua g.
    psoriasis g.
geometric
    g. mean concentration (GMC)
    g. mean titer (GMT)
geotrichosis
Geotrichum
GER
    gastroesophageal reflux
gerbil
Geref
Gerhardt disease
Gerhardt-Mitchell disease
geriatric

germ
    hair g.
    primary epithelial g.
    g. theory
German
    G. cockroach
    G. measles
    G. measles virus
germicidal
germicide
germinal
germinative
    g. cell
    g. time
germinativum
    stratum g.
Germiston virus
germline transcription
geroderma
gerontine
gerstaeckeri
    Triatoma g.
gestationis
    herpes g.
    hydroa g.
    impetigo g.
    prurigo g.
GF
    growth factor
GFR
    glomerular filtration rate
GG
    Slo-Phyllin G.
ggELISA
    glycoprotein-based enzyme-linked
    immunosorbent assay
Ghon complex
ghoul hand
Gianotti-Crosti
    G.-C. disease
    G.-C. syndrome
giant
    g. cell
    g. cell arteritis
    g. cell granuloma
    g. cell myositis
    g. cell tumor
    g. condyloma
    g. congenital nevus
    g. desert centipede
    g. desert centipede bite
    g. eccrine acrospiroma
    g. hive

g. lichenification
g. papillary conjunctivitis (GPC)
g. pigmented nevus
g. ragweed
g. urticaria
giantism
Giardia lamblia
Gibert disease
Giemsa stain
gift spot
Gila
G. monster
G. monster bite
Gilbert syndrome
Gillette Blue Blade
ginger
gingiva
gingival
g. fibromatosis
g. hyperplasia
g. lymphoma
gingivitis
acute necrotizing ulcerative g.
desquamative g.
ulcerative g.
gingivostomatitis
acute herpetic g.
herpetic g.
gio
cao g.
Girdlestone pseudarthrosis
Giroux-Barbeau syndrome
glabella
glabra
verruca g.
glabrata
Candida g.
Torulopsis g.
glabrate
glabrosa
tinea g.
glabrous
g. skin
gladiatorum
herpes g.

gland
apocrine g.
apocrine g.
apocrine sweat g.
axillary venom g.
ceruminous g.
cirrhotic lacrimal g.
coil g.
eccrine g.
eccrine sweat g.
ectopic sebaceous g.
holocrine g.
hyperplasia of sebaceous g.
Krause g.
lymph g.
meibomian g.
merocrine g.
Moll g.
oil g.
paired venom g.
parotid g.
salivary g.
sebaceous g.
stink g.
sweat g.
Zeis g.
glanders
glandular fever
glandularis
cheilitis g.
glans penis
glass
Wood g.
glebae
Acanthamoeba g.
glenoid labrum
Gliadin
Gliocladium fimbriatum
glioma
optic g.
gliomatous proliferation
global rating of pain
globi
globosum
Chaetomium g.
globulin
α_2 g.

NOTES

G

globulin *(continued)*
    alpha-2 g.
    antihuman g.
    antithymocyte g.
    β_{1F} g.
    β_{1C} g.
    β_{1E} g.
    γ g.
    gamma g.
    hepatitis B immune g. (H-
        BIG)
    human gamma g.
    immune serum g.
    intravenous immune g.
    intravenous immune serum g.
        (IVIG)
    pertussis immune g.
    placenta-eluted gamma g.
    respiratory syncytial virus IV
        immune g.
    RH$_o$(D) g.
    τ-g.
    tetanus immune g.
    vaccinia immune g.
    varicella-zoster immune g.
    zoster immune g.
α2-globulin
globus
glomangioma
glomangiomatosis
glomera (*pl. of* glomus)
glomerular
    g. eluate
    g. fibrosis
    g. filtration rate (GFR)
glomeruli
glomerulitis
glomerulonephritis
    acute hemorrhagic g.
    anti-basement membrane g.
    anti-basement membrane
        antibody-induced g.
    crescentic g.
    diffuse proliferative g.
    focal embolic g.
    immune complex g.
    lupus g.
    membranous g.
    poststreptococcal g.
    proliferative g.
glomus, pl. **glomera**
    g. body
    g. tumor

Glossina
    G. bite
glossitis, pl. **glossitides**
    g. areata exfoliativa
    atrophic g.
    benign migratory g.
    Candida g.
    median rhomboid g.
    migratory g.
    g. rhombica mediana
    rhomboid g.
glossodynia
    Candida g.
glossopyrosis
glossy
    g. skin
    g. tongue
glowing red lips
glucagon
    gut g.
glucagonoma syndrome
glucocorticoid (GC)
    intra-articular g.
    g. withdrawal syndrome
gluconate
    calcium g.
    chlorhexidine g.
glucoronidase
glucose
glucose-6-phosphatase deficiency
glucose-6-phosphate
    g.-p. dehydrogenase (G6PD)
glucuronate
    trimetrexate g.
glucuronic acid
glue
    bee g.
glutamate
    monosodium g.
α-glutathione S-transferase assay
gluten
    g. enteropathy
    g. intolerance
gluten-free diet
gluten-sensitive enteropathy
GLY
    glycerol
glycerin
glycerinated extract
glycerol (GLY)
    g. guaiacolate
Glycerol-T
glycine

glycine-rich
  g.-r. β-glycoprotein
  g.-r. β-glycoproteinase
glycocalyx
Glycofed
glycogen
  g. storage disease
glycogenolysis
glycol
  propylene g.
  salicylic acid and propylene g.
glycolysis
β-glycoprotein
  glycine-rich -g.
glycoprotein
  β₂-g. II
  pregnancy alpha-2 g. (PAG)
  pregnancy-associated g.
β-glycoproteinase
  glycine-rich -g.
glycoprotein-based enzyme-linked
  immunosorbent assay (ggELISA)
β₂-glycoprotein II
glycoproteinosis, pl. glycoproteinoses
glycopyrrolate
glycosaminoglycan (GAG)
  g. chain
glycoside
  cardiac g.
glycosphingolipidosis
glycyl-tRNA synthetase
Glycyphagus domesticus
Gm
  G. allotypes
  G. antigen
  factor G.
GMC
  geometric mean concentration
GM-CSF
  granulocyte-macrophage colony-
    stimulating factor
GMP
  guanosine monophosphate
GMT
  geometric mean titer
G-myticin topical
gnat bite

Gnathostoma
gnathostomiasis
GNB
  Gram-negative bacillus
gnotobiology
gnotobiota
gnotobiote
gnotobiotic
goat epithelium
goatpox
  g. virus
goat-serum-derived
goat's milk
goblet
  g. cell
  g. cell degranulation
  g. cell metaplasia
Goeckerman treatment
gold
  parenteral g.
  g. salts
  Selsun G.
  Selsun G. for Women
  g. sodium thioglucose
  g. sodium thiomalate
  g. therapy
goldenrod
gold-induced
  g.-i. aplasia
  g.-i. enterocolitis
golfer
  g. elbow
  g. skin
  g. skin
Golgi
  G. apparatus
  G. complex
Goltz-Gorlin syndrome
Goltz syndrome
gonadal dysgenesis
gonarthrosis
gondii
  Toxoplasma g.
gonococcal
  g. arthritis
  g. conjunctivitis

G

NOTES

gonococcal *(continued)*
  g. septicemia
  g. stomatitis
gono-opsonin
gonophage
gonorrhea
gonorrhoeae
  Neisseria g.
gonorrhoica
  macula g.
gonotoxemia
gonotoxin
Good antigen
Goodpasture syndrome
goose
  g. bump
  g. feather
  g. flesh, gooseflesh
gooseberry
gooseflesh *(var. of* goose flesh)
Gopalan syndrome
Gordofilm Liquid
gordonae
  Mycobacterium g.
Gordon phenomenon
Gorlin-Chaudhry-Moss syndrome
Gorlin-Goltz syndrome
Gorlin syndrome
Gorman syndrome
Gormel Creme
Göthlin test
Gottron
  G. papules
  G. sign
Gougerot
  pigmented purpuric lichenoid
    dermatitis of G.
Gougerot-Blum
  G.-B.-Blum disease
  G.-B. dermatosis
  G.-B. syndrome
Gougerot-Carteaud
  papillomatosis of G.-C.
  G.-C. syndrome
Gougerot-Sjögren disease
gout
  chronic tophaceous g.
  intercritical g.
  tophaceous g.
gouttes
  parapsoriasis en g.
Gower
  panatrophy of G.

gp110
  EBV glycoprotein g.
GPC
  giant papillary conjunctivitis
G6PD
  glucose-6-phosphate dehydrogenase
GP ib-IX complex
gradient
  alveolar-arterial oxygen g.
Gradle scissors
Graffi virus
graft
  AlloDerm universal dermal
    tissue g.
  allogeneic g.
  autogeneic g.
  autologous g.
  autoplastic g.
  heterologous g.
  heteroplastic g.
  heterospecific g.
  homologous g.
  homoplastic g.
  interspecific g.
  isogeneic g.
  isologous g.
  isoplastic g.
  Papineau g.
  syngeneic g.
  g. versus host (GVH)
  g. versus host disease
  g. versus host reaction
    (GVHR)
  white g.
  xenogeneic g.
grafting
  hair g.
Graham-Little-Piccardi-Lasseur
  syndrome
Graham Little syndrome
grain
  g. dust
  g. fever
  g. itch
Gram
  G. negative
  G. positive
  G. stain
grama grass
gramicidin
  neomycin, polymyxin b,
    and g.

Gram-negative
    G.-n. bacillus (GNB)
    G.-n. bacteremia
    G.-n. cocci
    G.-n. organism
    G.-n. rod
Gram-positive
    G.-p. bacillus
    G.-p. bacteremia
    G.-p. cocci
    G.-p. organism
    G.-p. rod
Gr antigen
granular
    g. cell
    g. cell layer
    g. cell myoblastoma
    g. cell tumor
    g. degeneration
    g. papulation
    g. vaginitis
granulation
    red g.
    g. tissue
granule
    azurophil g.
    Birbeck g.
    bismuth g.
    dextranomer g.
    Fordyce g.
    keratohyaline g.
    lamellar g.
    Langerhans cell g.
    membrane-coating g.
    Much g.
    Snaplets-FR G.
    sulfur g.
Granulex
granulocyte
    g. colony-stimulating factor (G-CSF)
    g. transfusion
granulocyte-macrophage colony-stimulating factor (GM-CSF)
granulocytic leukemia
granulocytopenia

granuloma
    actinic g.
    g. annulare
    beryllium g.
    bilharzial g.
    Candida g.
    caseating g.
    coccidioidal g.
    coli g.
    diaper g.
    elastolytic giant cell g.
    g. endemicum
    eosinophilic g.
    g. faciale
    fish tank g.
    g. fissuratum
    foreign body g.
    g. fungoides
    g. gangrenescens
    giant cell g.
    g. gluteale infantum
    infectious g.
    g. inguinale
    g. inguinale tropicum
    lethal midline g.
    lipoid g.
    lipophagic g.
    Majocchi g.
    metastatic g.
    midline lethal g.
    Miescher g.
    monilial g.
    g. multiforme
    necrotizing g.
    noncaseating g.
    oily g.
    palisading g.
    paracoccidioidal g.
    parasitic g.
    peripheral giant cell g.
    g. pudendi
    pyogenic g.
    g. pyogenicum
    reticulohistiocytic g.
    schistosome g.
    sea urchin g.
    silica g.

G

NOTES

granuloma *(continued)*
  swimming pool g.
  g. telangiectaticum
  trichophytic g.
  g. venereum
  zirconium g.
granulomatis
  Calymmatobacterium g.
  Donovania g.
granulomatosa
  cheilitis g.
  Miescher cheilitis g.
granulomatosis
  allergic g.
  Churg-Strauss g.
  g. disciformis et progressiva
  eosinophilic g.
  lethal midline g.
  limited Wegener g.
  lipid g.
  lymphomatoid g.
  midline g.
  g. rhinitis
  Wegener g.
granulomatous
  g. angiitis
  g. arteritis
  g. bacterial infection
  g. cheilitis
  g. cutaneous T-cell lymphoma
  g. dermal infiltrate
  g. disease
  g. foci
  g. hepatitis
  g. idiopathic arthritis
  g. inflammatory reaction
  g. pyoderma
  g. rosacea
  g. slack skin
  g. vasculitis
granulosis
  g. rubra nasi
granulosity
granulosum
  stratum g.
granulosus
  Echinococcus g.
granzymes
grapefruit
grasper
  nonsuction g.
grass
  alfalfa g.

Bahia g.
Bermuda g.
blue g.
brome g.
Canada blue g.
canary g.
common reed g.
crab g.
cultivated barley g.
cultivated corn g.
cultivated oat g.
cultivated rye g.
cultivated wheat g.
grama g.
Johnson g.
June g.
meadow fescue g.
meadow foxtail g.
orchard g.
perennial rye g.
g. pollen
g. pollen concentration
redtop g.
redtop A g.
salt g.
sorghum g.
sweet vernal g.
timothy g.
velvet g.
vernal g.
wild rye g.
Graves disease
gravidarum
  chloasma g.
  fibroma molle g.
  melasma g.
  striae g.
gravis
  icterus g.
  myasthenia g. (MG)
gravitational
  g. particle collection
  g. ulcer
gray patch tinea capitis
grease
  silicone g.
greasewood
Grecian Formula
green
  g. amaranth
  g. ash
  g. ash tree
  g. bean

g. coffee bean
malachite g.
g. monkey virus
g. pepper
Greenblatt
groove sign of G.
Greenhow disease
Greither syndrome
grenz
g. rays
g. ray therapy
Griesinger disease
Grifulvin V
grip, grippe
devil g.
Grisactin
G. Ultra
grisea
Madurella g.
griseofulvin
Grisolle sign
Gris-PEG
grocer's itch
groove
Harrison g.
nail g.
g. sign
g. sign of Greenblatt
transverse nasal g.
gross
g. lesion
G. leukemia virus
G. virus
Grossan nasal irrigator
ground
g. itch
g. substance
ground-glass
g.-g. appearance
g.-g. opacification
g.-g. pattern
groundsel tree
group
g. A beta-hemolytic
streptococcal infection
g. A beta-hemolytic
streptococcus (GABHS)

g. A carbohydrate antibody
g. agglutination
g. agglutinin
g. antigens
g. A streptococci
g. A streptococcus (GAS)
g. A streptococcus infection
blood g.
g. B streptococcus (GBS)
Contact Dermatitis Research G.
g. C rotavirus
cytophil g.
determinant g.
g. immunity
International Contact Dermatitis
Research G. (ICDRG)
Lewis Blood G.
Lutheran Blood G.
North American Contact
Dermatitis G. (NACDG)
g. reaction
retrovirus g.
support g.
g. 5 topical steroid
grouping
blood g.
chemical g.
Grover disease
growing season
growth
g. factor (GF)
g. hormone
g. phase
g. retardation
Gruber reaction
Gruber-Widal reaction
gryphosis
gryphotic
gryposis
g. unguium
GTP
guanosine triphosphate
guaiacolate
glycerol g.
Guaifed
G.-PD

G

NOTES

guaifenesin
  g. and phenylpropanolamine
  g., phenylpropanolamine, and
    phenylephrine
  g. and pseudoephedrine
  theophylline and g.
Guaifenex
  G.-DM
  G. LA
  G. PPA 75
  G. PSE
  G. PSE 120
  G. PSE 60
GuaiMAX-D
Guaipax
Guaitab
Guai-Vent/PSE
Guama virus
guanethidine
guanine
guanosine
  g. monophosphate (GMP)
  g. triphosphate (GTP)
guanylic acid
guar gum
Guarnieri bodies
Guaroa virus
Guiatex
Guiatuss PE
Guillain-Barré syndrome
guillermondii
  Candida g.
guinea
  g. corn yaws
  g. pig
  G. worm
  g. worm infection
Gulf War syndrome
gum
  guar g.
  karaya g.
  g. rash
  vegetable g.
gumma
  g. of tertiary syphilis
gummatous
  g. syphilid
  g. ulcer

gummosa
  scrofuloderma g.
gummy
Günther disease
gustatory
  g. hyperhidrosis
  g. rhinitis
gut-associated lymphoid tissue
  (GALT)
gut glucagon
guttata
  morphea g.
  parapsoriasis g.
  psoriasis g.
guttate
  g. hypomelanosis
  g. parapsoriasis
  g. psoriasis
guttering
  limbal g.
Guyon
  tunnel of G.
G/V
  penicilloyl G.
GVH
  graft versus host
  GVH disease
GVHR
  graft versus host reaction
G-well
  G.-w. Lotion
  G.-w. Shampoo
Gynecort
Gyne-Lotrimin
gypseum
  Microsporum g.
  Trichophyton g.
gypsy
  g. moth larva
  g. moth larva sting
gyrase
  DNA g.
gyrata
  cutis verticis g.
  psoriasis g.
gyrate
gyratum
  erythema g.

H
   H agglutinin
   H antigen
H-2
   H. antigen
   H. complex
H2
   H. blocker
   prostaglandin H. (PGH2)
HA
   hepatitis A
   hydroxyapatite
HA1 virus
HA2 virus
HAA
   hepatitis A antigen
   hepatitis-associated antigen
haarscheibe tumor
Haber syndrome
Haber-Weiss reaction
habit tic
habitus
   marfanoid h.
hackberry tree
HAE
   hereditary angioedema
haematobium
   Schistosoma h.
haemophilum
   Mycobacterium h.
Haemophilus
   H. ducreyi
   H. influenzae
   H. influenzae meningitis
   H. influenzae type b (HIB)
   H. parahaemolyticus
   H. parainfluenzae
   H. suis
Haffkine vaccine
Hafnia alvei
Hageman factor
Hailey-Hailey disease
Haines directory
hair
   animal h.
   axillary h.
   bamboo h.
   bayonet h.
   beaded h.
   bubble h.

   h. bulb
   burrowing h.
   h. cast
   club h.
   h. collar sign
   corkscrew h.
   cortex of h.
   cuticle of h.
   deer h.
   h. disk
   exclamation point h.
   h. fall
   h. follicle
   h. follicle mite
   h. follicle mite scabies
   h. follicle nevus
   Frey h.
   genital h.
   h. germ
   h. grafting
   horse h.
   ingrowing h.
   ingrown h.
   kinky h.
   knotted h.
   lanugo h.
   h. loss
   h. melanin
   moniliform h.
   nettling h.
   ringed h.
   Schridde cancer h.
   h. shaft
   stellate h.
   terminal h.
   h. transplant
   tuft of h.
   twisted h.
   vellus h.
   woolly h.
hairiness
   excessive h.
hair-like structure
hairy
   h. cell (HC)
   h. hamartoma
   h. leukoplakia
   h. mole
   h. nevus
Halberstaedter-Prowazek bodies

H

halcinonide
Halcion
Haldrone
Halfan
half-and-half
    h.-a.-h. fingernail
    h.-a.-h. nail
half-moon
    red h.-m.
Halfprin 81
Hallopeau
    acrodermatitis continua of H.
    H. disease
Hallopeau-Siemens epidermolysis
  bullosa
hallux
    h. valgus
    h. varus
halo
    anemic h.
    h. melanoma
    h. nevus
    purpuric h.
    red h.
halobetasol propionate
haloderma, halodermia
halodes
    Helminthosporium h.
halofantrine
    h. hydrochloride
Halog
    H. topical
halogen
    h. acne
halogenoderma
Halog-E topical
haloprogin
Halotex
    H. topical
Halotussin PE
Halprin 81
Halsted law
Haltran
hamartoma, pl. hamartomata
    Becker hairy h.
    hairy h.
Hamilton pseudophlegmon
Hamman-Rich syndrome
hammer toe, hammertoe
hamster
hand
    crab h.
    h. eczema

    edema of h.
    ghoul h.
    Marinesco succulent h.
    mechanic h.
    pulling boat h.
    trench h.
hand-and-foot syndrome
hand-foot-and-mouth
    h.-f.-a.-m. disease
    h.-f.-a.-m. disease virus
Handisol phototherapy device
Hand-Schüller-Christian disease
HANE
    hereditary angioneurotic edema
hanging skin
hang nail, hangnail
Hansen
    H. bacillus
    H. disease
Hantaan virus
Hantavirus
    H. infection
H_1 antihistamine
H_2 antihistamine
hapalonychia
haplotype
hapten
    conjugated h.
    h. inhibition of precipitation
haptene
Hapten-type reaction
haptoglobin
Harada syndrome
hard
    h. chancre
    h. corn
    h. keratin
    h. pad disease
    h. pad virus
    h. palate
    h. papilloma
    h. sore
    h. tick
    h. ulcer
hardening
harlequin
    h. fetus
    h. ichthyosis
Harrison groove
Harris pressure mat
Harter syndrome
Hartnup disease

harvest
    h. mite
    h. mite bite
Hashimoto
    H. disease
    H. thyroiditis
Hashimoto-Pritzker disease
hatchetti
    Acanthamoeba h.
Hauch
    ohne H.
HAV
    hepatitis A virus
    HAV RNA
Haverhill fever
Haversian system
Havrix
HAVRIX vaccine
hay
    h. asthma
    h. fever
Hayek oscillator
Hayfebrol Liquid
hazel
    witch h.
hazelnut tree
HB
    hepatitis B
    Recombivax H.
    Tagamet H.
HB$_e$, HBe
    hepatitis B$_e$
HB$_c$Ab, HBcAb
    antibody to hepatitis B core antigen
HB$_e$Ab, HBeAb
    antibody to hepatitis B e antigen
HB$_s$Ab, HBsAb
    antibody to hepatitis B surface
        antigen
HB$_c$Ag, HBcAg
    hepatitis B core antigen
HB$_s$Ag, HBsAg
    hepatitis B surface antigen
HBcAb (*var. of* HB$_c$Ab)
    antibody to hepatitis B core antigen
HbCO
    carboxyhemoglobin

HBe (*var. of* HB$_e$)
HBeAb (*var. of* HB$_e$Ab)
    antibody to hepatitis B e antigen
HBGF
    heparin binding growth factor
HBGF-1
    heparin binding growth factor-1
H-BIG
    hepatitis B immune globulin
    hepatitis B immunoglobulin
HBO
    hyperbaric oxygen
HbO$_2$
    oxyhemoglobin
HbOc/DTP vaccine
HbOC vaccine
HBsAb (*var. of* HB$_s$Ab)
    antibody to hepatitis B surface
        antigen
HBsAg (*var. of* HB$_s$Ag)
HBT Sleuth
HBV
    hepatitis B virus
    HBV bDNA signal
        amplification
    HBV DNA
    HBV DNA probe test
HC
    hairy cell
    hepatitis C
HC-1
    Anusol H.
HC-2.5%
    Anusol H.
HCA
    Orabase H.
HCl
    hydrochloride
    Cleocin H.
    doxepin H.
    fluoxetine H.
    hydroxyzine H.
    paroxetine H.
    pramoxine H.
    promethazine H.
    pseudoephedrine H.

NOTES

H

HCl *(continued)*
    sertraline H.
    valacyclovir H.
HCO₃
    bicarbonate
HCP
    hereditary coproporphyria
HCQ
    hydroxychloroquine
HCV
    hepatitis C virus
        RIBA HCV
        HCV by RIBA
        HCV RNA
HD
    hemodialysis
    hepatitis D
HDCV
    human diploid cell rabies vaccine
HDI
    isocyanate H.
HDV
    hepatitis D virus
HE
    hepatitis E
H&E
    hematoxylin and eosin
Head
    H. & Shoulders
    H. and Shoulders shampoo
head
    h. compression test
    h. distraction test
    h. lice
    h. louse
healed ulcer
healing
    fish-mouth h.
    wound h.
Health
    National Institute of H. (NIH)
health maintenance organization
  (HMO)
He antigen
hearing loss
heart
    h. antigen
    h. rate reserve (HRR)
heart-lung circuit
heartworm
heat
    h. exposure

    h. lamp
    prickly h.
    h. rash
    h. shock protein (HSP)
    h. urticaria
heat/moisture exchanger (HME)
heat-phenol inactivated vaccine
heavy chain
heavy-chain disease
Heberden node
Hebra
    H. disease
    H. prurigo
hebraeum
    Amblyomma h.
Heck syndrome
heel
    black h.
    cracked h.
Heelbo decubitus protector
Heerfordt syndrome
Heiner syndrome
HeLa cells
Helanthus
helicis
    chondrodermatitis nodularis
    chronica h.
Helicobacter
    ImmunoCard used for
    diagnosis of *H. pylori*
    H. mustelae
    H. pylori
heliopathy
heliotrope
    h. rash
Helisal rapid blood test
helix
    triple h.
HELLP
    hemolysis, elevated liver enzymes,
    low platelet
HELLP syndrome
helminth
helminthiasis
helminthic
    h. parasitic disease
Helminthosporium
    H. halodes
    H. savitum
Heloderma
    H. suspectum
    H. suspectum bite

heloma
    h. durum
    h. molle
helosis
helotomy
helper
    h. cell
    h. virus
helplessness
    learned h.
Helweg-Larssen syndrome
hemadsorption
    h. virus test
    h. virus type 1
    h. virus type 2
hemagglutinating
    h. antibody
    h. cold autoantibody
hemagglutination
    h. inhibition
    passive h. (PHA)
    reverse passive h.
    h. test
    viral h.
hemagglutinin
    influenza virus h.
hemangioendothelioma
    malignant h.
    spindle cell h.
hemangioma, pl. **hemangiomata**
    h. birthmark
    capillary h.
    cavernous h.
    deep h.
    involuting flat h.
    mixed h.
    h. planum extensum
    sclerosing h.
    senile h.
    spider h.
    strawberry h.
    superficial h.
    synovial h.
    verrucous h.
hemangioma-thrombocytopenia
    syndrome

hemangiomatosis
    Osler h.
    Parkes-Weber h.
    thrombocytopenic h.
    unilateral h.
hemangiomatous tissue
hemangiopericytoma
    benign h.
    borderline malignant h.
    malignant h.
hemarthrosis
hemathidrosis, hematidrosis
hematid
hematidrosis
hematogenous
    h. metastasis
hematologic
    h. disorder
    h. reaction
hematolysis
hematoma
    subungual h.
hematopoiesis
hematopoietic
    h. stem cell transplant
    h. system
hematotoxin
hematotropic
hematoxin
hematoxylin
    h. and eosin (H&E)
hematoxylin-eosin
hematoxyphilic inclusion
hematuria
hemiarthroplasty
    McKeever and MacIntosh h.
hemiatrophy
    progressive facial h.
    Romberg h.
hemidesmosome
hemidiaphoresis
hemidiaphragm
hemidrosis
hemidysplasia
    congenital h.
    unilateral h.
hemihidrosis

NOTES

H

hemihyperhidrosis
Hemiptera
hemithorax
hemoagglutination
hemoagglutinin
hemoantitoxin
hemochromatosis
hemocyanin
   keyhole limpet h.
hemocytometer
hemodialysis (HD)
hemodialysis-associated amyloidosis
hemoglobin
   h. C disease
   h. S disease
hemoglobinopathy
hemoglobinophilic
hemoglobinuria
   nocturnal h.
   paroxysmal cold h.
   paroxysmal nocturnal h. (PNH)
hemoglobinuric
   h. fever
   h. nephrosis
hemolysate
hemolysin
   α h.
   β h.
   bacterial h.
   cold h.
   heterophil h.
   immune h.
   natural h.
   specific h.
   h. unit
   warm-cold h.
hemolysinogen
hemolysis
   acute intravascular h.
   autoimmune h.
   β h.
   biologic h.
   conditioned h.
   h., elevated liver enzymes, low
     platelet (HELLP)
   h., elevated liver enzymes, low
     platelet count
   γ h.
   immune h.
   venom h.
   viridans h.
hemolytic
   h. anemia of newborn

   h. assay
   h. chain
   h. disease of newborn
   h. sickle cell disease
   h. streptococci
   h. uremic syndrome (HUS)
β-hemolytic streptococci
hemolyzation
hemolyze
hemopexin
hemophagocytic syndrome
hemophagocytosis
hemophil
hemophilia
   acquired h.
hemophiliac patient
hemophilic arthropathy
hemopoietic factor
hemoprecipitin
hemoptysis
hemorrhage
   intra-alveolar h.
   intraventricular h.
   petechial h.
   pulmonary h.
   punctate h.
   retinal h.
   splinter h.
hemorrhagic
   h. bulla
   h. cystitis
   h. dengue
   h. diathesis
   h. edema
   h. exudative erythema
   h. fever
   h. fever with renal syndrome
   h. gangrene
   h. lesion
   h. pian
   h. pyoderma gangrenosum
   h. rash
   h. smallpox
   h. telangiectasia
hemorrhagica
   purpura h.
   scarlatina h.
   urticaria h.
   variola h.
hemorrhagicus
   lichen h.
hemorrhagins

hemosiderin
  h. deposition
hemosiderin-laden macrophage
hemosiderosis
  idiopathic pulmonary h.
  pulmonary h.
  synovial h.
hemostasis
  chemical h.
hemostatic
  h. agent
  h. collodion
  h. disorder
hemothorax, pl. hemothoraces
  catamenial h.
hemotoxic
hemotoxin
  cobra h.
hemotropic
hemp
  western water h.
Hemril-HC Uniserts
Hendersonula
  H. toruloidea
Henle-Koch pustulate
Henle layer
henna
  extract of h.
Henoch purpura
Henoch-Schönlein
  H.-S. purpura (HSP)
  H.-S. syndrome (HSS)
  H.-S. vasculitis
henselae
  Bartonella h.
  Rochalimaea h.
HEPA
  high-efficiency particulate air
  high efficiency particulate arresting
  HEPA filter
Hepadnaviridae
Hepandrin
heparin
  h. binding growth factor
  (HBGF)

  h. binding growth factor-1
  (HBGF-1)
  h. sulfate
heparinization
hepatic porphyria
hepatitic
hepatitis
  h. A (HA)
  h. A antigen (HAA)
  h. A arthritis
  anicteric virus h.
  h.-associated antigen (HAA)
  autoimmune chronic h.
  h. A vaccine
  h. A virus (HAV)
  h. B (HB)
  h. B$_e$ (HB$_e$, HBe)
  h. B arthritis
  h. B core antigen (HB$_c$Ag, HBcAg)
  h. B DNA detection
  h. Be antigen
  h. B immune globulin (H-BIG)
  h. B immunoglobulin (H-BIG)
  h. B surface antigen (HB$_s$Ag, HBsAg)
  h. B vaccine
  h. B viral DNA assay
  h. B virus (HBV)
  h. C (HC)
  cholangiolitic h.
  cholestatic h.
  chronic active h. (CAH)
  h. contagiosa canis
  h. C RNA detection
  h. C virus (HCV)
  h. C virus antibody detection
  h. D (HD)
  delta antigen h.
  h. D virus (HDV)
  h. E (HE)
  epidemic h.
  equine serum h.
  h. E virus (HEV)
  granulomatous h.
  h. G virus (HGV)

NOTES

H

181

hepatitis *(continued)*
    infectious h. (IH)
    infectious canine h.
    long incubation h.
    lupoid h.
    mouse h.
    murine h.
    NANB h.
    non-A non-B h.
    serum h. (SH)
    short incubation h.
    transfusion h.
    viral h.
    h. virus
    virus A h.
hepatits B e
hepatobiliary disease
hepatoerythropoietic porphyria
hepatolenticular degeneration
hepatolysin
hepatomegaly
hepatosplenic tuberculosis
hepatosplenomegaly
hepatotoxic
hepatotoxicity
hepatotoxin
hepatoxicity
Hep-B-Gammagee
Heptavax immunization
herald patch
herd
    h. immunity
hereditaria
    alopecia h.
hereditarium
    erythema palmare h.
hereditary
    h. angioedema (HAE)
    h. angioneurotic edema
    (HANE)
    h. arthro-ophthalmopathy
    h. cardiopathic amyloidosis
    h. coproporphyria (HCP)
    h. hemorrhagic telangiectasia
    h. hemorrhagic telangiectasis
    h. multiple trichoepithelioma
    h. sensory radicular neuropathy
    h. spherocytosis
    h. vascular disorder
    h. vibratory angioedema
heredopathia atactica
polyneuritiformis

heres
    Scolopendra h.
heritable
    h. connective tissue disease
    h. disorder
Herlitz
    H. epidermolysis bullosa
    H. syndrome
Hermal
Hermansky-Pudlak
    H.-P. syndrome
    H.-P. syndrome type IV
    H.-P. syndrome type VI
hernia
    diaphragmatic h.
herniated presacral fat pad
herpangina
    h. pharyngitis
herpes
    h. B encephalomyelitis
    h. catarrhalis
    h. circinatus bullosus
    h. cornea
    h. desquamans
    h. digitalis
    h. facialis
    h. febrilis
    h. generalisatus
    genital h.
    h. genitalis
    h. gestationis
    h. gladiatorum
    h. iris
    h. labialis
    neonatal h.
    h. progenitalis
    h. simplex
    h. simplex conjunctivitis
    h. simplex encephalitis
    h. simplex infection
    h. simplex recurrens
    h. simplex virus (HSV)
    h. simplex virus arthritis
    h. simplex virus type II
    traumatic h.
    h. virus
    h. whitlow
    h. zoster (HZ)
    h. zoster generalisatus
    h. zoster infection
    h. zoster ophthalmicus
    h. zoster oticus

h. zoster varicellosus
h. zoster virus
herpes simplex virus type I
Herpesviridae
herpesvirus
   canine h.
   caprine h.
   h. hominis
   human h. 1–7 (HHV)
   suid h.
   h. type 1
herpetic
   h. angina
   h. fever
   h. gingivostomatitis
   h. infection
   h. keratitis
   h. keratoconjunctivitis
   h. meningoencephalitis
   h. paronychia
   h. ulcer
   h. whitlow
   zoster sine h.
herpeticum
   eczema h.
herpetiform
   h. aphtha
herpetiforme
   hydroa h.
herpetiformis
   dermatitis h. (DH)
   epidermolysis bullosa
    simplex h.
   impetigo h.
   morphea h.
herpetoid
Herpetoviridae
Herpetovirus
herpetovirus
   canine h.
   caprine h.
Herplex Ophthalmic
herringbone pattern
Hertoghe sign
Herxheimer reaction
Hess test

heteroagglutinin
heteroantibody
heteroantiserum
heterochromia
heterocyclic antidepressant
heterocytotropic
   h. antibody
heterodermic
heterogenetic
   h. antibody
   h. antigen
heterogenic, heterogeneic
   h. antigen
   h. enterobacterial antigen
heterogenote
heterogenous vaccine
heterograft
heterokeratoplasty
heterologous
   h. antiserum
   h. desensitization
   h. graft
   h. protein
   h. serotype
heterology
heterolysin
heterolysis
heterolytic
hetero-osteoplasty
heteropathy
heterophil, heterophile
   h. antibody
   h. antigen
   h. hemolysin
heteroplasia
   osseous h.
heteroplastic
   h. graft
heteroplastid
heteroplasty
heterospecific
   h. graft
heterotransplantation
heterotrichosis
heterovaccine therapy
heterozygous

NOTES

H

HEV
  hepatitis E virus
  high endothelial venules
HEVI
  hibernal epidemic viral infection
hexacetonide
  triamcinolone h.
hexachlorophene
Hexadnovirus
Hexadrol
  Decadron and H.
  H. Phosphate
hexahydrate
  aluminum chloride h.
hexamer
hexamethylmelamine
hexon
  h. antigen
Hfr, HFR
  high frequency of recombination
  Hfr strain
HGH
  human growth hormone
HGPRT
  hypoxanthine-guanine
  phosphoribosyltransferase
  HGPRT deficiency
HGV
  hepatitis G virus
HH6
HHV
  human herpesvirus 1–7
HIB
  Haemophilus influenzae type b
**hibernal epidemic viral infection
  (HEVI)**
hibernoma
Hibiclens topical
Hibistat topical
HibTITER
Hib-TT vaccine
HI-CAL VM bar
hiccup, hiccough
hickory
  shagbark h.
  h. tree
Hi-Cor
  H.-C.-1.0
  H.-C.-2.5
hidden nail skin
hidebound disease
hidradenitis
  h. axillaris of Verneuil

  eccrine h.
  neutrophilic eccrine h.
  h. suppurativa
hidradenoma
  clear cell h.
  cystic h.
  nodular h.
  papillary h.
  h. papilliferum
  poroid h.
  solid h.
hidroa
hidroacanthoma simplex
hidrocystoma
  eccrine h.
hidromeiosis
hidropoiesis
hidropoietic
hidrorrhea
hidrosadenitis
hidroschesis
hidrosis
hidrotic
  h. ectodermal dysplasia
hiemalis
  acrodermatitis h.
  dermatitis h.
  erythrokeratolysis h.
  prurigo h.
  pruritus h.
high
  h. dose tolerance
  h. efficiency particulate
    arresting (HEPA)
  h. endothelial venule cell
  h. endothelial venules (HEV)
  h. frequency oscillation
  H. Frequency Oscillatory
    ventilator
  h. frequency positive pressure
    ventilation
  h. frequency of recombination
    (Hfr, HFR)
  h. frequency transduction
  h. liquid content
  h. lung volume
high-arched palate
**high-efficiency particulate air
  (HEPA)**
high-egg-passage vaccine
high-frequency jet ventilation
**high-grade small noncleaved cell
  malignant lymphoma**

high-resolution computed tomography (HRCT)
hilar
  h. adenopathy
  h. lymphadenopathy
hindfoot
  h. splint
Hinton test
hip
  h. deflexion
  snapping h.
Hippocratic
  H. countenance
  H. face
  H. facies
  H. finger
  H. look
  H. nail
  H. visage
Hippocratica
  facies H.
hirci
  barbula h.
Hirschowitz syndrome
Hirst spore trap
hirsute
hirsuties
hirsutism
  Apert h.
  constitutional h.
  idiopathic h.
hirtellous
hirudiniasis
Hismanal
HISS
  human immune status survey
Histaject injection
Histalet
  H. Forte Tablet
  H. Syrup
Histalet X
histaminase
histamine
  h. flush
  h. liberator

  h. phosphate
  h. shock
histamine-releasing factor (HRF)
Histatrol
Hista-Vadrin Tablet
histidinemia
histidyl-tRNA synthetase
histiocyte
  alveolar infiltration by h.
  interstitial infiltration by h.
  palisading h.
histiocytic
  h. cytophagic panniculitis
  h. lymphoma
  h. response
histiocytoma
  fibrous h.
  generalized eruptive h.
  malignant fibrous h.
histiocytosis
  acute disseminated h.
  atypical h.
  benign cephalic h.
  cephalic h.
  chronic h.
  focal h.
  indeterminate cell h.
  juvenile xanthogranuloma h.
  Langerhans cell h.
  malignant h.
  multifocal h.
  nodular non-X h.
  regressing atypical h.
  sinus h.
  skin-limited h.
  h. X
  h. Y
histochemical
histocompatibility
  h. antigen
  h. antigen class I
  major h.
  h. testing
histoid leprosy
histoincompatibility

NOTES

H

histologic
  h. change
  h. lesion
histological
histology
  joint h.
histolytica
  Ameba h.
  Entamoeba h.
histone
histone-DNA antibody
Histoplasma
  H. capsulatum
  H. duboisii
histoplasmin
histoplasmin-latex test
histoplasmosis
  African h.
  cutaneous h.
history
  relevant sting h.
histotope
histotoxic
HIV
  human immunodeficiency virus
  HIV DNA amplification assay
  HIV DNA PCR test
  HIV encephalopathy
  HIV neutralizing antibodies
  HIV protease inhibitor
HIV-1
  human immunodeficiency virus-1
HIV-2
  human immunodeficiency virus-2
Hivagen antibody test
HIV-associated
hive
  giant h.
Hivid
HIVIG
HLA
  human leukocyte antigen
  human lymphocyte antigen
  HLA allele
  HLA class 1 associated
    disease
  HLA complex
  HLA Cw6
  HLA intercellular interaction
  HLA typing
HLA-129
HLA-A
HLA-A11

HL-A antigens
HLA-B
HLA-B8
HLA-B13
HLA-B17
HLA-B27
HLA-C
HLA class 1
HLA-DP
HLA-DQ
HLA-DR
HLA-DR3
  H.-D. gene
HLA-DR4
HLA-DRB and -DRQ DNA typing
HLA-DRw4
HLA-DRw52
HLA-E
HLA-F
HLA-G
HM-175
HME
  heat/moisture exchanger
  Tracheolife HME
HMG-CoA
  3-hydroxy-3-methylglutaryl
    coenzyme A
  HMG-CoA reductase inhibitor
HMO
  health maintenance organization
HMS
  hypothetical mean strain
  HMS Liquifilm Ophthalmic
Ho antigen
hobnail tongue
Hodgkin
  H. disease
  H. lymphoma
hog
  h. cholera
  h. cholera vaccine
  h. cholera virus
Hollister medial adhesive bandage
Hollister-Stier Laboratory
holocrine gland
holothurin
homatropine hydrobromide
home cleaning product
homeopathy
homeoplasia
homeoplastic
homeotherapy
homing receptor

hominis
Actinobacillus h.
Actinomyces h.
Dermatobia h.
herpesvirus h.
Mycoplasma h.
Pentatrichomonas h.
poliovirus h.
Sarcoptes h.
homme rouge
homocystinuria
homocytotropic
h. antibody
h. reaction
homogeneous
homogenous
homograft
h. reaction
homoioplasia
homolog
homologous
h. antigen
h. antiserum
h. desensitization
h. graft
h. serotype
h. serum jaundice
homology
h. of chain
DNA h.
h. of strand
homolysin
homolysis
homophil
homoplastic graft
homotransplantation
homozygous
honeycomb
h. ringworm
h. tetter
Hong Kong
H. K. foot
H. K. influenza
H. K. toe
hoof-and-mouth disease
hookworm
cat h.

Hoover sign
Hopf
acrokeratosis verruciformis of H.
hops
hordeolum
Horder spot
horizontal
h. growth phase
h. section
h. transmission
Hormodendron, Hormodendrum
H. compactum
H. pedrosoi
hormonal changes
hormone
adrenocorticotropic h. (ACTH)
corticotropin-releasing h. (CRH)
growth h.
human growth h. (HGH)
immunoreactive h.
melanocyte-stimulating h. (MSH)
α-melanocyte-stimulating h. (α-MSH)
β-melanocyte-stimulating h.
β-melanocytic-stimulating h.
polypeptide h.
thymic h.
horn
cicatricial h.
cutaneous h.
nail h.
sebaceous h.
warty h.
hornbeam
Horner syndrome
hornet
h. sting
white-faced h.
yellow h.
hornification
horny
h. cell layer
h. layer
h. spine
horripilation

NOTES

H

187

horror autotoxicus
horse
   h. hair
   h. serum
horsefly, horse fly
   h. bite
horsepox
   h. virus
horses
   infectious arteritis virus of h.
hortae
   Piedraia h.
hospital
   h. fever
   h. gangrene
hospital-acquired infection
host
   accidental h.
   amplifier h.
   dead-end h.
   h. defects
   graft versus h. (GVH)
   humoral h.
   h. immunity
   immunocompromised h.
   reservoir h.
   h. response
host-generated neutrophils
  recruitment
host-immune process
hot
   h. comb alopecia
   h. gangrene
Hotchkiss-McManus technique
hotfoot
hound-dog facies
hourglass
house
   h. dust
   h. dust mite
   h. dust mite F
   h. dust mite P
   h. fly
housefly
housemaid knee
Houssay animal
Howell-Evans syndrome
HP
   hypersensitivity pneumonitis
H.P. Acthar Gel
HPV
   human papillomavirus
   human parvovirus

HRCT
   high-resolution computed
   tomography
   HRCT scan
HRF
   histamine-releasing factor
   HRF deficiency
HRR
   heart rate reserve
HS
   hyperplastic synovium
HSP
   heat shock protein
   Henoch-Schönlein purpura
   hypersensitivity pneumonitis panel
   mycobacteria HSP
HSS
   Henoch-Schönlein syndrome
HSV
   herpes simplex virus
   Mollaret HSV
H-tetanase
HTLV
   human T-cell leukemia/lymphoma
   virus
   human T-cell leukemia virus
   human T-cell lymphotrophic virus
HTLV-I
   human T-cell lymphotrophic virus
   type I
HTLV-II
   human T-cell lymphotrophic virus
   type II
HTLV-III
   human T-cell lymphotrophic virus
   type III
Hu antigen
huff cough
human
   h. anti-CMV antibody
   CD4, immunoglobulin G,
   recombinant h.
   chickenpox immune globulin
   (h.)
   h. cloned DNA
   cytomegalovirus immune
   globulin intravenous, h.
   h. diploid cell rabies vaccine
   (HDCV)
   h. embryonic lung fibroblast
   h. gamma globulin
   h. growth hormone (HGH)
   h. herpesvirus 1–7 (HHV)

h. immune status survey
(HISS)
h. immunodeficiency virus
(HIV)
h. immunodeficiency virus-1
(HIV-1)
h. immunodeficiency virus-2
(HIV-2)
h. immunodeficiency virus
antigen testing
h. immunodeficiency virus
DNA amplification
h. leukemia-associated antigens
h. leukocyte antigen (HLA)
h. lymphocyte antigen (HLA)
measles immune globulin (h.)
h. measles immune serum
h. monocyte chemoattractant
protein-1
h. normal immunoglobulin
h. orf virus
h. papillomavirus (HPV)
h. papillomavirus infection
h. parvovirus (HPV)
h. parvovirus B19
h. pertussis immune serum
poliomyelitis immune globulin
(h.)
h. α1-proteinase inhibitor
rabies immune globulin, h.
rabies immune globulin (h.)
h. RD
h. recombinant
deoxyribonuclease
h. scarlet fever immune serum
h. serum
specific immune globulin (h.)
h. T-cell leukemia/lymphoma
virus (HTLV)
h. T-cell leukemia virus
(HTLV)
h. T-cell lymphotrophic virus
(HTLV)
h. T-cell lymphotrophic virus
type I (HTLV-I)
h. T-cell lymphotrophic virus
type II (HTLV-II)

h. T-cell lymphotrophic virus
type III (HTLV-III)
tetanus immune globulin, h.
humanus
Pediculus h.
Humatin
Humatrope
humectant
Humibid
H.-LA
humidified oxygen
humidifier
h. fever
h. lung
humidity
humid tetter
humoral
h. defects
h. host
h. immunity
h. immunity status panel
hump
buffalo h.
dowager h.
Hunter
H. mucopolysaccharidosis
H. syndrome
hunterian chancre
hunting
h. phenomenon
h. reaction
Hunt syndrome
Huriez syndrome
Hurler
H. disease
H. syndrome
Hurler-Scheie
H.-S. mucopolysaccharidosis
H.-S. syndrome
HUS
hemolytic uremic syndrome
Hutchinson
freckle of H.
melanotic freckle of H.
H. sign
H. summer prurigo
H. teeth

NOTES

H

Hutchinson-Gilford
  H.-G. progeria
  H.-G. syndrome
Huxley layer
hyaline
  h. articular cartilage
  h. basement membrane
  h. degeneration
hyalinosis
  h. cutis et mucosa
  systemic h.
hyalinum
  Scytalidium h.
Hyalomma variegatum
hyaluronan
hyaluronate
hyaluronic acid
hybrid
  SV40-adenovirus h.
hybridization
  DNA h.
  in situ h.
  h. test
hybridoma
Hycodan
Hycomine
Hycort
Hycotuss
hydantoin anticonvulsant
hydantoin/EDTA
hydatid rash
Hyde disease
Hydeltrasol injection
Hydeltra-TBA injection
hydradenitis
hydradenoma
hydralazine
  h. syndrome
Hydramyn Syrup
hydrarthrosis
  intermittent h.
hydrate
hydration
  adequate h.
  vigorous h.
Hydrea
Hydrisinol
hydroa
  h. estivale
  h. febrile
  h. gestationis
  h. herpetiforme
  h. puerorum

  h. vacciniforme
  h. vesiculosum
hydrobromide
  homatropine h.
hydrocephalus
hydrochloric acid
hydrochloride (HCl)
  amantadine h.
  amitriptyline h.
  bacampicillin h.
  benzphetamine h.
  bupivacaine h.
  chloroguanide h.
  chloroprocaine h.
  chlorpromazine h.
  chlortetracyline h.
  ciprofloxacin h.
  clonidine h.
  cyclizine h.
  cyproheptadine h.
  cytarabine h.
  daunorubicin h.
  demeclocycline h.
  diphenhydramine h.
  diphenidol h.
  eflornithine h.
  ethambutol h.
  ethylnorepinephrine h.
  etidocaine h.
  fluoxetine h.
  halofantrine h.
  hydroxyzine h.
  isoxsuprine h.
  levocabastine h.
  lidocaine h.
  lomefloxacin h.
  mechlorethamine h.
  meclizine h.
  mefloquine h.
  mepivacaine h.
  minocycline h.
  Mustargen H.
  naftifine h.
  naloxone h.
  oxymetazoline h.
  oxytetracycline h.
  paroxetine h.
  phenoxybenzamine h.
  phenylephrine h.
  phenylpropanolamine h.
  pramoxine h.
  prazosin h.
  procaine h.

promethazine h.
propranolol h.
ranitidine h.
rimantadine h.
sertraline h.
spectinomycin h.
terbinafine h.
tetracaine h.
tetrahydrozoline h.
vancomycin h.
hydrochlorothiazide (HCTZ)
hydrocodone bitartrate
hydrocolloid dressing
Hydrocort
hydrocortisone
  h. acetate
  acetic acid, propanediol
    diacetate, and h.
  bacitracin, neomycin, polymyxin
    b, and h.
  benzoyl peroxide and h.
  h. butyrate
  chloramphenicol, polymyxin b,
    and h.
  clioquinol and h.
  colistin, neomycin, and h.
  iodoquinol and h.
  lidocaine and h.
  neomycin, polymyxin b,
    and h.
  oxytetracycline and h.
  polymyxin b and h.
  urea and h.
Hydrocortone
  H. Acetate
  H. Phosphate
hydrocystoma
hydrofluoroalkane-134a
  Proventil HFA
    (hydrofluoroalkane-134a)
hydrogel dressing
hydroid
  feather h.
hydrolysis of surfactant
hydrolyze
hydroperoxyeicosatetraenoic acid
Hydrophen

Hydrophiinae
hydrophila
  Aeromonas h.
hydrophilic polymer dressing
hydrophobia
hydrophobic
hydropic change in pneumocyte
hydroquinone
HydroSKIN
Hydro-Tex
hydroxide
  dysprosium ferric h.
  lactic acid with ammonium h.
  potassium h. (KOH)
5-hydroxyindoleacetic acid
α-hydroxy acid
hydroxyapatite (HA)
  h. chondrocalcinosis
  h. crystal deposition
hydroxychloroquine (HCQ)
  h. sulfate
  h. therapy
hydroxyeicosatetraenoic acid
hydroxyl
16-hydroxylated metabolite
hydroxylation
hydroxylysine
  h. content of collagen
3-hydroxy-3-methylglutaryl coenzyme
  A (HMG-CoA)
hydroxyprogesterone caproate
hydroxyproline
hydroxypropyl cellulose
hydroxyurea
hydroxyzine
  h. HCl
  h. hydrochloride
  theophylline, ephedrine, and h.
    (TEH)
hyfrecator
  Birtcher h.
Hy-Gestrone injection
hygiene
  bronchial h.
hygroma
  cystic h.
hygroscopicity

NOTES

H

Hylutin injection
Hymenoptera
   H. sting
   H. venom
   H. venom anaphylaxis
Hymenopterous vespid
hyomagnesemia
Hy-Pam
hyper
   h. IgE syndrome
   h. IgM syndrome
Hyperab
hyperabduction
hyperacanthosis
hyperacute rejection
hyperbaric
   h. oxygen (HBO)
   h. oxygen therapy
hyperbilirubinemia
hypercalcemia
   familial hypocalciuric h.
hypercalciuria
hypercapnia
   permissive h.
hypercarbia
hypercholesteremic xanthoma
hypercoagulable state
hypercortisolism
hypereosinophilia
hypereosinophilic syndrome
hyperephidrosis
hyperergia
hyperergic
   h. encephalitis
hyperesthesia
hypergammaglobulinemia
   h. of Waldenström
hypergammaglobulinemic purpura
hypergia
hypergic
hyperglobulinemia
hyperglobulinemic purpura
hypergranulosis
HyperHep
hyperhidrosis
   generalized h.
   gustatory h.
   h. oleosa
   primary h.
hyperhydration
hypericin
hyperidrosis

hyperimmune
   h. bovine colostrum IgC concentrate
   h. gamma globulin preparation
   h. serum
   h. state
hyperimmunization
hyperimmunoglobulinemia
   h. D syndrome
   h. E syndrome
hyperinfection
hyperinflation
hyperirritability
hyperirritable skin
hyperkalemia
hyperkeratinization
hyperkeratomycosis
hyperkeratosis, pl. hyperkeratoses
   h. congenita
   h. eccentrica
   epidermolytic h.
   h. figurata centrifuga atrophica
   focal acral h.
   h. follicularis et parafollicularis
   h. follicularis et parafollicularis in cutem penetrans
   generalized epidermolytic h.
   h. lenticularis perstans
   subungual h.
   h. subungualis
hyperkeratotic epidermis
hyperlinear palm
hyperlipemic xanthoma
hyperlipidemia
hyperlipoproteinemia
hypermelanosis
   linear and whorled nevoid h.
   nevoid h.
hypermobility
   h. syndrome
hyperonychia
hyperostosis
   diffuse idiopathic skeletal h. (DISH)
hyperostotica
   spondylosis h.
hyperparathyroidism
   secondary h.
hyperperistalsis
hyperphenylalaninemia
hyperpigmentation
   cutaneous h.
   mercury h.

metal h.
oral postinflammatory h.
postinflammatory h.
hyperplasia
angiolymphoid h.
benign h.
congenital sebaceous h.
fibrous h.
focal epithelial h.
gingival h.
inflammatory fibrous h.
intravascular papillary
endothelial h.
pseudoepitheliomatous h.
sebaceous h.
h. of sebaceous gland
senile sebaceous h.
synovial h.
hyperplastic
h. epidermis
h. mucus-secreting goblet cell
h. synovium (HS)
hyperprebetalipoproteinemia
hyperresponsiveness
bronchial h. (BHR)
hypersecretion
mucus h.
hypersensitiveness
hypersensitivity
h. angiitis
cell-mediated h.
contact h.
cutaneous basophil h. (CBH)
delayed h. (DH)
delayed-type h. (DTH)
drug h.
food h.
immediate h.
latex h.
h. pneumonitis (HP)
h. pneumonitis panel (HSP)
h. reaction
reaginic h.
h. skin testing
tuberculin-type h.
h. vasculitis
hypersensitization

hypersomnia
hypersplenism
hypersteatosis
hypersusceptibility
hypertelorism
ocular h.
hypertension
benign intracranial h.
chronic thromboembolic
pulmonary h. (CTEPH)
mild h.
primary pulmonary h. (PPH)
pulmonary h.
Hyper-Tet
hyperthyroidism
hypertonia
hypertrichiasis
hypertrichophrydia
hypertrichosis
h. lanuginosa
nevoid h.
h. partialis
h. universalis
hypertriglyceridemia
hypertrophic
h. cervical pachymeningitis
h. lichen planus
h. lymphoid follicle
h. osteoarthropathy
h. rosacea
h. scar
h. smooth muscle layer
h. tonsil
hypertrophica
acne h.
hypertrophicum
eczema h.
hypertrophicus
corneus h.
lichen corneus h.
lichen planus h.
lupus erythematosus h.
hypertrophy
submucosal gland h.
h. of tongue papilla
hypertylosis
hyperuricemia

NOTES

H

193

hyperuricuria
hypervaccination
hypervariable region
hyperventilation
    isocapnic h. (ISH)
hyperviscosity syndrome
hypervitaminosis
    h. A
    h. C
    h. D
    h. E
hyperzincuria
hypha, pl. hyphae
hyphal form
hypoadrenalism
hypobaric hypoxia
hypocapnia
hypochondriasis
    monosymptomatic h.
hypochromic
    h. normocytic anemia
hypocomplementemia
hypocomplementemic
    h. urticarial vasculitis
    h. vasculitis urticarial
        syndrome
hypoderm
hypodermatic
hypodermic
hypodermolithiasis
hypogammaglobinemia
hypogammaglobulinemia
    acquired h.
    primary h.
    secondary h.
    X-linked h.
hypoglycemia
hypogonadism
hypohidrosis
hypohidrotic
    h. ectodermal dysplasia
hypomelanosis
    congenital circumscribed h.
    guttate h.
    idiopathic guttate h.
    h. of Ito
hypomotility
    esophageal h.
hyponychium
hyponychon
hypoparathyroidism
    immunodeficiency with h.
hypophosphatasia

hypophosphatemia
hypophysitis
    lymphocytic h.
    lymphoid h.
hypopigmentation
    postinflammatory h.
hypopigmented
    h. macular eruption
    h. macule
hypopituitarism
hypoplasia
    cartilage-hair h.
    dermal h.
    focal dermal h.
    thymic h.
hypopyon
    h. iritis
hyposensitivity
hyposensitization
    oral h.
hypostaticum
    ulcus h.
hypostome
    barbed h.
HypoTears
    H. PF solution
    H. solution
hypotension
    orthostatic h.
hypothalamic-pituitary-adrenal
    system
hypothesis
    Saunders-Zwilling h.
hypothetical
    h. mean organism
    h. mean strain (HMS)
hypothyroidism
    idiopathic h.
hypotonia
hypotonicity
hypotonic solution
hypotrichiasis
hypotrichosis
hypoventilation
hypovitaminosis B
hypoxanthine-guanine
    h.-g. phosphoribosyltransferase
        (HGPRT)
    h.-g. phosphoribosyltransferase
        deficiency
hypoxemia
    arterial h.

REM sleep-related h.
rest h.
hypoxia
hypobaric h.
synovial h.
hypoxic vasoconstriction
Hyprogest injection
Hysone topical
hysterical reaction
hystriciasis

hystrix
ichthyismus h.
ichthyosis h.
HY-TEC automated allergy diagnostic system
Hytone
Hyzine-50
HZ
herpes zoster

NOTES

H

I
- I antigen
- I cell
- I pilus
- I region

I3
- prostacyclin I.

IA
- intra-articular

Ia+
- immune-associated antigen-positive macrophage

Ia antigen

IAHIA
- immune adherence immunosorbent assay

iatrogenic
- i. Cushing syndrome
- i. pneumothorax

IB
- Excedrin I.
- Midol I.
- Motrin I.
- Sine-Aid I.

Ibaraki virus

IBD
- inflammatory bowel disease

IBIDS
- ichthyosis plus BIDS
- IBIDS syndrome

IBR
- infectious bovine rhinotracheitis
- IBR virus

IBS
- inflammatory bowel syndrome
- irritable bowel syndrome

Ibuprin

ibuprofen
- Arthritis Foundation I.
- pseudoephedrine and i.

Ibuprohm

Ibu-Tab

IBV
- infectious bronchitis virus

IC
- inspiratory capacity

ICAM
- intercellular adhesion module

ICAM-1
- intercellular adhesion molecule-1

ICDRG
- International Contact Dermatitis Research Group

ice
- i. compress
- i. cube test
- dry i.

ice-pick type scar

ichthyismus
- i. exanthematicus
- i. hystrix

ichthyosiform
- i. dermatosis
- i. erythroderma

ichthyosis
- acquired i.
- autosomal dominant lamellar i.
- autosomal recessive i.
- congenital i.
- congenital erythrodermic i.
- i. congenita neonatorum
- i. corneae
- i. fetalis
- follicular i.
- i. follicularis
- harlequin i.
- i. hystrix
- i. intrauterina
- lamellar i.
- i. lethalis
- i. linearis circumflexa
- nacreous i.
- nonbullous congenital erythrodermic i.
- i. palmaris et plantaris
- i. plus BIDS (IBIDS)
- recessive X-linked i.
- i. scutulata
- i. sebacea
- i. sebacea corneae
- i. simplex
- i. spinosa
- i. uteri
- i. vulgaris
- X-linked i.

ichthyotic

icosahedral

icteric

icteroid

icterus
  acquired hemolytic i.
  i. gravis
  i. melas
  i. neonatorum
  i. praecox
ID
  immunodiffusion
  infecting dose
  infectious disease
IDA
  idiopathic destructive arthritis
idarubicin
IDDM
  insulin-dependent diabetes mellitus
identification
  i. bracelet
  i. tag
identity
  reaction of i.
  reaction of partial i.
idioagglutinin
idioheteroagglutinin
idioheterolysin
idioisoagglutinin
idioisolysin
idiolysin
idiopathic
  i. acute eosinophilic pneumonia
  i. atrophoderma
  i. atrophoderma of Pasini and Pierini
  i. calcinosis cutis
  i. clubbing
  i. cold agglutinin disease
  i. cold urticaria
  i. destructive arthritis (IDA)
  i. eczematous disease
  i. guttate hypomelanosis
  i. hirsutism
  i. hypereosinophilic syndrome (IHES)
  i. hypertrophic osteoarthritis
  i. hypothyroidism
  i. inflammatory myopathy
  i. late-onset eczema
  i. livedo reticularis
  i. lobular panniculitis
  i. panhypopituitarism
  i. panniculitis
  i. periostosis
  i. pulmonary fibrosis (IPF)
  i. pulmonary hemosiderosis
  i. roseola
  i. thrombocytopenic purpura (ITP)
  i. urticaria
idiopathica
  livedo reticularis i.
idiosyncrasy
idiosyncratic
  i. drug reaction
  i. sensitivity
idiotope
  set of i.'s
idiotype
  i. antibody
  i. autoantibody
  cross-reactive i.
idiotypic antigenic determinant
idoxuridine
id reaction
idrosis
IDSA
  Infectious Disease Society of America
iduronic acid
I:E
  inspiratory to expiratory ratio
IEF
  isoelectric focusing
IFA
  silver stain
IF-A
  inflammatory factor of anaphylaxis
IFN
  interferon
IFN-α
  interferon alpha
IFN-β
  interferon beta
IFN-γ
  interferon gamma
Ig
  immunoglobulin
IgA
  immunoglobulin A
  IgA antibody
  IgA deficiency
  IgA dermatosis
  IgA nephropathy
  serum IgA
IgD
  immunoglobulin D
IgE
  immunoglobulin E

IgE antibody
IgE radioallergosorbent test
total serum IgE
IgE-dependent immunologic drug reaction
IgE-mediated
    I.-m. food allergy
    I.-m. response
IgE-sensitized cell
IGF-1
    insulin-like growth factor 1
IgG
    immunoglobulin G
    IgG antibody
    IgG avidity test
    Candida albicans IgG
    IgG complex
    IgG RF
    IgG subclass determination
    IgG subclass level
    IgG titer
IgG4
    immunoglobulin G4
IgG-RF-complement aggregate
IgM
    immunoglobulin M
    IgM antibody
    IgM anticardiolipin antibody
    indirect enzyme immunoassay
      for anti-*Mycoplasma pneumoniae* IgM
    IgM nephropathy
    IgM RF
    serum IgM
ignea
    zona i.
ignis
    sacer i.
IH
    infectious hepatitis
IHES
    idiopathic hypereosinophilic syndrome
II
    Protropin I.

IL
    interleukin
IL-1–15
    interleukin-1–15
IL-1β cytokine
ILD
    interstitial lung disease
Ilhéus
    I. encephalitis
    I. fever
    I. virus
iliacus
iliopectineal bursitis
iliotibial band syndrome
Ilizarov external fixation
ill
    louping i.
illinition
illness
    environmental i.
    roseola-like i.
Ilosone Oral
Ilotycin Ophthalmic
ILVEN
    inflamed linear verrucous epidermal nevus
imaging
    laser Doppler perfusion i.
    magnetic resonance i. (MRI)
imbalance
    endocrine hormone i.
    protease-antiprotease i.
imbedded stinger
imbricata
    tinea i.
I-Methasone
imglucerase
imidazole
    i. carboxamide
imipenem
imipenem/cilastatin
imipramine
imiquimod

NOTES

Imitrex
    I. injection
    I. Oral
IM Jaws alligator forceps
immediate
    i. ˙allergy
    i. antigen release
    i. contagion
    i. hypersensitivity
    i. hypersensitivity reaction
    i. skin reactivity
    i. tanning
    i. telogen release
    i. transfusion reaction
immersion
    excessive water i.
    i. foot
    oil i.
immitis
    Coccidioides i.
    Dirofilaria i.
immobilizing antibody
immortalization
immune
    i. adherence
    i. adherence immunosorbent
      assay (IAHIA)
    i. adherence phenomenon
    i. adhesion test
    i. adsorption
    i. agglutination
    i. agglutinin
    i. complex
    i. complex assay
    i. complex clearance
    i. complex disease
    i. complex disorder
    i. complex glomerulonephritis
    i. complex immunologic drug
      reaction
    i. complex-mediated drug
      reaction
    i. complex nephritis
    i. complex vasculitis
    i. deficiency
    i. deviation
    i. globulin, intramuscular
    i. globulin, intravenous
    i. hemolysin
    i. hemolysis
    i. inflammation
    i. interferon
    i. memory

    i. opsonin
    i. paralysis
    i. precipitation
    i. protein
    i. response
    i. serum
    i. serum globulin
    i. surveillance
    i. system
    i. theory
    i. thrombocytopenia
immune-associated antigen-positive
    macrophage (Ia+)
immune-derived amyloidosis
immune-mediated
    i.-m. coagulation disorder
    i.-m. disease
    i.-m. membranous nephritis
immunifacient
immunity
    acquired i.
    active i.
    adoptive i.
    antiviral i.
    artificial active i.
    artificial passive i.
    bacteriophage i.
    cell-mediated i. (CMI)
    concomitant i.
    i. deficiency
    general i.
    group i.
    herd i.
    host i.
    humoral i.
    infection i.
    innate i.
    local i.
    maternal i.
    natural i.
    passive i.
    relative i.
    specific active i.
    specific passive i.
immunization
    active i.
    Heptavax i.
    passive i.
    i. requirement
    Standards for Pediatric I. (SPI)
    viral i.
immunize
immunoadjuvant

immunoagglutination
immunoassay
    antinuclear antibody screening
      by enzyme i.
    double antibody i.
    enzyme i. (EIA)
    enzyme-linked i. (EIA)
    ImmunoCard i.
    solid phase i.
    thin-layer i.
    urine myoglobin i.
immunoblast
immunoblot
immunoblotting
immunobullous disease
Immuno-C
ImmunoCard
    I. immunoassay
    I. used for diagnosis of
      Helicobacter pylori
immunochemical
    i. abnormalities
    i. assay
    i. relative
immunochemistry
immunocompetence
immunocompetent
    i. cell
    i. tissue therapy
immunocomplex
immunocompromised
    i. host
immunoconglutinin
immunocyte
immunocyte-derived amyloidosis
immunocytochemical
immunocytochemistry
immunodeficiency
    acquired i.
    combined i.
    common variable i. (CVI)
    common variable
      unclassifiable i.
    i. disease
    i. disorder
    i. electrophoresis
    phagocytic dysfunction i.

    phagocytic dysfunction
      disorders i.
    secondary i.
    severe combined i. (SCID)
    i. syndrome
    i. with hypoparathyroidism
immunodeficient
immunodepressant
immunodepressor
immunodiagnosis
immunodiffusion (ID)
    antinuclear antibody i.
    double i.
    radial i. (RID)
    single i.
    single radial i. (SRID)
    i. technique
immunoelectrophoresis
    crossed i. (CIE)
    quantitative i. (QIE)
    rocket i. (RIE)
    two-dimensional i.
immunoenhancement
immunoenhancer
immunoferritin
immunofluorescence
    i. analysis
    antinuclear antibody i.
    cytometric indirect i.
    i. finding
    i. method
    i. microscopy
    i. technique
immunofluorescent
    i. examination
    i. stain
immunogen
immunogenetics
immunogenic
immunogenicity
immunoglobulin (Ig)
    anti-D i.
    chickenpox i.
    i. domains
    i. G rheumatoid factor (IgG
      RF)
    hepatitis B i. (H-BIG)

NOTES

immunoglobulin *(continued)*
  human normal i.
  i. IV
  i. light chain-origin amyloid
    deposit (AL protein)
  measles i.
  monoclonal i.
  i. M rheumatoid factor (IgM
    RF)
  pertussis i.
  poliomyelitis i.
  rabies i.
  $RH_o(D)$ i.
  secretory i.
  i. supergene family
  tetanus i.
  varicella-zoster i. (VZIG)
immunoglobulin A (IgA)
immunoglobulin D (IgD)
immunoglobulin E (IgE)
immunoglobulin G (IgG)
immunoglobulin G4 (IgG4)
immunoglobulin M (IgM)
immunoglobulin-secreting cell
immunohematology
immunohistochemical
immunohistochemistry
  Ki-67 i.
immunologic
  i. complication
  i. contact urticaria
  i. disorder
  i. drug reaction
  i. feature
  i. high dose tolerance
  i. inflammatory disease
  i. organ damage
  i. pregnancy test
  i. response
  i. tolerance
immunological
  i. competence
  i. deficiency
  i. enhancement
  i. mechanism
  i. paralysis
  i. surveillance
  i. tolerance
immunologically
  i. activated cell
  i. competent cell
  i. privileged site
immunologist

immunology
immunometric technique
immunomodulator
immunomodulatory
immunopathology
immunoperoxidase
immunophenotype
immunopotentiation
immunopotentiator
immunoprecipitation
  i. assay
immunoproliferative disorder
immunoprophylaxis
immunopurging
  complement-mediated tumor
    cell i.
immunoradiometric assay
immunoreaction
immunoreactive
  i. hormone
  i. insulin (IRI)
immunoregulation
immunoregulatory defect
immunoselection
immunosorbent
immunosuppressant
immunosuppression
  TGF-induced i.
immunosuppressive
  i. agent
  i. drug
  i. therapy
immunosurveillance
immunosympathectomy
immunotherapy
  adoptive i.
  biological i.
  passive i.
  venom i.
immunotolerance
immunotransfusion
Immupath
Immuthiol
Imogam
Imovax
  I. Rabies intradermal vaccine
  I. Rabies intramuscular vaccine
impactor
  Cascade i.
  rotating air i.
  rotating arm i.
impaired neutrophil chemotaxis

impairment
  i., decreased fertility, short
     stature
  functional i.
  photosensitivity, ichthyosis,
     brittle hair, intellectual i.
  restrictive functional i.
impending respiratory failure
imperfecta
  dentinogenesis i.
  lethal osteogenesis i.
  osteogenesis i.
  severe deforming
     osteogenesis i.
  Sillence type II–IV
     osteogenesis i.
Imperfecti
  Fungi I.
impermeable
impetigines (*pl. of* impetigo)
impetiginization
impetiginize
impetiginous
  i. cheilitis
  i. syphilid
impetigo, pl. **impetigines**
  Bockhart i.
  i. bullosa
  bullous i.
  i. circinata
  i. contagiosa
  i. contagiosa bullosa
  i. eczematodes
  follicular i.
  i. furfuracea
  furfuraceous i.
  i. gestationis
  i. herpetiformis
  i. neonatorum
  nonbullous i.
  i. vulgaris
impingement
  i. sign
  i. syndrome
implant
  bovine collagen dermal i.
  collagen i.

  Medpor surgical i.
  Neer II i.
implantation cyst
importance
  allergic i.
improper repair of DNA
Imuran
in
  i. noma ulcer
  i. situ
  i. situ hybridization
  i. situ squamous cell
     carcinoma
  i. toto
  i. vitro
  i. vitro anergy
  i. vitro proliferative
     lymphocyte response
  i. vitro test
  i. vivo
  i. vivo reaction
inactivate
inactivated
  Japanese encephalitis virus
     vaccine, i.
  i. poliovirus vaccine (IPV)
  poliovirus vaccine, i.
  i. serum
inactivation
inactivator
  anaphylatoxin i.
inadvertent trauma
inaperturate
incarnati
  pili i.
incarnatus
  unguis i.
incentive spirometry
incision
  elliptical i.
incisional biopsy
incisor
  overriding maxillary i.
inclusion
  i. body
  i. body disease
  i. body encephalitis

NOTES

inclusion *(continued)*
    i. body myositis
    i. cell
    i. conjunctivitis virus
    i. cyst
    cytoplasmic i.
    i. dermoid
    hematoxyphilic i.
    Rocha-Lima i.
incognitus
    Mycoplasma i.
incognito
    scabies i.
    tinea i.
incompatibility
    ABO i.
incompatible
    i. blood transfusion reaction
incomplete
    i. agglutinin
    i. antibody
    i. antigen
    i. neurofibromatosis
incontinence of pigment
incontinentia
    i. pigmenti
    i. pigmenti achromians
increased sympathoadrenal activity
incrustation
incubation
    i. period
incubative stage
incubatory carrier
Indanyl carbenicillin
Inderal
    I. LA
indeterminate
    i. cell histiocytosis
    i. leprosy
index, gen. indicis, pl. indices, indexes
    American Rheumatism
      Association i.
    chemotherapeutic i.
    endemic i.
    Lansbury articular i.
    leukopenic i.
    metacarpal i.
    phagocytic i.
    Ritchie articular i.
    Singh i.
    splenic i.

    tension-time i.
    volume thickness i. (VTI)
India-rubber skin
indicanidrosis
indicator system
indices *(pl. of* index)
indicis *(gen. of* index)
indigenous
indinavir
    i. sulfate
indirect
    i. agglutination
    i. agglutination test
    i. assay
    i. Coombs test
    i. Coombs titer
    i. enzyme immunoassay for
      anti-*Mycoplasma pneumoniae*
      IgM
    i. fluorescent antibody
    i. fluorescent antibody test
    i. hemagglutination test
indium chloride scan
indium-labeled scanning
Indocin
    I. I.V. injection
    I. Oral
    I. SR Oral
indolent
    i. nonpitting edema
    i. papule
    i. ulcer
indomethacin
induced
    i. phagocytosis
    i. sensitivity
inducer cell
inducible skin color
induction
    lysogenic i.
    i. period
indurata
    acne i.
    tuberculosis cutis i.
indurated
    i. border
    i. papule
    i. welt
induration
    brawny i.
induratio penis plastica
indurativa
    tuberculosis cutis i.

induratum
 erythema i.
industrial smog
inertial
 i. suction sampler
infancy
 acropustulosis of i.
 capillary hemangioma of i.
 transient
  hypogammaglobulinemia of i.
infantile
 i. acropustulosis
 i. acute hemorrhagic edema of
  the skin
 i. colic
 i. digital fibroma
 i. eczema
 i. gastroenteritis
 i. gastroenteritis virus
 i. myofibromatosis
 i. purulent conjunctivitis
infantilis
 prurigo i.
 roseola i.
infants
 sudden unexpected death in i.
  (SUDI)
 sudden unexplained death in i.
  (SUDI)
infantum
 acrodermatitis papulosa i.
 dermatitis exfoliativa i.
 dermatitis gangrenosa i.
 granuloma gluteale i.
 lichen i.
 roseola i.
infarction
 diabetic muscle i. (DMI)
 myocardial i. (MI)
infarctive
 i. inflammatory disease
 i. lesion
infect
infected vascular gangrene
infecting dose (ID)
infection
 atypical mycobacterial i.

bacterial i.
beta hemolytic streptococci i.
Candida i.
candidal i.
chlamydial i.
chronic Epstein-Barr virus i.
"closed space" i.
congenital HIV i.
cross i.
cryptogenic i.
dermatophyte fungal i.
disseminated gonococcal i.
droplet i.
EBV i.
ectothrix i.
endemic fungal i.
endogenous i.
endothrix i.
enteroviral i.
environmental mycobacterial i.
focal, i.
fungal i.
fungous i.
granulomatous bacterial i.
group A beta-hemolytic
 streptococcal i.
group A streptococcus i.
guinea worm i.
Hantavirus i.
herpes simplex i.
herpes zoster i.
herpetic i.
hibernal epidemic viral i.
 (HEVI)
hospital-acquired i.
human papillomavirus i.
i. immunity
laryngeal i.
latent i.
lower respiratory tract i.
 (LRTI)
mass i.
mixed i.
mixed nail i.
mycobacterial i.
natural focus of i.
necrotizing i.

I

NOTES

infection *(continued)*
    nondermatophyte fungal i.
    nontuberculous mycobacterial i.
    nosocomial i.
    opportunistic i.
    opportunistic systemic fungal i.
    overwhelming
      postsplenectomy i. (OPSI)
    paravaccinia virus i.
    pneumococcal i.
    primary i.
    primary herpes simplex i.
    pyodermatous i.
    pyogenic i.
    recurrent i.
    repeated respiratory i.
    reservoir of i.
    rhinocerebral i.
    rickettsial i.
    scalp i.
    secondary i.
    Shigella i.
    spirochete i.
    Streptococcus i.
    subcutaneous fungal i.
    subcutaneous necrotizing i.
    superficial i.
    sycosiform fungous i.
    systemic fungal i.
    unusual opportunistic i.
    upper respiratory i. (URI)
    upper respiratory tract i. (URI)
    urinary tract i. (UTI)
    vaccinia i.
    varicella-zoster i.
    vesicular viral i.
    Vincent i.
    viral i.
    viral respiratory i.
    Western blot i.
    yeast i.
    zoonotic i.
infection-immunity
infectiosity
infectiosum
    ecthyma i.
    erythema i. (EI)
infectious
    i. arteritis virus of horses
    i. arthritis
    i. avian bronchitis
    i. bovine rhinotracheitis (IBR)
    i. bovine rhinotracheitis virus

    i. bronchitis virus (IBV)
    i. bulbar paralysis
    i. canine hepatitis
    i. disease (ID)
    i. ectromelia virus
    i. eczematoid dermatitis
    i. endocarditis
    i. granuloma
    i. hepatitis (IH)
    i. hepatitis virus
    i. mononucleosis
    i. nucleic acid
    i. papilloma of cattle
    i. papilloma virus
    i. perichondritis
    i. plasmid
    i. polyneuritis
    i. porcine encephalomyelitis
    i. porcine encephalomyelitis
      virus
    i. rhinitis
    i. wart
**Infectious Disease Society of
America (IDSA)**
infectiousness
infectiva
    polioencephalitis i.
infective
infectivity
inferior fornix
infest
infestation
    Cheyletiella i.
    environmental mite i.
    louse i.
    mite i.
    Pediculus humanus capitis i.
    Pthirus pubis i.
infiltrate
    diffuse pulmonary i.
    fixed pulmonary i.
    fluffy alveolar i.
    granulomatous dermal i.
    lymphoid i.
    patchy i.
    perivascular i.
    transient migratory i.
    transient pulmonary i.
infiltration
    lymphocytic i.
    peribronchiolar lymphocyte i.
infiltrative basal cell carcinoma
Infinity sensor

I

Inflamase
   I. Forte Ophthalmic
   I. Mild Ophthalmic
inflame
inflamed
   i. linear verrucous epidermal
      nevus (ILVEN)
   i. ulcer
inflammation
   acute i. (AI)
   allergic i.
   chronic i. (CI)
   chronic jejunal i.
   diffuse i.
   focal i.
   immune i.
   interstitial i.
   mucosal i.
   necrotizing scleritis with
      adjacent i.
   necrotizing scleritis without
      adjacent i.
   neutrophilic i.
   i. reaction
   urate-associated i.
inflammatory
   i. bowel disease (IBD)
   i. bowel syndrome (IBS)
   i. cell
   i. dermatosis
   i. disease
   i. edema
   i. factor of anaphylaxis (IF-A)
   i. fibrous hyperplasia
   i. macrophage
   i. plaque
   i. tinea capitis
   i. ulcer
inflorescence
influenza, pl. **influenzae**
   i. A
   avian i.
   i. B
   i. C
   equine i.
   Hong Kong i.
   sequela of i.

   Spanish i.
   swine i.
   i. virus
   i. virus hemagglutinin
   i. virus vaccine
Influenzavirus
infolded
infrapatellar bursitis
infriction
infundibulofolliculitis
   disseminated recurrent i.
   recurrent i.
infundibulum
ingestion
   L-tryptophan i.
ingestive
ingrowing
   i. hair
ingrown
   i. hair
   i. nail
inguinal
inguinale
   Epidermophyton i.
   granuloma i.
   lymphogranuloma i.
inguinalis
   tinea i.
Inhal-Aid bronchodilator
inhalant
   i. allergen
   i. allergen extract
inhalation
   Atrovent Aerosol I.
   i. breath unit
   NebuPent I.
   smoke i.
inhaled dander
inhaler
   AeroBid-M Oral Aerosol I.
   Beclovent Oral I.
   Beconase AQ Nasal I.
   Beconase Nasal I.
   Chiesi powder i.
   Diskhaler i.
   FOII powder i.
   Inhalet i.

NOTES

inhaler *(continued)*
  InspirEase i.
  Intal Oral I.
  metered-dose i. (MDI)
  Nebuhaler i.
  Orion i.
  Rondo i.
  Rotahaler i.
  Spinhaler i.
  Turbuhaler i.
  Vancenase AQ I.
  Vancenase Nasal I.
  Vanceril Oral I.
Inhalet inhaler
inherited
  i. epidermolysis bullosa
  i. patterned lentiginosis
inhibin
inhibiting antibody
inhibition
  allogeneic i.
  eicosanoid i.
  i. factor
  i. fluorescent antibody
  hemagglutination i.
  leukotriene i.
  prostaglandin synthesis i.
  xanthine i.
inhibitor
  angiogenesis i.
  C1 i.
  C1 esterase i.
  cysteine proteinase i.
  factor VIII:C i.
  functional C1 esterase i.
  HIV protease i.
  HMG-CoA reductase i.
  human α1-proteinase i.
  mast cell i.
  non-nucleoside reverse
    transcriptase i.
  phosphodiesterase i.
  phosphodiesterase isoenzyme i.
  polypeptide i.
  protease i.
  protein C1 esterase i.
  secretory leukoprotease i.
  synthesis i.
  tissue i.
  transcriptase i.
  α_1-trypsin i.
Initiative
  Children's Vaccine I. (CVI)

injectable
  i. collagen
  i. dye
injection
  Adlone i.
  Adrucil i.
  A-methaPred i.
  Amikin i.
  amphotericin B lipid
    complex i.
  AquaMEPHYTON i.
  Articulose-50 i.
  Bactocill i.
  Bena-D i.
  Benadryl i.
  Benahist i.
  Benoject i.
  Bicillin C-R i.
  Bicillin C-R 900/300 i.
  Bicillin L-A i.
  Brethine i.
  Bricanyl i.
  Bronkephrine i.
  Calciferol i.
  Carbocaine i.
  Ceredase i.
  Chlor-Pro i.
  Chlor-Trimeton i.
  Cipro i.
  collagen i.
  conjunctival i.
  Cophene-B i.
  Cortone Acetate i.
  Crysticillin A.S. i.
  Cytoxan i.
  Dehist i.
  depMedalone i.
  Depoject i.
  Depo-Medrol i.
  Depopred i.
  D.H.E. 45 i.
  Diflucan i.
  Dizac i.
  D-Med i.
  Doxychel i.
  Duralone i.
  Duralutin i.
  Duranest i.
  Floxin i.
  Foscavir i.
  Garamycin i.
  Histaject i.
  Hydeltrasol i.

I

Hydeltra-TBA i.
Hy-Gestrone i.
Hylutin i.
Hyprogest i.
Imitrex i.
Indocin I.V. i.
intra-articular i.
intralesional i.
intratendinous i.
Isocaine HCl i.
Jenamicin i.
Kantrex i.
Keflin i.
Kefurox i.
Kenalog i.
Key-Pred i.
Key-Pred-SP i.
Konakion i.
Levophed i.
Lyphocin i.
Medralone i.
Metro I.V. i.
Minocin IV i.
M-Prednisol i.
Nafcil i.
Nallpen i.
Nasahist B i.
ND-Stat i.
Nebcin i.
Neosar i.
Netromycin i.
Neupogen i.
Neut i.
Nordryl i.
Novocain i.
Nydrazid i.
Octocaine i.
Oraminic II i.
Ornidyl i.
Osmitrol i.
Pentacarinat i.
Pentam-300 i.
Permapen i.
Pfizerpen i.
Pfizerpen-AS i.
Phenazine i.
Phenergan i.

Polocaine i.
Pontocaine i.
Predaject i.
Predalone i.
Predcor i.
Predicort-50 i.
Prednisol TBA i.
Pro-Depo i.
Prodrox i.
Prometh i.
Prorex i.
Prostaphlin i.
Prothazine i.
Retrovir i.
Rifadin i.
Sandimmune i.
sensitizing i.
Solu-Medrol i.
Spectam i.
subcutaneous i.
Terramycin I.M. i.
Toposar i.
Toradol i.
Trobicin i.
Unipen i.
Ureaphil i.
Valium i.
Vancocin i.
Vancoled i.
VePesid i.
V-Gan i.
Vibramycin i.
Vumon i.
Wellcovorin i.
Wycillin i.
Zantac i.
Zetran i.
Zinacef i.
Zovirax i.
injury
   whiplash i.
innate immunity
inner
   i. canthus
   i. root sheath
innocent bystander cell
inoculability

NOTES

inoculable
inoculate
inoculating
inoculation
inoculum
inosinic
   i. acid
   i. acid dehydrogenase
inositol triphosphate
Inoviridae
INR
   International Normalization Ratio
insect
   i. bite
   biting i.
   i. sting
   i. sting kit
   i. virus
insecticide
insensible perspiration
insensitive sweat
insidious onset
insipidus
   nephrogenic diabetes i.
insolation
inspiratory
   i. capacity (IC)
   i. to expiratory ratio (I:E)
   i. positive airway pressure
   (IPAP)
InspirEase
   I. inhaler
Inspiron
instructive theory
instrument
   IOS immunodiagnostic
   testing i.
   ProLine endoscopic i.
insufficiency
   adrenal i.
   adrenocortical i.
insula
insulin
   i. allergy
   i. antagonist
   immunoreactive i. (IRI)
   i. reaction
   i. resistance
   single-peak pork i.

   i. skin test
   i. tumor
insulin-dependent diabetes mellitus
   (IDDM)
insulin-like growth factor 1 (IGF-1)
insusceptibility
intake
   caloric i.
Intal
   I. Nebulizer solution
   I. Oral Inhaler
integrin
   1 i.
   2 i.
   3 i.
integument
integumentary system
integumentum
interaction
   adhesin-receptor i.
   drug i.
   HLA intercellular i.
   T-cell-counter-receptor i.
intercellular
   i. adhesion module (ICAM)
   i. adhesion molecule-1 (ICAM-
   1)
   i. bridge
   i. machinery
   i. space
intercritical gout
interdigital
   i. maceration
interdigitalis
interface
   Monarch Mini Mask nasal i.
interference
   bacterial i.
interfering
   defective i. (DI)
interferon (IFN)
   i. alfa-2a
   i. alfa-2b
   i. alpha (IFN-α)
   antigen i.
   i. B-1b
   i. beta (IFN-β)
   fibroblast i.
   i. gamma (IFN-γ)
   i. gamma-1b
   immune i.
   leukocyte i.
   natural i. alfa

therapeutic i.
  i. therapy
interleukin (IL)
interleukin-1–15 (IL-1–15)
interleukin-2 adjunctive
  chemotherapy
interlobular septa
intermedia
  β-thalassemia i.
intermediate
  i. carcinoma
  i. filament
  i. leprosy
intermedius
  Streptococcus i.
intermetacarpal
intermittent
  i. hydrarthrosis
  i. mandatory ventilation
  i. positive pressure breathing
    (IPPB)
  i. sterilization
internal hair apparatus
International
  I. Contact Dermatitis Research
    Group (ICDRG)
  I. Normalization Ratio (INR)
internum
  erysipelas i.
interpalpebral fissure
interpapillary ridges
interphalangeal
  distal i. (DIP)
  i. joint
  proximal i. (PIP)
interplant
interplanting
interpretation
  patch test i.
interrogans
  Leptospira i.
interspecific graft
interstitial
  i. fibrosis
  i. infiltration by histiocyte
  i. inflammation

i. lung disease (ILD)
i. nephritis
interstitium
  lung i.
intertinctus
  strophulus i.
intertriginous
  i. area
  i. psoriasis
  i. region
intertrigo
  Candida i.
  diaper rash i.
  eczema i.
  erythema i.
  i. with ulceration
interzone
intestinal
  i. biopsy
  i. fluke
  i. lipodystrophy
  i. nematode
  i. polyp
  i. ulceration
intestinotoxin
intine
intolerance
  carbohydrate i.
  cow-milk protein i.
  disaccharide i.
  drug i.
  gluten i.
  lactose i.
intoxication
  anaphylactic i.
  bromide i.
  metal i.
intra-alveolar hemorrhage
intra-articular (IA)
  i.-a. glucocorticoid
  i.-a. injection
  i.-a. ossicles
  i.-a. tophi
intrabursal
intracellular
  i. digestion

I

NOTES

intracellular *(continued)*
i. edema
i. toxin
intractable
i. pyoderma
i. wheezing
intracutaneous
i. nevus
i. reaction
intracytoplasmic
intradermal
i. anesthetic
i. melanocyte
i. nevus
i. reaction
i. skin test
i. test concentration
IntraDop probe
intraepidermal
i. abscess
i. acanthoma
i. bulla
i. carcinoma
i. microabscess
i. microabscess of psoriasis
i. neutrophilic IgA dermatosis
i. nevus
i. vesiculation
intraepithelial
intragastral provocation under endoscopy (IPEC)
intralesional injection
intramural thrombi
intramuscular
immune globulin, i.
intraosseous
intrapsychic stress
intrasynovial complement level
intratendinous injection
intrauterina
ichthyosis i.
intravascular
i. endothelial proliferation
i. endothelial proliferative lesion
i. papillary endothelial hyperplasia
Intravenous
Fungizone I.
intravenous
i. fluids
i. immune globulin
immune globulin, i.

i. immune serum globulin (IVIG)
Rh immune globulin i. (RhIGIV)
intraventricular hemorrhage
intrinsic
i. asthma
i. muscle atrophy
introduction of cereal
Intron A
Intropin
intrusion
alpha wave i.
intubation
intussusception
inunct
inunction
inundation fever
InV
I. allotypes
I. group antigen
invaccination
invadens
aegleria i.
invaginata
trichorrhexis i.
invariant chain CS
invasion
angiolymphatic i.
stage of i.
invasive
i. aspergillosis
i. candidiasis
i. squamous cell carcinoma
invecta
Solenopsis i.
Inventory
Minnesota Multiphasic Personality I. (MMPI)
inversa
acne i.
inverse
i. anaphylaxis
i. ratio ventilation (IRV)
inverted follicular keratosis
inveterata
psoriasis i.
Invirase
involuting flat hemangioma
involution form
involvement
cardiovascular i.

juvenile rheumatoid arthritis with spinal i.
kidney i.
lung i.
nervous system i.
palm-sole i.
peripheral nerve i.
predominant DIP joint i.
psoriatic arthritis with spinal i.
renal i.
skin i.
T-cell i.
INVOS Cerebral Oximeter
Io
   I. moth larva
Iobid DM
ioderma
Iodex Regular
iodica
   purpura i.
iodide
   i. acne
   potassium i.
   saturated solution of potassium i. (SSKI)
iodine
   i. bush
   i. eruption
   radiolabeled i.
iodized collodion
iododerma
iodophor
iodoquinol
   i. and hydrocortisone
Iohist DM
Ionil
ionizing radiation
iontophoresis
iontophoretic unit
IOS immunodiagnostic testing instrument
IPAP
   inspiratory positive airway pressure
IPEC
   intragastral provocation under endoscopy

IPF
   idiopathic pulmonary fibrosis
I-Phrine Ophthalmic solution
IPOL
IPPB
   intermittent positive pressure breathing
ipratropium
   i. bromide
   i. bromide aerosol
IPV
   inactivated poliovirus vaccine
IRI
   immunoreactive insulin
iridescent virus
iridocyclitis
Iridoviridae
Iridovirus
iris
   erythema i.
   herpes i.
   lichen i.
   i. scissors
iritis
   hypopyon i.
   plastic i.
iron
   i. deficiency
   i. deficiency anemia
   i. storage disease
irradiate
irradiation
   therapeutic i.
irregular border
irrigator
   Grossan nasal i.
irritable bowel syndrome (IBS)
irritans
   Pulex i.
   Trombicula i.
irritant
   i. contact dermatitis
   i. contact urticaria
   i. hand dermatitis
   mild i.
   i. patch-test reaction

NOTES

irritant *(continued)*
    i. patch-test response
    primary i.
irritate
irritation
    i. fibroma
IRV
    inverse ratio ventilation
ischemia
    transient cerebral i.
ischemic
    i. ulcer
ischidrosis
ischiogluteal bursitis
Iscove modified Dulbecco medium
isethionate
    pentamidine i.
    piritrexim i.
ISH
    isocapnic hyperventilation
island
    i. disease
    i. fever
    i. of sparing
islet α-cell
isoagglutination
isoagglutinin
isoagglutinogen
isoallotypic determinants
isoantibody
isoantigen
Isocaine HCl injection
isocapnic
    i. condition
    i. hyperventilation (ISH)
Isoclor
isocoproporphyrin
isocyanate
    i. HDI
    i. MDI
    i. TDI
isocytolysin
Isodine
isoelectric
    i. focusing (IEF)
isoerythrolysis
Isoetharine
    Arm-a-Med I.
    Dey-Lute I.
isoetharine
isoflurane
isogeneic
    i. graft

isograft
isohemagglutination
isohemagglutinin
    saline i.
isohemolysin
isohemolysis
isoimmune
    i. neonatal neutropenia
    i. neonatal thrombocytopenia
isoimmunization
isokinetic
    i. collection
isolate
isolated dyskeratosis follicularis
isoleucyl-tRNA synthetase
isoleukoagglutinin
isologous
    i. graft
isolysin
isolysis
isolytic
isomeric response
isometric exercise
isomorphic
    i. effect
    i. phenomenon
    i. response
isoniazid
    rifampin and i.
isopathy
isophagy
isoplastic
    i. graft
isoprecipitin
isoprenaline
isopropyl alcohol
isoproterenol
    Arm-a-Med I.
    Dey-Dose I.
    Dispos-a-Med I.
    nebulized i.
    i. and phenylephrine
Isopto
    I. Atropine Ophthalmic
    I. Cetapred Ophthalmic
    I. Frin Ophthalmic solution
    I. Homatropine Ophthalmic
    I. Hyoscine Ophthalmic
    I. Plain solution
    I. Tears solution
isosensitize
isoserum treatment
Isospora belli

isosporiasis
isothiocyanate
    fluorescein i. (FITC)
isotransplantation
isotretinoin
isotype
isotypic
isoxsuprine hydrochloride
Ispaghula
israelii
    Actinomyces i.
issue
isthmic spondylolisthesis
isthmus
I-Sulfacet Ophthalmic
Isuprel
Italian
    I. cypress
    I. cypress tree
itch
    Absorbine Jock I.
    azo i.
    baker's i.
    barber's i.
    barn i.
    bath i.
    clamdigger's i.
    coolie i.
    copra i.
    Cortef Feminine I.
    Cuban i.
    dew i.
    dhobie i.
    frost i.
    grain i.
    grocer's i.
    ground i.
    jock i.
    jock strap i.
    kabure i.
    lumberman's i.
    mad i.
    Malabar i.
    i. mite
    Norway i.
    poultryman's i.
    prairie i.

    rice i.
    Saint Ignatius i.
    straw i.
    summer i.
    swamp i.
    swimmer's i.
    toe i.
    warehouseman's i.
    washerwoman's i.
    water i.
    winter i.
itching
    nasal i.
itchy
    i. red bump disease
    i. soft palate
    i. throat
Ito
    hypomelanosis of I.
    nevus of I.
    I. nevus
Ito-Reenstierna test
ITP
    idiopathic thrombocytopenic purpura
itraconazole
I-Tropine Ophthalmic
I.V.
    Pepcid I.
ivermectin
IVIG
    intravenous immune serum globulin
ivy
    poison i.
Ixodes
    I. cookei
    I. dammini
    I. dammini tick
    I. pacificus
    I. pacificus tick
    I. persulcatus
    I. ricinus
    I. ricinus wood tick
    I. scapularis
    I. spinipalpis
ixodiasis
ixodic
Ixodidae

NOTES

J5 lipopolysaccharide
jaagsiekte
Jaccoud arthropathy
jacket
    yellow j.
Jacquet erythema
Jadassohn
    anetoderma of J.
    J. epithelioma
    J. nevus
    nevus sebaceus of J.
Jadassohn-Lewandowski syndrome
Jadassohn-Pellizzari anetoderma
Jadassohn-Tièche nevus
jail fever
Jakob-Creutzfeldt disease
Jamestown Canyon virus (JCV)
Janeway lesion
Japanese
    J. B encephalitis
    J. B encephalitis virus
    J. cedar
    J. cedar tree
    J. encephalitis virus vaccine,
      inactivated
    J. lacquer tree
    J. river fever
    J. sargassum
japonica
    encephalitis j.
japonicum
    Schistosoma j.
Jarisch-Herxheimer reaction
jasmine
jaundice
    catarrhal j.
    homologous serum j.
jaw
    lumpy j.
    pincer j.
J chain
JCV
    Jamestown Canyon virus
JDMS
    juvenile dermatomyositis
JDMS/PM
    juvenile dermato/polymyositis
jeanselmei
    Exophiala j.
Jeanselme nodule

JEB
    junctional epidermolysis bullosa
jejuni
    Campylobacter j.
jelly
    Vaseline petroleum j.
jellyfish
    box j.
    Portuguese j.
    j. sting
Jenamicin injection
Jerne technique
Jessner
    lymphocytic infiltrate of J.
Jessner-Kanof disease
jet-bubble mechanism
jet nebulizer
JE-VAX
jeweler's forceps
JH
    J. gene
    J. virus
jigger
Jk antigen
Jobbins antigen
Job syndrome
jock
    j. itch
    j. strap itch
Joest bodies
John Bunn Mini-Mist nebulizer
johnin
Johnson
    J. grass
    J. smut
joint
    active j.
    apophyseal j.
    atlantoaxial j.
    Charcot j.
    Clutton j.
    coding j.
    j. congruence
    cricoarytenoid j.
    j. effusion
    facetal j.
    j. histology
    interphalangeal j.
    manubriosternal j.
    patellofemoral j.

J

joint *(continued)*
   j. protection training
   j. space narrowing
   sternoclavicular j.
   sternocostal j.
   subtalar j.
   j. swelling
   trochleo-ginglymoid j.
jojoba
Jojoba oil
Jones criteria
Jonston
   J. alopecia
   J. area
jordanis
   Legionella j.
josamycin
JR
   Aerolate J.
   Congess J.
JRA
   juvenile rheumatoid arthritis
   JRA rash
Js antigen
juccuya
judgment
   clinical j.
junction
   dermoepidermal j.
   j. nevus
   pannus-cartilage j.
junctional
   j. epidermolysis bullosa (JEB)
   j. nevus
   j. variant
June grass
jungle
   j. rot
   j. yellow fever

Junin virus
juniper
   j. mix
   j. mix tree
   Western j.
Jun proto-oncogene
Just Tears solution
jute
juvenile
   j. arthritis
   j. biotin deficiency
   j. chronic arthritis
   j. chronic polyarthritis
   j. colloid milium
   j. dermatomyositis (JDMS)
   j. dermato/polymyositis
      (JDMS/PM)
   j. elastoma
   j. hyalin fibromatosis
   j. melanoma
   j. palmo-plantar fibromatosis
   j. papillomatosis
   j. pityriasis rubra pilaris
   j. rheumatoid arthritis (JRA)
   j. rheumatoid arthritis with
      spinal involvement
   j. spring eruption
   j. xanthogranuloma
   j. xanthogranuloma histiocytosis
juvenilis
   verruca plana j.
juxta-articular
   j.-a. node
   j.-a. nodule
   j.-a. osteoporosis
juxtacrine
   j. stimulation

K
K antigen
K cell
killer cell
K virus
kabure itch
Kaffir pox
kala azar
Kalcinate
kale
kallak
kallikrein
basophil k.
plasma k.
Kaltostat alginate dressing
kanamycin
k. sulfate
kansasii
Mycobacterium k.
Kantrex
K. injection
K. Oral
Kaplan-Meier method
kapok
Kaposi
K. disease
K. sarcoma (KS)
K. varicelliform eruption
kappa
k. binding nuclear factor
k.-deleting element
k. light chain
karaya
k. gum
Kartagener syndrome
Kasabach-Merritt syndrome
Katayama fever
Kathon-CG
Kawasaki
K. disease (KD)
K. syndrome
Kayser-Fleischer ring
KD
Kawasaki disease
kD, kd, kdal
kilodalton
72-kD gelatinase
92-kD gelatinase
220-kD protein
kedani fever

Keflex
Keflin injection
Keftab
Kefurox injection
Kefzol
Kelev strain rabies virus
Kelley-Seegmiller syndrome
Kellgren-Lawrence stage
kellicotti
Paragonimus k.
keloid
acne k.
k. formation
keloidal
k. folliculitis
k. scarring
k. type scar
keloidalis
acne k.
folliculitis k.
keloidosis
Kenacort
K. Syrup
K. Tablet
Kenalog
K. injection
K. in Orabase
Kenicef
Kenonel
Kentucky bluegrass
Keralyt Gel
keratiasis
keratic
keratin
hard k.
nail k.
soft k.
keratinase
keratinization
ectopic k.
keratinize
keratinized
keratinocyte
dyskeratotic k.
keratinocytic adhesion
keratinous
k. cyst
k. material
k. sheet

K

keratitis
    k. deafness
    epithelial k.
    filamentary k.
    herpetic k.
keratitis-deafness cornification disorder
keratitis-ichthyosis-deafness (KID)
keratoacanthoma
    Ferguson-Smith k.
    multiple k.
    solitary k.
keratoangioma
keratoatrophoderma
keratoconjunctivitis
    epidemic k.
    herpetic k.
    k. sicca
    vernal k.
    virus k.
keratoconus
keratocyte
keratoderma
    k. blennorrhagica
    k. blennorrhagicum
    k. climacterica
    k. climactericum
    k. eccentrica
    epidermolytic palmoplantar k.
    lymphedematous k.
    mutilating k.
    k. palmaris et plantaris
    palmoplantar k. (PPK)
    k. plantare sulcatum
    punctate k.
    punctate porokeratotic k.
    k. punctatum
    senile k.
    k. symmetrica
    Unna-Thost k.
    Vorner variant of Unna-Thost k.
keratodermatitis
keratodermia
keratodermic sandal
keratodes
    erythema k.
keratoelastoidosis
    k. marginalis
keratogenesis
keratogenetic
keratogenous

keratohyaline
    k. granule
keratoid
    k. exanthema
keratolysis
    k. exfoliativa
    k. exfoliativa areata manuum
    pitted k.
    k. plantare sulcatum
keratolytic
    k. agent
keratoma
    k. disseminatum
    k. hereditarium mutilans
    k. malignum
    k. plantare sulcatum
    senile k.
keratomalacia
keratonosis
keratopachyderma
keratopathy
    band k.
    epithelial k.
keratoplastic
keratosa
    acne k.
keratose
keratosic cone
keratosis, pl. keratoses
    actinic k.
    arsenical k.
    k. blennorrhagica
    k. climactericum
    k. diffusa fetalis
    follicular k.
    k. follicularis
    k. follicularis contagiosa
    k. follicularis spinulosa decalvans
    inverted follicular k.
    k. labialis
    lichenoid k.
    k. lichenoides chronica
    lichen planus-like k.
    nevus follicularis k.
    k. nigricans
    oral k.
    k. palmaris et plantaris
    k. palmaris et plantaris of the Meleda type
    k. palmaris et plantaris of Unna-Thost
    k. palmoplantaris punctata

k. pilaris
k. pilaris atrophicans
k. pilaris atrophicans faciei
k. punctata
k. rubra figurata
seborrheic k.
senile k.
k. senilis
solar k.
stucco k.
tar k.
k. vegetans
keratotic
k. angioma
k. material
k. papule
keratouveitis
Keri moisturizer
kerion
Celsus k.
tinea k.
kerionic
kernicterus
keroid
kerotherapy
ketoconazole
ketoprofen
ketorolac
k. tromethamine
ketotifen
Ketron-Goodman disease
Kettle syndrome
keyhole limpet hemocyanin
Key-Pred
K.-P. injection
K.-P.-SP injection
KF-1 antigen
Ki-67
K. immunohistochemistry
K. marker detection
KI antigen
KID
keratitis-ichthyosis-deafness
KID syndrome
kidney
k. bean
k. involvement

Kienböck disease
Kiesselbach plexus
Kikuchi disease
Kilham rat virus
killer
k. cell (K cell, K cell)
natural k. (NK)
killing test
kilodalton (kD, kd, kdal)
45-k. protein
Kimura disease
kinase
creatinine k.
tyrosine k.
kinin
k. system
kininase
kinky
k. hair
k.-hair disease
k.-hair syndrome
Kinyoun stain
Kirby-Bauer agar
Kisenyi sheep disease virus
kissing
k. bug
k. bug bite
kit
Arrow pneumothorax k.
insect sting k.
Pro-Vent arterial blood
sampling k.
Quantikine ELISA k.
Screening Patch Test K.
Klebsiella
K. oxytoca
K. pneumoniae
K. rhinoscleromatis
Klein-Waardenburg syndrome
Klerist-D Tablet
Klinefelter syndrome
Klippel-Trenaunay syndrome
Klippel-Trenaunay-Weber syndrome
Klonopin
Km
K. allotype
K. antigen

K

NOTES

knee
  housemaid k.
  knock k.
knife
  chalazion k.
Knight-Taylor brace
knock knee
knotted hair
knuckle pad
Köbberling-Duncan disease
Köbner
  K. effect
  K. epidermolysis bullosa
  K. phenomenon
  K. reaction
Koch
  K. bacillus
  K. law
  K. old tuberculin
  K. phenomenon
  K. postulate
  K. pustulate
kochia
Koenen tumor
Kogoj
  K. pustule
  spongiform pustule of K.
KOH
  potassium chloride stain
  potassium hydroxide
  KOH examination
  KOH preparation
Köhler
  K. disease
  K. line
Kohn pore
koilonychia
Kolmer test
Konakion injection

Koongol virus
Koplik spot
Korean
  K. hemorrhagic fever
  K. hemorrhagic fever virus
Kostmann syndrome
Kotonkan virus
kra-kra (*var. of* craw-craw)
Kramer-Collins Spore trap
kraurosis
  k. vulva
Krause gland
Kromayer lamp
Kronofed
krusei
  Candida k.
Kruskal-Wallis test
KS
  Kaposi sarcoma
KT
  Orudis K.
Kulchitsky cell
kuru
Kurunegala ulcer
Kveim
  K. antigen
  K. test
Kveim-Stilzbach antigen
kwashiorkor
  marasmic k.
Kwell
  K. Cream
  K. Lotion
  K. Shampoo
Kyasanur
  K. Forest disease
  K. Forest disease virus
Kyrle disease

L
L doses
L unit of streptomycin
LA
long acting
lupus anticoagulant
Dalalone L.
Dexasone L.
Phenylfenesin L.
Solurex L.
Theoclear L.
La
L. antigen
L. Crosse virus
labial
l. herpes simplex virus
labialis
herpes l.
keratosis l.
myxadenitis l.
labium
Laboratory
colony-stimulating factor-developed by Venereal Disease Research L. (CSF-VDRL)
Hollister-Stier L.
Medical Research Council L.'s (MRCL)
Venereal Disease Research L.'s (VDRL)
labrum
glenoid l.
lacerate
laceration
Lachman test
Lac-Hydrin
Lacril Ophthalmic solution
lacrimal
Lacrisert
lactalbumin
alpha l.
β-lactam
β-lactamase
CAZ -l.
lactase
lactate
l. dehydrogenase
l. dehydrogenase virus

lactea
crusta l.
lactenin
lactic
l. acidosis
l. acid and sodium-PCA
l. acid with ammonium hydroxide
LactiCare
L.-HC
Lactinol
lactobacillary milk
Lactobacillus
L. acidophilus
L. casei
lactobin
lactoferrin
lactoglobulin
beta l.
lactose
l. intolerance
l. malabsorption
lacuna
lacunae
osteocyte l.
lacunata
Moraxella l.
LAD
leukocyte adhesion deficiency
Laelaps echidninus
LAF-3
leukocyte antigen factor-3
lag phase
laidlawii
Acholeplasma l.
LAK
lymphokine-activated killer cell
lake
venous l.
Lalonde hook forceps
la main en lorgnette
LAMB
lentigines, atrial myxoma, mucocutaneous myxomas, and blue nevi
LAMB syndrome
lamb
lambda light chain
lamblia
Giardia l.

L

223

lamb's quarter
lame foliacée
lamella
    cornoid l.
lamellar
    l. congenital ichthyosiform
      erythroderma
    l. dominant
    l. dyshidrosis
    l. exfoliation of the newborn
    l. granule
    l. ichthyosis
    l. plates
    l. scale
lamina
    basal l.
    cell l.
    l. densa
    l. fusca
    l. lucida
    l. propria
    l. splendens
laminated epithelial plug
laminin
Lamisil
    L. tablet
    L. topical cream
lamivudine
    l., Epivir (3TC)
lamp
    black light l.
    heat l.
    Kromayer l.
    quartz l.
    ultraviolet l.
    uviol l.
    Wood l.
Lamprene
Lanacort
Lan antigen
Lanaphilic topical
Lancefield classification
lancet
    Pharmacia l.
    Phazet l.
Landry-Guillain-Barré syndrome
Landry syndrome
Landschutz tumor
Lane disease
Langerhans
    L. cell
    L. cell granule
    L. cell histiocytosis
Langer line

Langer line
Langhans cell
Laniazid Oral
lanolin
lanolin, cetyl alcohol, glycerin, and
    petrolatum
Lanophyllin-GG
lanosum
    Microsporum l.
Lansbury articular index
lansingensis
    Legionella l.
lanuginosa
    acquired hypertrichosis l.
    hypertrichosis l.
lanuginous
lanugo
    l. hair
Lanvisone topical
lapinization
lapinized
larbish
large
    l. cell lymphoma
    l. vessel vasculitis
large, external transformation-
    sensitive fibronectin (LETS)
large-joint inflammatory arthritis
large-molecular-weight drug
large-plaque parapsoriasis
Lariam
Larsen grading system
larva, pl. larvae
    brown-tail moth l.
    l. currens
    gypsy moth l.
    Io moth l.
    l. migrans
larvalis
    porrigo l.
laryngeal
    l. edema
    l. infection
    l. papillomatosis
laryngotracheitis
    avian infectious l.
laryngotracheobronchitis
    acute l.
LaseAway
    Polytec PI L.
laser
    alexandrite l.
    argon l.
    argon pumped tunable-dye l.

carbon dioxide l.
CO_2 l.
copper bromide l.
copper vapor l.
l. Doppler perfusion imaging
l. Doppler velocimetry
dye l.
flashlamp-pumped pulsed-dye l.
  (FLPD, FPDL)
frequency doubled
  neodymium:yttrium-aluminum-
  garnet l.
gallium-aluminum-arsenide 904-
  nm l.
Nd:YAG l.
pulsed dye l. (PDL)
Q-switched Nd:YAG l.
ruby l.
Spectrum ruby l.
l. surgery
YAG l.
Lassa
  L. hemorrhagic fever
  L. virus
Lassar paste
lata
  condylomata l.
  fascia l.
late
  l. benign syphilis
  l. latent syphilis
  l. onset neurofibromatosis
  l. phase allergic reaction
  l. reaction
  l. respiratory systemic
    syndrome (LRSS)
latency
latens
  scarlatina l.
latent
  l. allergy
  l. infection
  l. microbism
  l. period
  l. rat virus
  l. stage
  l. syphilis

late-onset spondyloepiphyseal
  dysplasia
late-phase response
lateralis
  nevus unius l.
  onychia l.
lateral nail fold
lateris
  nevus unius l.
laterosporus
  Bacillus l.
latex
  l. agglutination
  l. agglutination test
  l. fixation reaction
  l. fixation test
  l. hypersensitivity
  l. particle agglutination
  l. RIA panel
Laticaudinae
Latrodectus
  L. mactans
  L. mactans antivenom
  L. mactans bite
LATS
  long-acting thyroid stimulator
lattice fiber
latticework
latum
  condyloma l.
Laugier-Hunziger syndrome
laurel fever
LAV
  lymphadenopathy-associated virus
lava bean
lavage
  bronchoalveolar l. (BAL)
law
  Behring l.
  Farr l.
  Halsted l.
  Koch l.
  Marfan l.
  l. of priority
  Profeta l.
Lawrence-Seip syndrome

L

NOTES

225

laxa
    cutis l.
layer
    barrier l.
    basal cell l.
    Bowman l.
    cornified l.
    granular cell l.
    Henle l.
    horny l.
    horny cell l.
    Huxley l.
    hypertrophic smooth muscle l.
    malpighian l.
    mushroom-hook l.
    palisade l.
    prickle cell l.
    squamous cell l.
lazarine leprosy
Lazaro
    mal de San L.
LazerSporin-C Otic
LBT
    lupus band test
L-canavaline
LCD
    liquor carbonis detergens
LCMV
    lymphocytic choriomeningitis virus
LCR-based HLA typing
LCV
    leukocytoclastic vasculitis
LD
    lethal dose
LDA-1 antigen
LDH agent
L+ dose
LE
    lupus erythematosus
        LE cell
        discoid LE
        LE factor
        LE phenomenon
Le
    L. antigen
lead
    12-l. electrocardiogram
    l. poisoning
    l. stomatitis
leaflet
    mitral l.
    tricuspid valvular l.
leaf litter

learned helplessness
lectin
lectularius
    Cimex l.
Ledercillin VK Oral
leek
leg
    Barbados l.
    elephant l.
Legg-Calvé-Perthes disease
Legionella
    L. anisa
    L. birminghamensis
    L. bozemanii
    L. cincinnatiensis
    L. dumoffii
    L. feeleii
    L. jordanis
    L. lansingensis
    L. longbeachae
    L. maceachernii
    L. micdadei
    L. oakridgensis
    L. pneumophila
legionellosis
Legionnaire disease
legume
Leiner disease
leiodermia
leiomyoma
    l. cutis
    uterine l.
leiomyosarcoma
leiotrichous
Leishmania
    L. donovani
    L. orientalis
    L. tropica
leishmaniasis
    acute cutaneous l.
    American l.
    anergic l.
    anthroponotic cutaneous l.
    antimonial drug therapy for l.
    chronic cutaneous l.
    cutaneous l.
    diffuse cutaneous l.
    disseminated cutaneous l.
    dry cutaneous l.
    lupoid l.
    mucocutaneous l.
    nasopharyngeal l.
    New World l.

Old World l.
pseudolepromatous l.
l. recidivans
rural cutaneous l.
l. tegumentaria diffusa
l. tropica
urban cutaneous l.
visceral l.
wet cutaneous l.
zoonotic cutaneous l.
leishmanid
leishmanin test
leishmaniosis
leishmanoid
dermal l.
post-kala azar dermal l.
lemic
Lemierre disease
lemon
length
restriction fragment l.
Lennert lymphoma
lens
lenscale
lens-induced uveitis
lenticula
lenticular
l. syphilid
lenticulopapular
lentigines (*pl. of* lentigo)
l., atrial myxoma, mucocutaneous myxomas, and blue nevi (LAMB)
l., electrocardiographic defects, ocular hypertelorism, pulmonary stenosis, abnormalities of genitalia, retardation of growth, deafness (LEOPARD)
lentiginosis
centrofacial l.
generalized l.
inherited patterned l.
l. profusa
lentiginous
lentigo, pl. **lentigines**
genital l.

l. maligna
nevoid l.
nevus spilus l.
PUVA-induced l.
senile l.
l. senilis
simple l.
l. simplex
solar l.
Touraine centrofacial l.
lentil
Lentivirinae
lentivirus
lentogenic
leonine facies
leontiasis
LEOPARD
lentigines, electrocardiographic defects, ocular hypertelorism, pulmonary stenosis, abnormalities of genitalia, retardation of growth, deafness
LEOPARD syndrome
leopard
l. skin
leper
Lepidoglyphus destructor
Lepidoptera
lepidosis
Leporipoxvirus
lepothrix
lepra
l. bacillus
l. cells
leprae
Mycobacterium l.
leprid
leprologist
leprology
leproma
lepromatous
l. leprosy
l. nodule
l. reaction
lepromin
l. reaction
l. test

NOTES

227

leprosarium
leprose
leprosery
leprostatic
leprosum
    erythema nodosum l.
leprosus
    pemphigus l.
leprosy
    anesthetic l.
    articular l.
    borderline l.
    dimorphous l.
    dry l.
    histoid l.
    indeterminate l.
    intermediate l.
    lazarine l.
    lepromatous l.
    Lucio l.
    macular l.
    maculoanesthetic l.
    Malabar l.
    mixed l.
    mutilating l.
    neural l.
    nodular l.
    paucibacillary l.
    smooth l.
    trophoneurotic l.
    tuberculoid l.
leprotic
leprotica
    alopecia l.
leprous
leptochroa
leptodermic
Leptospira interrogans
leptospirosis
Leptothrix
Leptotrombidium akamushi
Lesch-Nyhan syndrome
Leser-Trélat sign
lesion
    acneform l.
    angioinvasive l.
    angioproliferative l.
    annular l.
    l. arrangement
    blanchable red l.
    blue-gray l.
    brown-black l.
    bullous l.

bullous skin l.
Bywaters l.
l. color
l. configuration
l. consistency
cutaneous l.
dermal l.
l. distribution
Division (I–IV) l.
eczematous l.
elementary l.
erysipelas-like skin l.
l. evolution
firm l.
genital papulosquamous l.
genitourinary l.
gross l.
hemorrhagic l.
histologic l.
infarctive l.
intravascular endothelial
    proliferative l.
Janeway l.
lichenified l.
linear l.
l. margination
medium l.
l. morphology
nickel and dime l.
nonblanchable, abnormally
    colored l.
nummular l.
ocular l.
oil drop l.
osseous l.
osteolytic bone l.
papulopustular l.
papulosquamous l.
papulovesicular l.
polypoid l.
precancerous l.
primary l.
proliferative l.
pruritic l.
pulmonary l.
purpuric l.
pustular l.
pyodermatous skin l.
reticular l.
rolled shoulder l.
satellite l.
scaling l.
scaling skin-colored l.

secondary l.
l. size
skin l.
skin-colored l.
slope shouldered l.
smooth l.
smooth skin-colored l.
soft l.
special l.
square shouldered l.
l. surface characteristic
target l.
traumatic l.
ulcer l.
varicelliform l.
vasculitic l.
venular l.
vesicobullous l.
vulvar l.
weeping l.
white l.
yellow l.
lethal
l. chondrodysplasia
l. dose (LD)
l. midline granuloma
l. midline granulomatosis
l. osteogenesis imperfecta
lethalis
epidermolysis bullosa l.
ichthyosis l.
lethargica
encephalitis l.
LETS
large, external transformation-
sensitive fibronectin
Letterer-Siwe disease
lettuce
Leu-3+ helper T cell
leu-CAM
leukocyte cell adhesion molecule
leucin
Leucomax
leucovorin
l. calcium
leukapheresis
leukasmus

leukemia
adult T-cell l. (ATL)
aleukemic l.
B-cell l.
B-cell lymphocytic l.
chronic T-cell l.
cutaneous B-cell lymphocytic l.
l. cutis
feline l.
l. of fowls
granulocytic l.
lymphocytic l.
monocytic l.
murine l.
myeloid l.
null cell l.
primary cutaneous B-cell
lymphocytic l.
secondary cutaneous B-cell
lymphocytic l.
T-cell l.
T-cell lymphocytic l.
thymus-derived l.
leukemid
Leukeran
leukin
leukoagglutinin
leukocidin
leukocytactic
leukocytaxia
leukocyte
l. adhesion deficiency (LAD)
l. antigen factor-3 (LAF-3)
l. attachment assay
l. cell adhesion molecule (leu-
CAM)
l. chemotaxis
l. common antigen
l. concentrate
l. factor antigen-1 (LFA-1)
l. histamine release
l. histamine release test
l. interferon
polymorphonuclear l. (PML)
leukocyte-poor preparation
leukocytoclastic vasculitis (LCV)
leukocytolysin

L

NOTES

leukocytolysis
leukocytolytic
leukocytosis
leukocytosis-promoting factor
leukocytotactic
leukocytotaxia
leukocytotoxin
leukoderma
    acquired l.
    l. acquisitum centrifugum
    chemical l.
    l. colli
    contact l.
    patterned l.
    syphilitic l.
leukodermatous
leukodermia
leukoencephalitis
    acute epidemic l.
    subacute sclerosing l.
leukoencephalopathy
    progressive multifocal l. (PML)
leukokeratosis
    l. oris
leukolysin
leukolysis
leukolytic
leukonecrosis
leukonychia
    apparent l.
    partial l.
leukopathia
    acquired l.
    l. unguis
leukopenia
leukopenic
    l. factor
    l. index
leukoplakia
    Candida l.
    candidal l.
    hairy l.
    oral hairy l.
    l. vulva
leukoplakic vulvitis
leukoplasia
leukorrhea
LeukoScan diagnostic agent
leukosialin
leukosis
    avian l.
    enzootic bovine l.
    fowl l.

leukotactic
leukotaxia
leukotaxine
leukotaxis
leukotoxin
leukotrichia
    l. annularis
leukotrichous
leukotriene
    l. antagonist
    l. B4 (LTB4)
    l. C
    l. E
    l. inhibition
    l. reduction
    l. regulation
Leukovirus
Leutrol
levamisole
levarterenol bitartrate
Levay antigen
level
    Clark l.
    fibrinogen l.
    free salicylate l.
    IgG subclass l.
    intrasynovial complement l.
    peak serum l.
    serum complement l.
    specific IgE antibody l.
    total serum IgE l.
Lever 2000
Leviviridae
levocabastine hydrochloride
levofloxacin
levonorgestrel
Levophed
    L. injection
Lewandowski
    nevus elasticus of L.
    rosacea-like tuberculid of L.
Lewandowski-Lutz
    epidermodysplasia verruciformis
    of L.-L.
Lewis
    L. Blood Group
    L. X oligosaccharide
Lf
    L. dose
LFA
    lymphocyte function-associated
    antigen

LFA-1
  leukocyte factor antigen-1
  lymphocyte function antigen-1
LFT
  liver function test
L-glutathione
LGV
  lymphogranuloma venereum
LH 7:2 antigen
l'homme rouge
liasis
Liatest C4b-BP test
liberator
  histamine l.
Librium
lice (*pl. of* louse)
  body l.
  End L.
  head l.
  pubic l.
Lice-Enz
lichen
  l. agrius
  l. albus
  l. amyloidosis
  l. annularis
  l. chronicus simplex
  l. corneus hypertrophicus
  l. hemorrhagicus
  l. infantum
  l. iris
  l. myxedematosus
  myxedematous l.
  l. nitidus
  l. nuchae
  l. obtusus
  l. obtusus corneus
  l. pilaris
  l. pilaris seu spinulosus
  l. planopilaris
  l. planus
  l. planus annularis
  l. planus et acuminatus
  atrophicans
  l. planus follicularis
  l. planus hypertrophicus
  l. planus-like keratosis

  l. planus pemphigoid
  l. planus verrucosus
  l. ruber
  l. ruber acuminatus
  l. ruber moniliformis
  l. ruber planus
  l. ruber verrucosus
  l. sclerosis et atrophicus
  (LS&A) ˹sclerosus˺
  l. sclerosus
  sclerosus l.
  l. sclerosus et atrophicans
  l. sclerosus scleroatrophy
  l. scrofulosorum
  l. scrofulous
  l. simplex chronicus (LSC)
  l. spinulosus
  l. striatus
  l. striatus epidermal nevus
  l. strophulosus
  l. syphiliticus
  l. trichophyticus
  tropical l.
  l. tropicus
  l. urticatus
  Wilson l.
lichenification
  giant l.
lichenified
  l. dermatitis
  l. lesion
  l. plaque
licheniformis
  Bacillus l.
lichenization
lichenoid
  l. acute pityriasis
  l. amyloidosis
  chronica parapsoriasis l.
  l. chronic dermatosis
  l. eczema
  l. eruption
  l. keratosis
  parapsoriasis l.
  pityriasis l.
  tuberculosis cutis l.
lichen-type scale

L

NOTES

licorice
Lida-Mantle HC topical
Lidex
    L. topical
Lidex-E topical
lidocaine
    bacitracin, neomycin, polymyxin
    B, and l.
    l. and epinephrine
    l. hydrochloride
    l. and hydrocortisone
LidoPen
ligamentosa
    spondylitis ossificans l.
ligament of Struthers
ligamentum nuchae
ligand
    addressing l.
    tissue l.
light
    Bili l.
    l. chain
    l. exposure
    long-wavelength ultraviolet l.
    (UVA)
    l. microscopy
    midrange spectrum
    ultraviolet l.
    midrange-wavelength
    ultraviolet l. (UVB)
    l. scatter technique
    l. treatment
    ultraviolet l.
    Wood l.
lignieresii
    Actinobacillus l.
lilac tree
lima bean
limb
    l. defects
    l. pain
limbal guttering
limbus, pl. limbi
lime
liminal
liminaris
    alopecia l.
limitation of exposure
limited
    l. progressive systemic
    sclerosis
    l. Wegener granulomatosis

limnophilus
    Paederus l.
Limulus lysate assay
lincomycin
lincosamide
Lindane
lindane
Lindner bodies
line
    Beau l.
    Blaschko l.
    cell l.
    cement l.
    Dennie l.
    Dennie-Morgan l.
    established cell l.
    Futcher l.
    Köhler l.
    Langer l.
    Mees l.
    Morgan l.
    Muerhrcke l.
    Muerhrcke l.
    Pastia l.
    pigmentary demarcation l.
    Sergent white l.
    tram l.
    Voigt l.
    white l.
linea, pl. lineae
    l. alba
    l. albicans
    l. nigra
linear
    l. atrophoderma of Moulin
    l. atrophy
    l. distribution
    l. epidermal nevus
    l. focal elastosis
    l. IgA bullous dermatosis
    l. IgA bullous disease
    l. lesion
    l. lichen planus
    l. nevus
    l. petechia
    l. porokeratosis
    l. progressive systemic
    sclerosis
    l. scleroderma
    l. scleroderma variant
    l. streaking
    l. teleangiectases

l. and whorled nevoid
   hypermelanosis
linearis
   morphea l.
lines of cleavage
lingua
   l. geographica
   l. plicata
   l. scrotalis
linguae
   exfoliatio areata l.
   nigrities l.
   pityriasis l.
   tylosis l.
lingula
liniment
lining
   synovial l.
linker
   tonofilament-cytoplasmic
      plaque l.
   transmembrane l.
linnaean system of nomenclature
linoleic acid
Linomide
linter
   cotton l.
Lioresal
LIP
   lymphocytic interstitial pneumonitis
lip cosmetic
lipedematous alopecia
lipid
   l. granulomatosis
   l. liquid crystal
   neutral l.
   l. storage disease
lipide
lipid-free cleanser
lipoatrophia annularis
lipoatrophy
   annular l.
   postinfection l.
   semicircular l.
lipocortin
lipodermatosclerosis

lipodystrophy
   acquired generalized l.
   acquired partial face-sparing l.
   congenital total l.
   intestinal l.
   partial l.
   partial face-sparing l.
5-lipogenase
lipogranulomatosis
   l. subcutanea
lipoid
   l. dermatoarthritis
   l. granuloma
   l. pneumonia
   l. proteinosis
lipoidica
   necrobiosis l.
lipoidosis
   l. cutis et mucosa
lipoma·
   l. arborescens
   atypical l.
   pleomorphic l.
   spindle cell l.
   synovial l.
lipomatodes
   nevus l.
lipomatosis
   benign symmetric l.
   mediastinal l.
   multiple symmetric l.
lipomatosus
   nevus l.
lipomelanic reticulosis
lipomelanotic
Liponyssus bacoti
lipophagic granuloma
lipopolysaccharide
   J5 l.
   l. vaccine
lipoprotein
   l. polymorphism
liposarcoma
liposomal doxorubicin
liposome
liposuction

L

NOTES

lipotrophy
    semicircular l.
lipovaccine
Lipovnik virus
lipoxin
lipoxygenase
lips
    cracked l.
    dry l.
    glowing red l.
    pseudocolloid of l.
Lipschütz ulcer
Lipsorex
lipstick
liquefaction
    l. degeneration
    l. necrosis
Liqui-Caps
    Vicks 44 Non-Drowsy Cold &
      Cough L.-C.
liquid
    Anaplex L.
    bland aerosolized l.
    Chlorafed L.
    l. ethyl chloride
    Gordofilm L.
    Hayfebrol L.
    l. human serum
    Lotrimin AF Spray L.
    l. nitrogen (LN$_2$)
    Occlusal-HP L.
    Rhinosyn L.
    Rhinosyn-PD L.
    Ryna L.
    Sudafed Plus L.
liquidambar
Liquid Pred Oral
Liquifilm
    L. Forte solution
    L. Tears
    L. Tears solution
Liqui-Gels
    Robitussin Severe
      Congestion L.-G.
Liquiprin
LiquiVent
liquor carbonis detergens (LCD)
Lisch nodule
lissotrichic
Listeria monocytogenes
listeriosis
litmus paper

litter
    leaf l.
Little League elbow
Live
    Bacillus Calmette-Guérin L.
    TICE Bacillus Calmette-
      Guérin L. (TICE BCG)
live
    measles virus vaccine, l.
    l. oak
    l. oak tree
    l. oral polio vaccine
    l. oral poliovirus vaccine
    rubella virus vaccine, l.
    l. vaccine
    varicella virus vaccine l.
livedo
    l. pattern
    l. patterned disease
    l. racemosa
    l. reticularis
    l. reticularis idiopathica
    l. reticularis symptomatica
    l. telangiectatica
    l. vasculitis
livedoid
    l. dermatitis
liver
    l. disease
    l. function test (LFT)
    l. palm
    l. spot
livid
lividity
livido
    lupus l.
livor
Livostin
    L. Ophthalmic
lizard
LMC
    lymphocyte-mediated cytotoxicity
LN
    lupus nephritis
LN$_2$
    liquid nitrogen
LNPF
    lymph node permeability factor
loa
    Filaria l.
loaiasis
lobar bronchus
lobenzarit disodium

loblolly
  l. pine
  l. pine tree
Lobo disease
lobomycosis
lobster
lobular panniculitis
local
  l. anaphylaxis
  l. immunity
  l. reaction
localized
  l. albinism
  l. angiokeratoma
  l. cutaneous amyloidosis
  l. granuloma annulare
  l. mucocutaneous candidiasis
  l. neurodermatitis
  l. pagetoid reticulosis
  l. pemphigoid of Brunsting-Perry
  l. progressive systemic sclerosis
  l. pustular psoriasis
  l. scleroderma
  l. vitiligo
loci (*pl. of* locus)
Locoid
locomotor ataxia
loculation
locus, pl. **loci**
locust
  black l.
lod
  logarithm of odds
lodgepole
  l. pine
  l. pine tree
Lodine
Lo dose
lodoxamide tromethamine
Loesche classification
Loewenthal reaction
Löffler syndrome
Lofgren syndrome
logarithmic phase
logarithm of odds (lod)

logit transformation
loiasis
Loiasis filariasis
Lolium
  L. perenne (Lol p)
  L. perenne allergen
Lol p
  Lolium perenne
Lol p allergen (I-III)
Lombardy
  L. poplar tree
lomefloxacin
  l. hydrochloride
lomustine
Lone Star tick
long
  l. incubation hepatitis
  l. terminal repeat sequences (LTR)
long acting (LA)
long-acting thyroid stimulator (LATS)
longbeachae
  Legionella l.
longior
  Tyroglyphus l.
longitudinal melanonychia
long-wavelength ultraviolet light (UVA)
look
  Hippocratic l.
loop
  l. diuretic
loose
  l. anagen hair syndrome
  l. body
  l. skin
loperamide
lophate
Loprox
Lopurin
Lorabid
loracarbef
loratadine
  l. and pseudoephedrine
lorgnette
  la main en l.

L

NOTES

Loroxide
loss
    chronic blood l.
    eyebrow l.
    eyelash l.
    hair l.
    hearing l.
    powered air l. (PAL)
    weight l.
lotion
    A/T/S l.
    calamine l.
    G-well L.
    Kwell L.
    Lotrimin AF L.
    Panscol L.
    Scabene L.
    Tinver L.
    triamcinolone l. (TAL)
Lotrimin
    L. AF Cream
    L. AF Lotion
    L. AF Powder
    L. AF solution
    L. AF Spray Liquid
    L. AF Spray Powder
Lotrisone
Lou Gehrig disease
Louis-Bar syndrome
louping
    l. ill
    l.-ill virus
louse, pl. **lice**
    body l.
    clothes l.
    crab l.
    head l.
    l. infestation
    pubic l.
    scalp l.
louse-borne relapsing fever
lousiness
lousy
Lovibond
    L. angle
    L. profile sign
Loviride
low
    l. flow rate
    l. frequency transduction
    l. plasma albumin
    l. urine pH
low-air-loss bed

low-egg-passage vaccine
Löwenstein-Jensen agar
lower respiratory tract infection
    (LRTI)
low-grade fever
Loxosceles
    L. reclusa
    L. reclusa bite
lozenge
    zinc gluconate l.
Lr dose
LRSS
    late respiratory systemic syndrome
LRTI
    lower respiratory tract infection
LS&A
    lichen sclerosis et atrophicus
LSC
    lichen simplex chronicus
L-selectin
LTB4
    leukotriene B4
LTR
    long terminal repeat sequences
L-tryptophan
    L.-t. ingestion
Lu antigen
lubricant
lubricant/emollient
    Bag Balm l.
    Udder Butter l.
lubrication
    skin l.
lubricin
Lubriderm
    L. moisturizer
LubriTears solution
lucent cleft
lucida
    lamina l.
lucidum
    stratum l.
Lucilia
Lucio
    L. leprosy
    L. leprosy phenomenon
Lucké
    L. adenocarcinoma
    L. carcinoma
    L. virus
lucotherapy
Ludwig angina
Luer-Lok syringe

lues
luetic mask
Lufyllin
Lukes-Collins classification
lumberman's itch
lumbricoides
    Ascaris *l.*
lumpy
    l. jaw
    l. skin disease
lunata
    Curvularia *l.*
lunate
lunate-capitate
lung
    bird-breeder's l.
    butterfly l.
    diffuse interstitial fibrosis of
      the l.
    l. disease
    farmer's l.
    humidifier l.
    l. interstitium
    l. involvement
    malt-worker's l.
    mushroom-worker's l.
    thresher's l.
lunula, pl. lunulae
    diffusion of the l.
    l. unguis
Lunyo virus
lupiform
lupinosa
    porrigo l.
lupoid
    l. hepatitis
    l. leishmaniasis
    l. sycosis
    l. ulcer
luposa
    tuberculosis cutis l.
lupous
lupus
    l. anticoagulant (LA)
    l. band test (LBT)
    chilblain l.
    cutaneous l.

discoid l.
drug-induced l.
    l. erythematodes
    l. erythematosus (LE)
    l. erythematosus cell
    l. erythematosus cell test
    l. erythematosus hypertrophicus
    l. erythematosus, neonatal
    l. erythematosus panniculitis
    l. erythematosus profundus
    l. erythematous-like rash
    l. glomerulonephritis
    l. livido
    l. lymphaticus
    l. miliaris disseminatus faciei
    l. mutilans
neonatal l.
    l. nephritis (LN)
    l. papillomatosus
    l. pernio
    l. profundus
    l. profundus/panniculitis
    l. sebaceous
    l. serpiginosus
    l. superficialis
    l. syndrome
    l. tuberculosus
    l. verrucosus
    l. vulgaris
lupus-like syndrome
lusitaniae
    Candida *l.*
Lutheran Blood Group
Lutzomyia
LVG
    lymphogranuloma venereum
lwoffi
    Acinetobacter *l.*
lycopenemia
Lyell
    L. disease
    L. syndrome
Lymantria
    L. dispar
    L. dispar sting
Lyme
    L. arthritis

L

NOTES

Lyme *(continued)*
  L. borreliosis
  L. disease
  L. disease DNA detection
  L. disease (stage 1–3)
lymhaticus
lymph
  l. cell
  l. gland
  l. node
  l. node biopsy
  l. node permeability factor
    (LNPF)
  vaccine l.
lymphadenitis
  necrotizing l.
  regional granulomatous l.
  tuberculosis l.
lymphadenoma
lymphadenomatosis
lymphadenopathy
  angioblastic l.
  angioimmunoblastic l. (AIL)
  dermatopathic l.
  drug-induced l.
  hilar l.
lymphadenopathy-associated virus
  (LAV)
lymphadenosis
  benign l.
  l. benigna cutis
  l. cutis benigna
lymphangiectasia
lymphangiectasis
lymphangiectatica
  pachyderma l.
lymphangiectodes
lymphangioleiomyomatosis
lymphangioma
  l. capillare varicosum
  cavernous l.
  l. circumscriptum
  solitary simple l.
  l. superficium simplex
lymphangiomyomatosis
lymphangitis
  penile sclerosing l.
  sclerosing l.
lymphapheresis
lymphatic malformation
lymphatics
  dermal l.

lymphaticus
  lupus l.
  nevus l.
lymphedema
  chronic hereditary l.
  primary l.
  secondary l.
lymphedematous keratoderma
lymphoblastoma
lymphocytapheresis
B-lymphocyte
lymphocyte
  B l.
  cytotoxic T l. (CTL)
  l. function antigen-1 (LFA-1)
  l. function assay
  l. function-associated antigen
    (LFA)
  l. homing receptor
  sensitized l.
  l. serine esterase
  T l.
  l. transformation
  transformed l.
  tumor-infiltrating l. (TILS)
lymphocyte-mediated cytotoxicity
  (LMC)
lymphocytic
  l. choriomeningitis virus
    (LCMV)
  l. disease
  l. hypophysitis
  l. infiltrate of Jessner
  l. infiltration
  l. infiltration of the skin
  l. interstitial pneumonitis (LIP)
  l. leukemia
lymphocytoma
  Borrelia l.
  l. cutis
lymphocytopenia
lymphocytosis
  diffuse infiltrative l.
  l. syndrome
lymphocytotoxic antibody
lymphoderma
lymphoepithelioid lymphoma
lymphogenous metastasis
Lymphogranuloma
  L. venereum conjunctivitis
lymphogranuloma
  l. inguinale
  l. venereum (LGV, LVG)

l. venereum antigen
l. venereum virus
lymphogranulomatosis
l. benigna
l. maligna
lymphohistiocytic
lymphoid
l. cell
l. hypophysitis
l. infiltrate
lymphokine
l.-activated killer cell (LAK)
production of l.
lympholeukocyte
lymphoma
adult T-cell l.
African Burkitt l.
angiocentric l.
angiodestructive l.
B-cell l.
Burkitt l.
cutaneous B-cell l.
cutaneous T-cell l. (CTCL)
gingival l.
granulomatous cutaneous T-cell l.
high-grade small noncleaved cell malignant l.
histiocytic l.
Hodgkin l.
large cell l.
Lennert l.
lymphoepithelioid l.
malignant l.
MALT l.
non-Hodgkin l. (NHL)
peripheral T-cell l.
primary cutaneous B-cell l.
primary cutaneous T-cell l.
pseudomalignant l.
pulmonary l.
retrovirus-associated l.
secondary cutaneous B-cell l.
signet ring l.
subcutaneous T-cell l.
T-cell l.

lymphoma-leukemia
adult T-cell l.-l.
lymphomatoid
l. granulomatosis
l. papulosis
lymphomatosis
avian l.
fowl l.
ocular l.
visceral l.
lymphopathia
l. venereum
lymphopenia
lymphopenic thymic dysplasia
lymphoplasmacytapheresis
lymphoplasmacytic
lymphoproliferative disease
lymphoreticular disorder
lymphoreticulosis
benign inoculation l.
lymphostatic verrucosis
lymphotoxicity
lymphotoxin
LYOfoam dressing
lyophilized extract
lyophilized immunoglobulin G
Lyphocin injection
lysate
lyse
lysin
lysinogen
lysinogenic
lysis
endothelial l.
lysogen
lysogenesis
lysogenic
l. bacterium
l. induction
l. strain
lysogenicity
lysogenization
lysogeny
lysosomal
l. enzyme
l. proteinase
lysosome

L

NOTES

lysosomotropic anti-malarial drug
lysozyme
    tear l.
lyssa
Lyssavirus
lysyl oxidase
Lyt antigens

lytic
    l. enzyme
Lytta
    L. vesicata
    L. vesicata sting
lytta
lyze

M
M antigen
M protein
M1
streptococcal M.
2M
A 2M
2-microglobulin-origin
amyloid deposit
M3
streptococcal M.
MA
monoarthritis
MAB
monoclonal antibody
MAC
membrane attack complex
membranolytic attack complex
Mycobacterium avium complex
Mycobacterium avium-intracellulare
maceachernii
Legionella m.
macerate
macerated
maceration
interdigital m.
plantar m.
machination
machine
CPM m.
G5 massage and percussion m.
Respitrace m.
machinery
intercellular m.
Machupo virus
MacMARCKS protein
Macrobid
macrocheiria, macrochiria
macrochilia
macrocytase
macrodactylia
Macrodantin
macroglobulin
α2-m.
macroglobulinemia
Waldenström m.
macroglossia
macrolabia
macrolide antimicrobial agent
macromelia

macromolecule
bacterial m.
matrix m.
macronychia
macrophage
activated m.
alveolar m.
armed m.
associated m.
dendritic m.
hemosiderin-laden m.
immune-associated antigen-
positive m. (Ia+)
inflammatory m.
m. inflammatory protein (MIP)
m. migration inhibition test
system of m.
macrophage-activating factor (MAF)
macrophagocyte
macroscopic
m. agglutination test
mactans
Latrodectus m.
macula, pl. maculae
m. atrophica
m. cerulea
m. gonorrhoica
mongolian m.
Saenger m.
macular
m. amyloidosis
m. atrophy
m. erythema
m. leprosy
m. purpura
m. rash
m. syphilid
maculata
pityriasis m.
maculation
maculatum
atrophoderma m.
macule
atrophic m.
evanescent m.
hypopigmented m.
maculoanesthetic leprosy
maculoerythematous
maculopapular rash
maculopapule

maculosa
    urticaria m.
Madajet XL local anesthesia
madarosis
Madelung disease
madescent
madidans
mad itch
madre
    buba m.
Madura
    M. boil
    M. foot
madurae
    Actinomadura m.
Madurella
    M. grisea
    M. mycetomi
maduromycosis
maedi
    m. virus
MAF
    macrophage-activating factor
mafenide acetate
Maffucci syndrome
Magellan Monitor
maggot
    Congo floor m.
magnesium sulfate
magnetic resonance imaging (MRI)
magnus
    Peptostreptococcus m.
MAI
    Mycobacterium avium-intracellulare
    MAI bacteremia
maintenance dose
Majocchi
    M. disease
    M. granuloma
    M. purpura
    purpura annularis telangiectodes
      of M.
major
    m. agglutinin
    aphthae m.
    Babesia m.
    m. basic protein
    erythema multiforme m.
    m. histocompatibility
    m. histocompatibility complex
      (MHC)
    thalassemia m.
    variola m.

major histocompatibility complex
    class I
makeup
    Covermark corrective m.
mal
    m. de Cayenne
    m. de los pintos
    m. de Meleda
    m. de San Lazaro
    m. perforans
    m. perforant
Malabar
    M. itch
    M. leprosy
malabarica
    phlegmasia m.
malabsorption
    fat m.
    lactose m.
malachite green
malaise
malakoplakia
malaleuca tree
malar
    m. butterfly rash
    m. erythema
    m. rash (MR)
malaria
    apocrine m.
    cerebral m.
    m. prophylaxis
    therapeutic m.
malariae
    Plasmodium m.
Malassezia
    M. furfur
    M. ovalis
malayi
    Brugia m.
male
    m. pattern alopecia
    m. pattern baldness
maleate
    azatadine m.
    brompheniramine m.
    chlorpheniramine m.
    dexchlorpheniramine m.
    methysergide m.
malformation
    arteriovenous m. (AVM)
    capillary m.
    lymphatic m.
    venous m.

Malherbe
    calcifying epithelioma of M.
    epithelioma of M.
maligna
    lentigo m.
    lymphogranulomatosis m.
    onychia m.
    papulosis atrophicans m.
    scarlatina m.
    variola m.
malignancy
    myositis with m.
    systemic m.
malignant
    m. acanthosis nigricans
    m. angioendotheliomatosis
    m. atrophic papulosis
    m. bubo
    m. catarrhal fever
    m. catarrhal fever virus
    m. catarrh of cattle
    m. degeneration
    m. down
    m. dyskeratosis
    m. fibrous histiocytoma
    m. hemangioendothelioma
    m. hemangiopericytoma
    m. histiocytosis
    m. lentigo melanoma
    m. lymphoma
    m. melanoma
    m. melanoma in situ
    m. mole syndrome
    m. neoplasia
    m. neoplastic disease
    m. papillomatosis
    m. papillomatosis of Degos
    m. peripheral nerve sheath
    tumor
    m. progression
    m. pustule
    m. pyoderma
    m. smallpox
    m. systemic mastocytosis
    m. transformation
    m. tumor

maligne
    papulose atrophicante m.
malignum
    keratoma m.
malingering
mallei
    Malleomyces m.
mallein
malleinization
Malleomyces
    M. mallei
    M. pseudomallei
mallet toe
malnutrition
    episodic m.
Maloney leukemia virus
malpighian layer
malpighii
    stratum m.
MALT
    mucosa-associated lymphoid tissue
    MALT lymphoma
malt
Malta fever
maltase
    acid m.
Maltese cross
maltophilia
    Stenotrophomonas m.
    Xanthomonas m.
malt-worker's lung
malum
    m. perforans
    m. perforans pedis
Malvern analyzer
mamanpian
mammary
    m. cancer virus of mice
    m. Paget disease
    m. tumor virus of mice
mammillitis
    bovine herpes m.
    bovine ulcerative m.
    bovine vaccinia m.
Manchurian hemorrhagic fever
Mancini technique

M

NOTES

mandibulae
  torus m.
mandibular torus
Mandol
maneuver
  Apley m.
  Proetz m.
  Valsalva m.
mange
  demodectic m.
  follicular m.
  sarcoptic m.
mango dermatitis
manifestation
  allergic m.
  clinical m.
  cutaneous m.
  mucocutaneous m.
  presenting clinical m.
mannequin
mannitol
Mann-Whitney U test
man-of-war
  Portuguese m.-o.-w.
Mansonella
  M. ozzardi
  M. streptocerca
mansoni
  Schistosoma m.
mansonii
  Cladosporium m.
Manson pyosis
Mantadil
M₁ antigen
Mantoux
  M. pit
  M. test
manubriosternal joint
manum
manus
  tinea m.
  tinea pedis et m.
manuum
  keratolysis exfoliativa areata m.
maple
  box elder m.
  red m.
  sugar m.
  m. tree
Maranox
marasmic kwashiorkor
marasmus
Marax

Marbaxin
marble skin
Marburg
  M. virus
  M. virus disease
Marcaine
marcescens
  Serratia m.
Marcillin
Marek
  M. disease
  M. disease virus
Marezine
Marfan
  M. law
  M. syndrome
marfanoid
  m. habitus
  m. hypermobility syndrome
margarine disease
marginal band
marginalis
  alopecia m.
  keratoelastoidosis m.
marginata
  alopecia m.
margination
  lesion m.
marginatum
  eczema m.
  erythema m.
Marie-Strümpell disease
marine
  m. animal sting
Marinesco-Sjögren syndrome
Marinesco succulent hand
Marinol
marinum
  Mycobacterium m.
Marjolin ulcer
mark
  beauty m.
  dhobie m.
  ecchymotic m.
  erythematous m.
  port-wine m.
  strawberry m.
  Unna m.
  washerman's m.
marked localized reaction
marker
  allotypic m.
  cell m.

cell surface m.
genetic m.
pan T-cell m.
solid-tumor m.
tumor m.
market men disease
markings
bronchovascular m.
marks
stretch m.
Marmine Oral
marmorata
cutis m.
marmorated
marmorization
marmoset virus
marneffei
Penicillium m.
Maroteaux-Lamy
M.-L. mucopolysaccharidosis
M.-L. syndrome
Marseilles fever
Marshall syndrome
marsh elder
marsupialization
Marthritic
mascara
solvent-based m.
water-based m.
maschalephidrosis
maschalyperidrosis
mask
luetic m.
Neutrogena Acne M.
PEP m.
m. of pregnancy
Swiss Therapy eye m.
tropical m.
masked virus
Mason-Pfizer virus
masoprocol
m. cream
masque biliaire
MASS
mitral valve prolapse, aortic

anomalies, skeletal changes, and
skin changes
MASS syndrome
mass
m. infection
m. median aerodynamic
diameter (MMD)
Masson
M. intravascular endothelial
proliferation
M. pseudoangiosarcoma
mast
m. cell
m. cell inhibitor
m. cell proteinase
Mastadenovirus
mastectomy
radical m.
Mastisol
mastitis
bovine m.
mastocyte
mastocytoma
mastocytosis
benign systemic m.
cutaneous m.
diffuse cutaneous m.
malignant systemic m.
papular m.
systemic m.
telangiectatic systemic m.
mastoiditis
Masugi nephritis
mat
m. burn
Harris pressure m.
material
absorbent gelling m. (AGM)
cross-reacting m.
Epicel skin graft m.
keratinous m.
keratotic m.
test m.
maternal immunity
matrilysin
matrix
m. component

M

NOTES

245

matrix *(continued)*
  distal nail m.
  extracellular m. (ECM)
  m. macromolecule
  m. metalloproteinase (MMP)
  m. metalloproteinase-2 (MMP-2)
  m. metalloproteinase-3 (MMP-3)
  m. metalloproteinase-7 (MMP-7)
  m. metalloproteinase-8 (MMP-8, MMP-9)
  m. metalloproteinase-10 (MMP-10)
  nail m.
  proximal nail m.
matter
  particulate m.
mattress
  AkroTech m.
  convoluted foam m.
  vinyl-alternating air m.
maturation
  affinity m.
mature bacteriophage
max
  VO_2 m.
  maximal oxygen consumption
Maxair Autohaler
Maxaquin Oral
Max-Caro
Maxidex
Maxiflor
  M. topical
maximal
  m. oxygen consumption (VO_2 max)
  m. ventilation (MV)
  m. voluntary ventilation (MVV)
maximum
  m. breathing capacity (MBC)
  M. Strength Desenex Antifungal Cream
  M. Strength Nytol
  m. temperature
Maxi-Myst
  M.-M. bronchodilator
Maxipime
Maxitrol Ophthalmic
Maxivate
Maxivent

Mayaro virus
mayfly, may fly
maynei
  Euroglyphus m.
Mayo
  M. classification of rheumatoid elbow
  M. modified total elbow arthroplasty
mazamorra
Mazzotti
  M. reaction
  M. test
MBC
  maximum breathing capacity
  minimal bactericidal concentration
McArdle disease
McCune-Albright syndrome
MCF
  monocyte chemotactic factor
McKeever and MacIntosh hemiarthroplasty
McKenzie test
McKusick
  oculocerebral syndrome of Cross and M.
McMurray sign
McNemar
  M. test
  M. test of significance
MCP-1
  monocyte chemoattractant protein-1
m-cresyl acetate
MCTD
  mixed connective tissue disease
MDI
  metered-dose inhaler
  isocyanate MDI
MDR-TB
  multi-drug-resistant tuberculosis
MDS
  myelodysplastic syndrome
meadow
  m. fescue
  m. fescue grass
  m. foxtail
  m. foxtail grass
  m. grass dermatitis
meal
  rye m.
  soybean m.
mean forced expiratory flow during the middle of FVC ($FEF_{25-75\%}$)

measles
    atypical m.
    m. convalescent serum
    German m.
    m. immune globulin (human)
    m. immunoglobulin
    modified m.
    m., mumps, and rubella
      vaccine (MMR)
    m., mumps and rubella
      vaccines, combined
    m. and rubella vaccines,
      combined
    three-day m.
    tropical m.
    m. virus
    m. virus vaccine
    m. virus vaccine, live
measles,
measles-mumps-rubella (MMR)
measures
    CD4+ m.
Measurin
meatus
mebendazole
mechanica
    acne m.
mechanical
    m. abrasion
    m. pleurodesis
    m. vector
    m. ventilation (MV)
    m. ventilator
    m. vessel blockage
mechanic hand
mechanism
    m. of action
    defense m.
    immunological m.
    jet-bubble m.
mechanoblister
mechanobullous disease
mechlorethamine hydrochloride
Mecholyl skin test
Meclan topical
meclizine hydrochloride
meclocycline sulfosalicylate

meclofenamate sodium
Meclomen Oral
media
    acute otitis m. (AOM)
    chronic otitis m.
    otitis m.
    pneumococcal otitis m.
    radiographic contrast m.
      (RCM)
    secretory otitis m.
median
    m. raphe cyst of the penis
    m. rhomboid glossitis
    m. survival time (MST)
mediana
    glossitis rhombica m.
mediastinal
    m. amyloidosis
    m. lipomatosis
mediastinoscopy
mediate contagion
mediation
    fibroblast m.
mediator
    vasoactive m.
Medical
    M. Dynamics 5990 needle
      arthroscope
    M. Research Council (MRC)
    M. Research Council
      Laboratories (MRCL)
medical therapy
medicamentosa
    acne m.
    alopecia m.
    dermatitis m.
    dermatosis m.
    rhinitis m.
    stomatitis m.
    urticaria m.
medicamentosus
medicinal eruption
medicine
    Reese's Pinworm M.
    sports m.
Medi-Facts system

M

NOTES

Medihaler
    M.-Epi
    M. Ergotamine
    M.-Iso
Medimist
Medi-Mist nebulizer
medinensis
    Dracunculus m.
Mediplast Plaster
Medipren
Medi-Quick Topical Ointment
Mediterranean
    M. exanthematous fever
    M. fever
medium
    dermatophyte test m. (DTM)
    Dulbecco m.
    Iscove modified Dulbecco m.
    m. lesion
    Sabouraud m.
    Thayer-Martin m.
medi virus
Medlar bodies
Medpor surgical implant
Medralone injection
Medrol
    M. Dosepak
    M. Oral
medrysone
medulla
Mees
    M. line
    M. stripes
MEF
    middle ear fluid
mefenamic acid
mefloquine
    m. hydrochloride
Mefoxin
Megabombus
Megabombus **sting**
Megace
megacins
megaloblastic
megalonychia
megalonychosis
Megalopyge
    M. opercularis
    M. opercularis sting
megaterium
    Bacillus m.
megestrol acetate
meglumine diatrizoate enema study

meibomian
    m. gland
    m. gland dysfunction
Meinicke test
Meissner corpuscle
mekongi
    Schistosoma m.
Melacine vaccine
melanidrosis
melanin
    hair m.
    m. synthesis
    m. transfer
    white m.
melaninogenica
    Prevotella m.
melanism
melanoacanthoma
    oral m.
melanoblast
melanoblastoma
melanocarcinoma
melanocomous
melanocyte
    intradermal m.
β-melanocyte-stimulating hormone
melanocyte-stimulating hormone
    (MSH)
α-melanocyte-stimulating hormone
    (α-MSH)
melanocytic nevus
melanoderma
    m. cachecticorum
    m. chloasma
    parasitic m.
    racial m.
    Riehl m.
    senile m.
melanodermatitis
melanodermia
melanodermic
melanogenesis
melanohidrosis
melanoid
melanoleukoderma
    m. colli
melanoma
    acral lentiginous m.
    amelanotic m.
    benign juvenile m.
    desmoplastic malignant m.
    halo m.
    juvenile m.

malignant m.
malignant lentigo m.
minimal deviation m.
nodular m.
nodular malignant m.
subungual m.
superficial malignant m.
superficial spreading m.
m. warning sign
melanomatosis
melanomatous
melanonychia
longitudinal m.
m. striata
melanopathy
melanophage
melanophore
melanoplakia
melanoprotein
melanosis
m. circumscripta precancerosa
m. corii degenerativa
m. diffusa congenita
generalized m.
neonatal pustular m.
neurocutaneous m.
oculodermal m.
pustular m.
Riehl m.
transient neonatal pustular m.
melanosity
melanosome
melanotic
m. carcinoma
m. freckle
m. freckle of Hutchinson
m. progonoma
m. whitlow
melanotrichous
melas
icterus m.
melasma
m. gravidarum
m. universale
melatonin
Meleda
mal de M.

Meleney
chronic undermining ulcer
of M.
M. gangrene
M. ulcer
melioidosis
Melkersson-Rosenthal syndrome
mellifera
Apis m.
mellitus
diabetes m.
insulin-dependent diabetes m.
(IDDM)
non-insulin-dependent
diabetes m. (NIDDM)
Meloidae
melorheostosis
melphalan
Melzer reagent
membrane
antiglomerular basement m.
(anti-GMB)
m. attack complex (MAC)
basal cell m.
basement m.
bronchial mucous m.
Bruch m.
collodion m.
croupous m.
false m.
m. filter
focal rupture of basement m.
hyaline basement m.
mucous m.
PAN m.
plasma m.
semi-impermeable m.
Seprafilm bioresorbable m.
synovial m.
tympanic m. (TM)
membrane-coating granule
membranolytic attack complex
(MAC)
membranous
m. glomerulonephritis
m. nephropathy

M

NOTES

memory
 B-cell m.
 immune m.
MEN ⁻
 multiple endocrine neoplasia
 multiple endocrine neoplasms
 MEN syndrome
Menadol
Mendelson syndrome
Mengo
 M. encephalitis
 M. virus
Meni-D
méningéale
 tache m.
meningeal stage
meningioma
 cutaneous m.
meningitic streak
meningitidis
 Neisseria m.
meningitis, pl. meningitides
 bacterial m. (BM)
 cerebrospinal m.
 epidemic cerebrospinal m.
 Haemophilus influenzae m.
 meningococcal m.
meningocele
 atretic m.
meningococcal
 m. arthritis
 m. meningitis
 m. polysaccharide vaccine,
  groups A, C, Y and W-135
 m. vaccine
meningococcemia
 acute m.
meningoencephalitis
 acute primary hemorrhagic m.
 biundulant m.
 herpetic m.
 mumps m.
meningo-oculofacial angiomatosis
meningosepticum
 Flavobacterium m.
meningovasculitis
meniscus, pl. menisci
Menkes kinky hair syndrome
menocelis
Menomune-A/C/Y/W-135
menopausal flushing
menstrual acne
mentagra

mentagrophytes
 Trichophyton m.
menthol
 camphorated m.
meperidine
Mephyton Oral
mepivacaine
 m. hydrochloride
Mepron
meralgia ʿparesthetica
merbromin
2-mercaptoethane sulphonate sodium
 (mesna)
6-mercaptopurine (6-MP)
mercurial stomatitis
mercuric oxide
mercurochrome
mercury
 m. arc
 m. hyperpigmentation
 m. poisoning
meridian
Merkel
 M. cell
 M. cell carcinoma
 M. cell tumor
Merkel-Ranvier
 tactile cell of M.-R.
Merlenate topical
merocrine gland
meropenem
merosin
merozygote
Merrem
Mersol
Merthiolate
Meruvax II
mesalamine
Mesalt dressing
mesenchymal
 m. cell
 m. tissue
mesenchyme
 synovial m.
mesenteric vasculitis
meshwork
 coagulation m.
mesna
 2-mercaptoethane sulphonate sodium
mesoderm
mesodermal
 m. dysplasia
 m. nevus
mesogenic

mesophilic
mesosyphilis
mesothelioma
mesquite tree
mesylate
    bitolterol m.
    delavirdine m.
    dihydroergotamine m.
    saquinavir m.
Metabisulfite
metabolic
    m. acidosis
    m. alteration
    m. bone disease
    m. disorder
    m. study
metabolism
    amino acid m.
    copper m.
    phenylalanine m.
    tyrosine m.
metabolite
    arachidonic acid m.
    16-hydroxylated m.
    oxygen m.
metacarpal index
metacarpophalangeal (MP)
metachromasia
metaguazone
metal
    m. fume fever
    m. hyperpigmentation
    m. intoxication
metalloenzyme
metalloproteinase
    matrix m. (MMP)
    punctated m.
metalloproteinase-2
    matrix m. (MMP-2)
metalloproteinase-3
    matrix m. (MMP-3)
metalloproteinase-7
    matrix m. (MMP-7)
metalloproteinase-8
    matrix m. (MMP-8, MMP-9)
metalloproteinase-10
    matrix m. (MMP-10)

metalloscopy
Metamucil
metaphyseal
metaphysis, pl. metaphyses
metaplasia
    goblet cell m.
metaplastic mucus-secreting cell
Metaprel
metaproterenol
    Arm-a-Med M.
    Dey-Dose M.
    m. sulfate
metaraminol bitartrate
Metasep
metastasis
    biochemical m.
    hematogenous m.
    lymphogenous m.
    tumor, node, m. (TNM)
metastatic
    m. calcinosis cutis
    m. granuloma
    m. mumps
metatarsalgia
metatypical carcinoma
Metazoa
metazoal parasite
metazoonosis
Metchnikoff theory
meter
    Assess peak flow m.
    Astech peak flow m.
    Mini-Wright peak flow m.
    peak flow m.
    Pocketpeak peak flow m.
    TruZone peak flow m.
metered-dose inhaler (MDI)
methacholine
    m. bronchoprovocation
    challenge
    m. challenge
    m. chloride
    m. chloride skin test
methenamine
methicillin-resistant *Staphylococcus aureus* (MRSA)
methicillin sodium

M

NOTES

methionine
methocarbamol
method
 Dick m.
 disk sensitivity m.
 double antibody m.
 immunofluorescence m.
 Kaplan-Meier m.
 Ouchterlony m.
 prick-test m.
 Ranawat triangle m.
 Schick m.
 volumetric m.
methotrexate (MTX)
methoxsalen
methoxycinnamate and oxybenzone
methoxypsoralen
5-methoxypsoralen (5-MOP)
8-methoxypsoralen (8-MOP)
methyldopa
methylmethacrylate
methylprednisolone
 m. acetate
 pulse m.
methylxanthine
methysergide maleate
Meticorten Oral
Metimyd Ophthalmic
Metreton Ophthalmic
MetroGel
Metro I.V. injection
metronidazole
Mexican tea
mexiletine
Mezlin
mezlocillin
 m. sodium
MG
 myasthenia gravis
MHA-TP
 microhemagglutination-*Treponema pallidum*
 MHA-TP test
MHC
 major histocompatibility complex
 chromosome 6, class III M.
 M. restriction
MI
 myocardial infarction
Miacalcin
Mibelli
 angiokeratoma of M.
 M. disease

 porokeratosis of M.
 M. porokeratosis
MIC
 minimal inhibitory concentration
 minimum inhibitory concentration
micaceous scale
Micanol
Micatin
 M. topical
micdadei
 Legionella m.
mice
 mammary cancer virus of m.
 mammary tumor virus of m.
 New Zealand m.
 pneumonia virus of m. (PVM)
 SCID m.
 severe combined
  immunodeficient m.
 transgenic m.
miconazole
Micro
 M. Mist nebulizer
 M. Plus spirometer
microabscess
 intraepidermal m.
 Munro m.
 m. of mycosis fungoides
 Pautrier m.
 m. of psoriasis
microangiopathic hemolytic anemia
microaspiration
microbe
microbial
 m. associates
 m. genetics
 m. persistence
 m. vitamin
microbic
microbicidal
microbicide
microbid
microbiologic
microbiologist
microbiology
microbiotic
microbism
 latent m.
microceras
 Dermatophagoides m.
microcontaminant
MicroDigitrapper
 M.-HR

M.-S
M.-V
microemulsion
cyclosporine m.
microevolution
microfibril
microfilaria
degenerated m.
microfocus, pl. **microfoci**
MicroGard
microglobulin
2-m.
β$_2$-m.
2-m.-origin amyloid deposit (A 2M)
micrognathia
microhemagglutination
microhemagglutination-*Treponema pallidum* (MHA-TP)
m. test
microheterogeneity
microimmunofluorescence test (MIF)
microNefrin
micronychia
microorganism
micropapular tuberculid
microphage
microphagocyte
Micropolyspora faeni
Micropore tape
microscope
electron m. (EM)
microscopic
m. agglutination test
m. polyangiitis
microscopically controlled surgery
microscopy
darkfield m.
electron m.
immunofluorescence m.
light m.
microshaver
Stryker m.
microspherule
microspore
Microsporidia
microsporidia diagnostic procedure

microsporidiosis
microsporosis
Microsporum, Microsporon
M. audouinii
M. canis
M. canis, var distortum
M. felineum
M. ferrugineum
M. fulvum
M. furfur
M. gypseum
M. lanosum
M. minutissimum
M. nanum
Microsulfon
microti
Babesia m.
microtrauma
postexertional m.
Microtrombidium
microvascular abnormality
microvesicle
Microviridae
MID
minimal infecting dose
midazolam
benzodiazepine m.
middle
m. ear
m. ear fluid (MEF)
midfoot
midge
m. bite
nimitti m.
midline
m. granulomatosis
m. lethal granuloma
Midol
M. IB
M. PM
midpoint skin test
midrange
m. spectrum ultraviolet light
m.-wavelength ultraviolet light (UVB)
Midrin

M

NOTES

Miescher
  M. cheilitis granulomatosa
  M. elastoma
  M. granuloma
MIF
  microimmunofluorescence test
  migration-inhibitory factor
migrans
  annulus m.
  cutaneous larva m.
  erysipelas m.
  erythema m. (EM)
  erythema chronicum m.
  erythema nodosum m.
  larva m.
  ocular larma m.
  spiruroid larva m.
  ulcus m.
  visceral larva m.
migration
  m. inhibition test
  m. inhibitory factor test
migration-inhibitory factor (MIF)
migratory glossitis
Mikulicz
  M. aphtha
  M. disease
mild
  m. hypertension
  m. irritant
  silver protein, m.
milia (*pl. of* milium)
Milian
  M. disease
  M. erythema
miliaria
  m. alba
  apocrine m.
  m. crystallina
  m. profunda
  pustular m.
  m. pustulosa
  m. rubra
miliaris
  acne m.
  acne necrotica m.
  tuberculosis cutis m.
  variola m.
miliary
  m. acne
  m. fever

  m. papular syphilid
  m. tuberculosis
milium, pl. milia
  colloid m.
  milia cyst
  juvenile colloid m.
  pinhead-sized milia
  pinpoint-sized milia
milk
  acidophilus m.
  cow's m.
  m. crust
  m. factor
  goat's m.
  lactobacillary m.
  m. scall
  soy m.
  m. tetter
milkers'
  m. node
  m. nodule
  m. nodule virus
milk-induced colitis
milkpox
Miller-Fisher variant
miller's asthma
millet seed
mill fever
millipede sting
millipore
milphosis
Milroy disease
Milton disease
Milwaukee shoulder syndrome
mimicry
  molecular m.
mineralocorticoid
mineral oil
mineral-related nutritional disorder
miniature scarlet fever
Min-I-Jet
minimal
  m. bactericidal concentration
    (MBC)
  m. deviation melanoma
  m. dose possible
  m. infecting dose (MID)
  m. inhibitory concentration
    (MIC)
  m. lethal dose (MLD)
  m. pigment (MP)
  m. reacting dose (MRD)

minimal-pigment oculocutaneous albinism
minimum
   m. inhibitory concentration (MIC)
   m. temperature
MiniOX
   M. 1000
   M. 1A oxygen analyzer
Minipress
Miniscope MS-3
Mini Thin Asthma Relief
Mini-Wright peak flow meter
mink
   enteritis of m.
   m. enteritis virus
Minnesota Multiphasic Personality Inventory (MMPI)
Minocin
   M. IV injection
   M. Oral
minocycline
   m. hydrochloride
minor
   m. agglutinin
   aphthae m.
   erythema multiforme m.
   variola m.
minoxidil
Mintezol
minus
   Spirillum m.
minute
   alveolar ventilation per m.
   oxygen consumption per m. (VO$_2$)
   physiological dead space ventilation per m.
   m. ventilation
minutissimum
   Corynebacterium m.
   Microsporum m.
miostagmin reaction
MIP
   macrophage inflammatory protein
mirabilis
   Proteus m.

Mirchamp sign
miscellaneous reaction
misoprostol
missense mutation
Mist
   Bronkaid M.
   Primatene M.
Mitchell disease
mite
   m. bite
   m. control
   dust m.
   elevator grain dust m.
   hair follicle m.
   harvest m.
   house dust m.
   m. infestation
   itch m.
   pyroglyphid m.
   scabietic m.
   soybean grain dust m.
   m. typhus
   wheat grain dust m.
mitis
   prurigo m.
mitochondria
mitogen
   pokeweed m. (PWM)
mitogenesis
mitogenetic
mitogenic
mitoguazone
mitral
   m. leaflet
   m. valve prolapse
   m. valve prolapse, aortic anomalies, skeletal changes, and skin changes (MASS)
Mitsuda
   M. antigen
   M. reaction
   M. test
mix
   juniper m.
mixed
   m. aerobic/anaerobic abscess
   m. agglutination

M

NOTES

mixed *(continued)*
    m. agglutination reaction
    m. agglutination test
    m. asthma
    m. chancre
    m. connective tissue disease
      (MCTD)
    m. feather
    m. hemangioma
    m. infection
    m. leprosy
    m. lymphocyte culture (MLC)
    m. lymphocyte culture reaction
    m. lymphocyte culture test
    m. nail infection
    m. seborrheic-staphylococcal
      blepharitis
    m. tumor
    m. tumor of skin
mixed-linker PCR (ML-PCR)
mixing
    phenotypic m.
Miyagawa bodies
mizolastine
mizoribine
Mkar disease
MLC
    mixed lymphocyte culture
    MLC test
MLD
    minimal lethal dose
ML-PCR
    mixed-linker PCR
3MM
    Whatman 3MM
MMD
    mass median aerodynamic diameter
MMP
    matrix metalloproteinase
MMP-2
    matrix metalloproteinase-2
MMP-3
    matrix metalloproteinase-3
MMP-7
    matrix metalloproteinase-7
MMP-8
    matrix metalloproteinase-8
MMP-9
    matrix metalloproteinase-8
MMP-10
    matrix metalloproteinase-10

MMPI
    Minnesota Multiphasic Personality
      Inventory
MMR
    measles-mumps-rubella
    measles, mumps, and rubella vaccine
    MMR vaccine
M-M-R II
MM virus
MNSs antigen
MoAb
    monoclonal antibody
Mobiluncus
moccasin
    m. foot
    m. snake bite
modified
    m. measles
    m. smallpox
module
    CO-Oximeter m.
    intercellular adhesion m.
      (ICAM)
mofetil
    mycophenolate m.
mohair
Mohs
    M. chemosurgery
    M. fresh-tissue technique
    M. micrographic surgery
moist
    m. gangrene
    Nasal M.
    m. papule
    m. tetter
    m. wart
Moi-Stir
Moisture
    M. Ophthalmic Drops
Moisturel
    M. moisturizer
moisture vapor transmission rate
    (MVTR)
moisturizer
    Aqua Care m.
    Betadine First Aid Antibiotics
    + m.
    body m.
    Eucerin m.
    Eucerin Plus m.
    facial m.
    Keri m.
    Lubriderm m.

Moisturel m.
Nivea m.
occlusive m.
RoEzIt skin m.
topical m.
Vaseline Intensive Care m.
Mokola virus
mold
    m. aeroallergen
    Alternaria m.
    m. control
    m. spore
mole
    atypical m.
    hairy m.
    spider m.
molecular mimicry
molecule
    accessory m.
    adhesion m.
    cell adhesion m. (CAM)
    effector m.
    endothelial-leukocyte
      adhesion m. (E-LAM)
    leukocyte cell adhesion m.
      (leu-CAM)
    multideterminant m.
    vascular cell adhesion m.
molecule-1
    endothelial leukocyte
      adhesion m. (ELAM-1)
    intercellular adhesion m.
      (ICAM-1)
molgramostim
Mollaret HSV
molle
    fibroma m.
    heloma m.
    papilloma m.
Moll gland
mollusciformis
    verruca m.
molluscoid neurofibroma
molluscous
molluscum
    m. body
    m. contagiosum

m. contagiosum virus
m. corpuscle
m. fibrosum
m. sebaceum
m. verrucosum
Moloney
    M. test
    M. virus
molt
mometasone furoate
Monarch Mini Mask nasal
    interface
monarthritis
monarticular
Mondor disease
mongolian
    m. macula
    m. spot
mongolism
monilated
monilethrix
Monilia albicans
Moniliaceae
monilial
    m. granuloma
moniliasis
moniliform
    m. hair
moniliforme
    Fusarium m.
moniliformis
    lichen ruber m.
    Streptobacillus m.
moniliid
Monistat
    M.-Derm topical
    M. Vaginal
monitor
    Digitrapper MkIII sleep m.
    EcoCheck oxygen m.
    Magellan M.
    NoxBOX m.
    Pick and Go m.
    TINA m.
    VenTrak respiratory
      mechanics m.

M

NOTES

monitoring
    pulse oximetry m. (POM)
monkey
    m. B virus
    m. epithelium
monkeypox
    m. virus
monk's cowl
monoarthritis (MA)
monoarticular arthritis of unknown etiology
monoassociated
monobactam
monobenzone
monochromatic light source
Monocid
monoclonal
    m. antibody (MAB, MoAb)
    m. antibody to CD4, 5a8
    m. autoantibody
    m. B-cell neoplasm
    m. gammopathy
    m. immunoglobulin
    m. peak
    m. protein
    m. protein, skin
monocyte
    m. chemoattractant protein-1 (MCP-1)
    m. chemotactic factor (MCF)
monocyte-derived neutrophil chemotactic factor
monocyte-macrophage system
monocytic leukemia
monocytogenes
    Listeria *m.*
monocytopoiesis
    factor-inducing m.
monocytosis
    avian m.
monodisperse
    m. aerosol
Monodox Oral
monoecious
Mono-Gesic
monohydrate
    cefadroxil m.
    cephalexin m.
monoinfection
monokine
monoleptic fever
monomer
monomeric

monomers
    Actin m.
monomicrobic
monomorphous
mononeuritis
    m. multiplex
mononuclear
    m. cell
    m. phagocyte system (MPS)
mononucleosis
    infectious m.
monooxygenase pathway
monophonic wheeze
monophosphate
    adenosine m. (AMP)
    cyclic adenosine m. (cAMP)
    cyclic guanosine m.
    cyclic nucleotides adenosine m.
    guanosine m. (GMP)
monoplast
monoplastic
monorecidive
    m. chancre
monosodium
    m. glutamate
    m. urate (MSU)
    m. urate crystal
Monosporium apiospermum
monosymptomatic hypochondriasis
monosyphilide
monotherapy
monovalent
    m. antiserum
monoxide
    carbon m.
    diffusing capacity for carbon m. (DLCO)
Monro
    foramen of M.
Monsel solution
monster
    Gila m.
Monterey
    M. cypress
    M. cypress tree
montevideo
    Salmonella *m.*
Monurol
moon facies
5-MOP
    5-methoxypsoralen
8-MOP
    8-methoxypsoralen

Moraxella
   M. catarrhalis
   M. conjunctivitis
   M. lacunata
morbilli
morbilliform
   m. basal cell carcinoma
   m. eruption
Morbillivirus
   equine M.
morbus
   m. Darier
Morgan
   M. fold
   M. line
Morganella morganii
morganii
   Morganella m.
morning stiffness
morphe
morphea
   m. acroterica
   m. alba
   generalized m.
   m. guttata
   m. herpetiformis
   m. linearis
   m. pigmentosum
   subcutaneous m.
   m. variant
morpheaform basal cell carcinoma
morphine
   m. sulfate
morphologic classification
morphology
   dendritic m.
   lesion m.
   stellate m.
morphometric
morphonuclear
Morquio
   M. mucopolysaccharidosis
   M. syndrome
Morrow-Brown needle
morsicatio buccarum
mortality
mortification

mortified
Morton neuroma
mosaic
   m. fungus
   m. wart
Moschcowitz disease
mosquito
   m. bite
   m. forceps
mosquito-borne disease
mossy foot
moth
   m. patch
moth-eaten
   m.-e. alopecia
   m.-e. baldness
mother yaw
motion
   active range of m.
   continuous passive m. (CPM)
   pain on m.
   passive m.
   m. sickness
motor
   m. neuron weakness
   m. neuropathy
motorized cutter
Motrin
   M. IB
   M. IB Sinus
mottled
   m. opacities
   m. rarefaction
mottling
   netlike m.
moulage
mould
Moulin
   linear atrophoderma of M.
moult
mountain
   m. cedar
   m. cedar tree
mouse
   m. encephalomyelitis
   m. encephalomyelitis virus
   m. epithelium

M

NOTES

mouse *(continued)*
   m. hepatitis
   m. hepatitis virus
   m. leukemia virus
   m. mammary tumor virus
   nude m.
   m. parotid tumor virus
   m. poliomyelitis
   m. poliomyelitis virus
   m. serum
   m. serum protein (MSP)
   m. thymic virus
   m. urine
   m. urine protein (MUP)
mousepox
   m. virus
mouth
   burning m.
   dry m.
   m. erythema multiforme
   painful m.
   scabby m.
   sore m.
   trench m.
movement
   alpha nonrapid eye m. (alpha-NREM)
   nonrapid eye m. (nonREM, NREM)
   periodic leg m. (PLM)
   rapid eye m. (REM)
moxa
moxalactam
Moxam
moxibustion
Moynahan syndrome
MP
   metacarpophalangeal
   minimal pigment
6-MP
   6-mercaptopurine
MPO
   myeloperoxidase
M-Prednisol injection
MPS
   mononuclear phagocyte system
   myofascial pain syndrome
MPT
   multiple-parameter telemetry
   multiple puncture test
MR
   malar rash
   multicentric reticulohistiocytosis

MRC
   Medical Research Council
MRCL
   Medical Research Council Laboratories
MRD
   minimal reacting dose
MRI
   magnetic resonance imaging
MRSA
   methicillin-resistant *Staphylococcus aureus*
M-R-VAX II
MS-3
   Miniscope M.
MS-1 agent
MS-2 agent
MSH
   melanocyte-stimulating hormone
   α-MSH
      α-melanocyte-stimulating hormone
   β-MSH
MSP
   mouse serum protein
MST
   median survival time
MSU
   monosodium urate
MTB
   Mycobacterium tuberculosis
MTC
   multilocular thymic cyst
MTD
   Mycobacterium Tuberculosis Direct
      MTD Test
MTP-PE
MTX
   methotrexate
Mu antigen
mucate
   acetaminophen and isometheptene m.
Mucha-Habermann
   M.-H. disease
   M.-H. syndrome
Much granule
mucicarmine stain
mucin
   m. clot test
mucinoid

mucinosa
    alopecia m.
mucinosis, pl. **mucinoses**
    cutaneous focal m.
    follicular m.
    papular m.
    plaque-like cutaneous m.
    reticular erythematous m.
      (REM)
mucinous
    m. cyst
    m. degeneration
mucocele
mucociliary
    m. clearance
mucocutaneous
    m. candidiasis
    chronic m.
    m. disease
    m. leishmaniasis
    m. lymph node syndrome
    m. manifestation
    m. sporotrichosis
Muco-Fen-LA
mucogenicum
    Mycobacterium m.
mucoid
    m. degeneration
    m. exopolysaccharide
mucolytic
Mucomyst
mucopolysaccharide
mucopolysaccharidosis,
   pl. **mucopolysaccharidoses**
    Hunter m.
    Hurler-Scheie m.
    Maroteaux-Lamy m.
    Morquio m.
    Sanfilippo m.
    Scheie m.
    Sly m.
    type I–VII m.
mucopurulent
Mucor
    M. racemosus
mucormycosis
mucosa, pl. **mucosae**

hyalinosis cutis et m.
lipoidosis cutis et m.
oral m.
reddening of oropharyngeal m.
ulceration of oral m.
upper respiratory tract m.
mucosa-associated lymphoid tissue
   (MALT)
mucosal
    m. disease
    m. disease virus
    m. inflammation
    m. neuroma
mucositis
    genital plasma cell m.
    plasma cell m.
Mucosol
mucosum
    stratum m.
mucous
    m. cyst
    m. desiccation
    m. membrane
    m. membrane ulceration
    m. papule
    m. patch
    m. plaque
    m. plug
    m. plugging
    m. stool
mucous-membrane pemphigoid
mucus
    m. hypersecretion
    oyster mass of m.
    thick and sticky m.
mud fever
Muerhrcke
    M. band
    M. line
    M. sign
Muerto Canyon virus
mugwort
Muir-Torre syndrome
mulberry
    black m.
    paper m.
    m. rash

M

NOTES

mulberry *(continued)*
   red m.
   m. spot
   white m.
multicentric reticulohistiocytosis (MR)
multideterminant molecule
multidigit dactylitis
multi-drug-resistant tuberculosis (MDR-TB)
multifactorial
multifidus
multifocal
   m. histiocytosis
   m. Langerhans cell
multiforme
   atypical erythema m.
   bullous erythema m.
   chronic erythema m.
   drug-associated erythema m.
   erythema m.
   granuloma m.
   mouth erythema m.
   oral erythema m.
   postherpetic erythema m.
multiformis
   dermatitis m.
multigemini
   pili m.
multi-infection
multilocular
   m. thymic cyst (MTC)
multilocularis
   Echinococcus m.
multinucleated giant cell
multipartial
multiple
   m. benign cystic epithelioma
   m. chemical sensitivity
   m. drug allergy syndrome
   m. endocrine neoplasia (MEN)
   m. endocrine neoplasms (MEN)
   m. epiphyseal dysplasia
   m. hamartoma syndrome
   m. hereditary hemorrhagic telangiectasis
   m. idiopathic hemorrhagic sarcoma
   m. keratoacanthoma
   m. lentigines syndrome
   m. mucosal neuroma
   m. mucosal neuroma syndrome

   m. myeloma
   m. myositis
   m. neuroma
   m. puncture test (MPT)
   m. puncture tuberculin test
   m. sclerosis
   m. sulfatase deficiency
   m. sulfatase deficiency syndrome
   m. symmetrical lipomatosis
   m. trichoepithelioma
multiple-parameter telemetry (MPT)
multiplex
   mononeuritis m.
   m. steatocystoma
   steatocystoma m.
   xanthoma m.
multisegmented
Multitest test
multivalent
   m. vaccine
multivariant
multocida
   Pasteurella m.
mummification
   m. necrosis
mumps
   m. meningoencephalitis
   metastatic m.
   m. sensitivity test
   m. skin test antigen
   m. virus
   m. virus vaccine
   m. virus vaccine, live, attenuated
Mumpsvax
Munchausen syndrome
Munro
   M. abscess
   M. microabscess
MUP
   mouse urine protein
mupirocin
   m. ointment
muramyl-tripeptide
Murex Suds
muriform
murine
   m. hepatitis
   m. leukemia
   m. sarcoma virus
   M. solution
   m. typhus

murmur
Carey Coombs m.
Murocel Ophthalmic solution
muromonab-CD3
Murray
M. test
M. Valley encephalitis (MVE)
M. Valley encephalitis virus
M. Valley rash
Murutucu virus
muscle
accessory m.
arrectores pilorum m.
arrector pili m.
m. biopsy
bronchial smooth m.
sacrospinalis m.
sternocleidomastoid m.
m. weakness
Muscle-Wells syndrome
musculamine
muscular dystrophy
musculotendinous
m. damage
m. unit
mushroom dust
mushroom-hook layer
mushroom-worker's lung
musician's overuse syndrome
mussel
blue m.
mustard
nitrogen m.
yellow m.
Mustargen Hydrochloride
mustelae
.*Helicobacter m.*
mutagen
frame-shift m.
mutant ˋ
conditional-lethal m.
conditionally lethal m.
suppressor-sensitive m.
temperature-sensitive m.
mutation
addition-deletion m.
frame-shift m.

missense m.
point m.
reading-frame-shift m.
transition m.
transversion m.
mutilans
arthritis m.
keratoma hereditarium m.
lupus m.
psoriatic arthritis m.
mutilating
m. keratoderma
m. keratoderma of Vohwinkel
m. leprosy
MV
maximal ventilation
mechanical ventilation
MVE
Murray Valley encephalitis
MVE virus
MVTR
moisture vapor transmission rate
MVV
maximal voluntary ventilation
myalgia
eosinophilic m.
epidemic m.
Myambutol
Myapap Drops
myasthenia gravis (MG)
Mycelex
M.-G
M. troche
mycelium
mycetoma
Bouffardi black m.
Bouffardi white m.
Brumpt white m.
Carter black m.
Nicolle white m.
Vincent white m.
mycetomi
Madurella m.
mycid
Mycifradin
M. Sulfate Oral
M. Sulfate topical

M

NOTES

Mycitracin topical
mycobacteria
  m. HSP
mycobacterial
  m. abscess
  m. infection
mycobacteriosis
  environmental m.
Mycobacterium
  M. abscessus
  M. avium
  M. avium complex (MAC)
  M. avium-intracellulare (MAC, MAI)
  M. balnei
  M. chelonae
  M. fortuitum
  M. gordonae
  M. haemophilum
  M. kansasii
  M. leprae
  M. marinum
  M. mucogenicum
  M. peregrinum
  M. phlei
  M. smegmatis
  M. thermorisistable
  M. tuberculosis (MTB)
  M. tuberculosis detection
  M. Tuberculosis Direct (MTD)
  M. ulcerans
  M. vaccae
  M. xenopi
Mycobutin
mycodermatitis
Mycogen II topical
Mycolog-II topical
mycology
Myconel topical
mycophage
mycophenolate mofetil
Mycoplasma
  M. faucium
  M. genitalium
  M. hominis
  M. incognitus
  M. pneumoniae
mycoplasma
  m. disease
  m. IgM titer
  m. pneumonia of pigs
mycoplasmal pneumonia
mycosis, pl. mycoses

  m. cutis chronica
  deep m.
  m. framboesioides
  m. fungoides
  m. fungoides d'emblée
  opportunistic systemic m.
  pulmonary m.
  rare m.
  subcutaneous m.
mycostatic
Mycostatin
  M. Oral
  M. topical
mycotic
mycovirus
Mydfrin Ophthalmic solution
mydriatic
myelin-associated glycoprotein antibody detection
myelitic enterovirus
myelitis
  transverse m.
myeloblastic protein
myeloblastosis
  avian m.
myelodysplastic syndrome (MDS)
myeloid
  m. leukemia
  m. stem cell
myeloma
  m. growth factor
  multiple m.
  plasma cell m.
myelomatosis
myelonecrosis
myeloperoxidase (MPO)
  m. deficiency
myeloproliferative disease
myeloradiculopolyneuronitis
myiasis
  botfly facultative m.
  botfly obligate m.
  creeping m.
  facultative m.
  obligate m.
  m. oestruosa
  subcutaneous m.
  wound m.
Myminic Expectorant
myoadenylate deaminase deficiency
myoblast

myoblastoma
    granular cell m.
myocardial infarction (MI)
myocarditis
    clinical m.
Myochrysine
myoclonus
    nocturnal m.
myocyte
    Anitschkow m.
myoD
myoepithelioma
myoepithelium
myofascial pain syndrome (MPS)
myofibrils
myofibromatosis
    infantile m.
myogenic
    m. paralysis
myoglobin
    quantitative immunoassay for
      urine m.
    m. release
myoglobinuria
myoma
myonecrosis
    clostridial m.
myopathy
    drug-related m.
    idiopathic inflammatory m.
    steroid m.
    vacuolar m.
myophosphorylase deficiency
myosin
myositis
    acute disseminated m.
    childhood m.
    eosinophilic m.
    epidemic m.
    giant cell m.
    inclusion body m.

    multiple m.
    nodular m.
    orbital m.
    m. ossificans
    overlap m. (OVLP)
    m. with malignancy
myositis-associated autoantibody
myosynovitis
Myoviridae
Myphetapp
myringitis
    m. bulbosa
    bullous m.
myringodermatitis
myringotomy with aspiration
myrmecia
    m. wart
myrmekiasm
myrtle
    wax m.
Mytrex
    M. F topical
myxadenitis labialis
myxedema
    circumscribed m.
    generalized m.
    pretibial m.
myxedematosus
    lichen m.
myxedematous
    m. arthropathy
    m. lichen
myxoid cyst
myxolipoma
myxoma
    cardiocutaneous m.
    nerve sheath m.
myxomatosis
    m. virus
myxomatous degeneration
myxovirus

M

NOTES

N
nitrogen
nabumetone
NACDG
North American Contact Dermatitis
Group
N-acetylcysteine
N-acetylneuraminic acid
nacreous ichthyosis
nadolol
NADPH oxidase
Naegeli syndrome
Naegleria fowleri
NAEP
National Asthma Education Program
naeslundii
Actinomyces n.
naevoid (*var. of* nevoid)
naevus (*var. of* nevus)
NAF
neutrophil activating factor
nafate
cefamandole n.
Nafcil injection
nafcillin
n. sodium
naftifine
n. hydrochloride
Naftin
N. cream
N. topical
Naga sore
nail
azure lunula of n.
n. biting
brittle n.
n. change
clubbing of n.
n. clubbing
convex n.
egg shell n.
n. fold
n. fold capillaroscopy
n. fold capillary loop
abnormality
geographic stippling of n.
n. groove
half-and-half n.
hang n.
Hippocratic n.

n. horn
ingrown n.
n. keratin
n. matrix
Ony-Clear N.
parrot-beak n.
pincer n.
n. pit
pitted n.
n. pitting
pitting of n.
n. plate
n. polish
racket n.
ram horn n.
reedy n.
ringworm of n.
n. root
shell n.
splitting n.
spoon n.
Terry n.
n. wall
yellow n.
nailbed
nail fold
nail-patella-elbow syndrome
nail-patella syndrome
Nairobi sheep disease virus
naive B cell
naked
n. tubercle
n. virus
Naldecon
N.-EX Children's Syrup
Naldelate
Nalebuff classification
Nalfon
Nalgest
nalidixic acid
Nallpen injection
naloxone hydrochloride
Nalspan
NAME
nevi, atrial myxoma, myxoid
neurofibromas, and ephelides
NAME syndrome
NANB
non-A non-B
NANB hepatitis

Nanophyetus salmincola
nanum
   Microsporum n.
NAP
   neutrophil activating protein
nape nevus
Naphcon-A
napkin rash
Naprelan
Naprosyn
naproxen
   n. sodium
naris, pl. nares
narium
narrowing
   joint space n.
Nasabid
Nasacort
Nasahist B injection
nasal
   n. antigen challenge test
   n. canthus
   n. congestion
   n. itching
   N. Moist
   n. mucosal ulceration
   n. polyp
   n. provocation test
   n. scraping
   n. smear
   n. turbinates
   Tyzine N.
   n. verge
Nasalcrom
   N. Nasal solution
Nasalide
   N. Nasal Aerosol
Nasarel
nasi
   alae n.
   granulosis rubra n.
Nasik vibrio
nasoantral window
nasociliary
nasolabial fold (NLF)
nasopharyngeal
   n. aspirate (NPA)
   n. biopsy
   n. carcinoma
   n. leishmaniasis
   n. ulcer
nasopharyngoscopy

Natacyn Ophthalmic
natamycin
National
   N. Asthma Education Program
   (NAEP)
   N. Center for Health Statistics
   (NCHS)
   N. Committee for Clinical
   Laboratory Standards
   (NCCLS)
   N. Immunization Program
   (NIP)
   N. Institute of Arthritis,
   Musculoskeletal and Skin
   Disorders (NIAMS)
   N. Institute of Health (NIH)
   N. Vaccine Advisory
   Committee (NVAC)
native
   n. anergy
   n. type anti-DNA antibody
natural
   n. anergy
   n. antibody
   n. focus of infection
   n. hemolysin
   n. immunity
   n. interferon alfa
   n. killer (NK)
   n. killer cell
   n. killer cell stimulating factor
   (NKSF)
Naturale
   Tears N.
Nature's Tears solution
nausea
   epidemic n.
navy bean
NCCLS
   National Committee for Clinical
   Laboratory Standards
NCHS
   National Center for Health Statistics
NCS
   nerve conduction study
ND
   Newcastle disease
   ND virus
Nd
   neodymium
ND-Stat injection

Nd:YAG
neodymium:yttrium-aluminum-
garnet
Nd:YAG laser
Nebcin injection
Nebraska calf scours virus
Nebuhaler inhaler
nebules
Ventolin n.
nebulin
nebulization
nebulize
nebulized
n. bronchodilator
n. isoproterenol
nebulizer
Aerochamber n.
AeroSonic personal
ultrasonic n.
AeroTech II n.
DeVilbiss Pulmon-Aid n.
jet n.
John Bunn Mini-Mist n.
Medi-Mist n.
Micro Mist n.
Pulmo-Aide n.
Respirgard II n.
Schuco 2000 n.
Shuco-Myst n.
Twin Jet n.
ultrasonic n.
Wright n.
NebuPent
N. Inhalation
NEC
necrotizing enterocolitis
Necator americanus
neck
n. dermatitis
fiddler n.
necklace
Casal n.
n. of pearls
n. of Venus
necrobiosis
n. lipoidica
n. lipoidica diabeticorum

necrobiotic
n. xanthogranuloma
necrogenic
n. tubercle
n. wart
necrogenica
verruca n.
necrolysis
toxic epidermal n. (TEN)
necrolytic migratory erythema
necrosis
acute retinal n. (ARN)
aseptic n.
aspirin-induced papillary n.
avascular n. (AVN)
central fibrinoid n.
coumarin n.
fat n.
fibrinoid n.
liquefaction n.
mummification n.
neutrophilic n.
papillary n.
progressive outer retinal n.
(PORN)
subcutaneous fat n.
traumatic fat n.
necrotic
n. arachnidism
n. center
n. pocket
n. tissue
n. ulcer
necrotica
acne n.
dermatitis nodularis n.
necrotisans
sycosis nuchae n.
necrotizing
n. angiitis
n. enterocolitis (NEC)
n. fasciitis
n. granuloma
n. infection
n. lymphadenitis
n. scleritis with adjacent
inflammation

N

NOTES

necrotizing *(continued)*
  n. scleritis without adjacent
    inflammation
  n. sialometaplasia
  n. vasculitis
nectary of floral unit
nedocromil
  n. sodium
needle
  Allerprick n.
  n. arthroscopy
  n. biopsy
  Colorado microdissection n.
  Morrow-Brown n.
  Osterballe precision n.
  Parker-Pearson n.
  Pricker n.
  Stallerpointe n.
  Wyeth bifurcated n.
needlestick
Neer II implant
Neethling virus
negative
  n. anergy
  n. control test
  Gram n.
  n. nevus
  n. patch test
  n. phase
  n. reaction
  n. schick test
  n. strand virus
NegGram
Negishi virus
Negri
  N. bodies
  N. corpuscles
Neisseria
  N. gonorrhoeae
  N. meningitidis
  N. meningitidis B
nelfinavir
Nellcor Symphony N-3000 pulse
  oximeter
Nelson syndrome
nematocyst
  venom-bathed n.
nematode
  filarial n.
  intestinal n.
neo-angiomatous
neoantigen
Neo-Cortef topical

NeoDecadron
  N. Ophthalmic
Neo-Dexameth Ophthalmic
neodymium (Nd)
neodymium:yttrium-aluminum-garnet
  (Nd:YAG)
Neofed
neoformans
  Cryptococcus n.
  Saccharomyces n.
Neo-fradin Oral
neomembrane
Neomixin topical
neomycin
  n. dermatitis
  n. and polymyxin b
  n., polymyxin b, and
    dexamethasone
  n., polymyxin b, and
    gramicidin
  n., polymyxin b, and
    hydrocortisone
  n., polymyxin b, and
    prednisolone
  n. sulfate
neonatal
  n. acne
  n. anemia
  n. biotin deficiency
  n. calf diarrhea virus
  n. candidiasis
  n. herpes
  n. herpes simplex virus
  n. lupus
  n. lupus erythematosus (NLE)
  lupus erythematosus, n.
  n. pustular melanosis
  n. systemic candidiasis
  n. tyrosinemia
neonate
neonatorum
  acne n.
  adiponecrosis subcutanea n.
  anemia n.
  blennorrhea n.
  dermatitis exfoliativa n.
  edema n.
  erythema toxicum n.
  ichthyosis congenita n.
  icterus n.
  impetigo n.
  ophthalmia n.
  pemphigus n.

scleredema n.
sclerema n.
seborrhea squamosa n.
Neopap
neoplasia
malignant n.
multiple endocrine n. (MEN)
vulvar intraepithelial n.
neoplasm
monoclonal B-cell n.
multiple endocrine n.'s (MEN)
plasma cell n.
neoplastic
n. cell
n. disease
neoplastica
acrokeratosis n.
alopecia n.
neopterin
Neoral
N. Oral
Neosar injection
Neospora canium
Neosporin
N. Cream
N. Ophthalmic Ointment
N. Ophthalmic solution
N. Topical Ointment
NeoSynalar
Neo-Synephrine Ophthalmic solution
Neo-Tabs Oral
Neothylline
Neotricin HC Ophthalmic Ointment
neovascularization
nephelometry
nephritic factor
nephritis, pl. nephritides
acute n.
acute interstitial n.
anti-basement membrane n.
anti-kidney serum n.
immune complex n.
immune-mediated
membranous n.
interstitial n.
lupus n. (LN)
Masugi n.

scarlatinal n.
serum n.
silent lupus n.
streptococcal n.
transfusion n.
tuberculous n.
tubulointerstitial n.
nephrocaps
nephrogenic diabetes insipidus
nephrolithiasis
nephrolysin
nephrolysis
nephrolytic
nephropathia epidemica
nephropathy
amyloidotic n.
Berger IgA n.
IgA n.
IgM n.
membranous n.
urate n.
nephrosis
hemoglobinuric n.
toxic n.
nephrotoxic
nephrotoxicity
nephrotoxin
NERDS
nodules, eosinophilia, rheumatism,
dermatitis, and swelling
NERDS syndrome
nerve
n. compression-degeneration
syndrome
n. conduction study (NCS)
n. conduction velocity
n. deafness
n. entrapment
n. entrapment syndrome
n. growth factor (NGF)
n. growth factor antiserum
peripheral n.
phrenic n.
n. sheath
n. sheath myxoma
sinuvertebral n.
vagus n.

N

NOTES

Nervocaine
nervorum
    vasa n.
nervosa
    onychalgia n.
    purpura n.
    rhinitis n.
nervous
    n. exhaustion
    n. system
    n. system involvement
Nesacaine
    N.-MPF
nests of nevus cells
Netherton syndrome
netilmicin sulfate
netlike mottling
Netromycin injection
netted pattern
nettle
    n. rash
Nettleship disease
Nettleship-Falls ocular albinism
nettling hair
Neucalm
Neufeld
    N. capsular swelling
    N. reaction
Neumann disease
Neupogen
    N. injection
neural
    n. leprosy
    n. theory
    n. tissue
neuralgia
    postherpetic n. (PHN)
    red n.
neural-mediated flushing
neuraminidase
α$_2$-neuraminoglycoprotein
neurapraxia
neurasthenia
neuridine
neurilemmoma, neurolemmoma
neuriticum
    atrophoderma n.
neuritis
    optic n.
    peripheral n.
neuroallergy
neuroarthropathy
neurocirculatory asthenia

neurocutaneous
    n. melanosis
    n. syndrome
neurocysticercosis
neurodegenerative disease
neurodermatitic
neurodermatitis
    circumscribed n.
    disseminated n.
    genital n.
    localized n.
    nodular n.
neurodermatosis
neuroectodermal defect
neuroendocrine tumor
neurofibroma
    molluscoid n.
    pacinian n.
    plexiform n.
neurofibromatosis
    abortive n.
    central type n.
    classic n.
    incomplete n.
    late onset n.
    segmental n.
    n. (types 1-8)
    variant n.
neurofibrosarcoma
neurolemmoma (var. of
    neurilemmoma)
neuro-leprosy
neurologic
    n. disorder
    n. genodermatosis
neurolymphomatosis gallinarum
neurolysin
neuroma
    n. cutis
    encapsulated n.
    Morton n.
    mucosal n.
    multiple n.
    multiple mucosal n.
    palisaded encapsulated n.
    plexiform n.
    Verneuil n.
neuromatosa
    elephantiasis n.
neuromelanin
neuromyopathy
    peripheral n.
neuronevus

neuronophage
neuronophagia
neuropathic
   n. amyloidosis
   n. arthropathy
   n. foot
neuropathy
   asymmetric peripheral
     sensory n.
   entrapment n.
   hereditary sensory radicular n.
   motor n.
   posterior interosseous n.
neuropeptide
neuropsychiatric
   n. disease
   n. symptom
neurorelapse
neuroretinitis
Neurospora sitophila
neurosyphilis
neurothekeoma
neurotica
   alopecia n.
neurotic excoriation
neurotoxin
   eosinophil-derived n.
neurotrophic ulcer
neurotropic virus
neurovaccine
neurovirus
Neut injection
neutral
   n. lipid
   n. lipid storage
   n. lipid storage disease
   n. protease
   n. proteinase
neutralization
   serum n.
   n. test
   viral n.
neutralizing (Nt)
   n. antibody
Neutrexin

Neutrogena
   N. Acne Mask
   N. T/Derm
neutropenia
   autoimmune n.
   cyclic n.
   isoimmune neonatal n.
neutrophil
   n. activating factor (NAF)
   n. activating protein (NAP)
   n. antibody and transfusion
     reaction
   n. chemotactant factor
   n. chemotaxis
   n. elastase
   polymorphonuclear n. (PMN)
neutrophil-activating peptide-1
neutrophilic
   n. eccrine hidradenitis
   n. inflammation
   n. intraepidermal IgA
     dermatosis
   n. necrosis
neutrophils
nevi (*pl. of* nevus)
nevirapine
nevocyte
nevoid, naevoid
   n. anomaly
   n. basal cell carcinoma
   n. basal cell carcinoma
     syndrome
   n. elephantiasis
   n. hyperkeratosis of nipple and
     areola
   n. hypermelanosis
   n. hypertrichosis
   n. lentigo
   n. telangiectasia
nevolipoma
nevose
nevoxanthoendothelioma
nevus, naevus, pl. nevi
   acquired n.
   acquired melanocytic n.
   n. anemicus
   n. angiectodes

N

NOTES

nevus *(continued)*
n. arachnoideus
n. araneus
nevi, atrial myxoma, myxoid
  neurofibromas, and ephelides
  (NAME)
balloon cell n.
basal cell n.
bathing-trunk n.
Becker n.
blue n.
blue rubber-bleb nevi
capillary n.
n. cavernosus
n. cell, A-type
n. cell, B-type
n. cell, C-type
cellular blue n.
comedo n.
comedones epidermal n.
n. comedonicus
common n.
compound n.
congenital n.
connective tissue n.
dysplastic n.
n. elasticus of Lewandowski
epidermal n.
epidermic-dermic n.
epithelial n.
epithelioid cell n.
faun tail n.
n. fibrosus
flame n.
n. flammeus
n. flammeus nuchae
n. follicularis keratosis
n. fuscoceruleus
n. fuscoceruleus
  acromiodeltoideus
n. fuscoceruleus
  ophthalmomaxillaris
garment n.
giant congenital n.
giant pigmented n.
hair follicle n.
hairy n.
halo n.
inflamed linear verrucous
  epidermal n. (ILVEN)
intracutaneous n.
intradermal n.
intraepidermal n.

Ito n.
n. of Ito
Jadassohn n.
Jadassohn-Tièche n.
junction n.
junctional n.
lentigines, atrial myxoma,
  mucocutaneous myxomas, and
  blue nevi (LAMB)
lichen striatus epidermal n.
linear n.
linear epidermal n.
n. lipomatodes
n. lipomatosus
n. lymphaticus
melanocytic n.
mesodermal n.
nape n.
negative n.
nevus-cell n.
n. ophthalmomaxillaris
oral epithelial n.
organoid n.
Ota n.
n. of Ota
n. papillomatosus
pigmented hair epidermal n.
n. pigmentosus
n. pigmentosus et pilosus
n. pilosus
n. sanguineus
scarf n.
n. sebaceous
n. sebaceus of Jadassohn
speckled lentiginous n.
spider n.
n. spilus
n. spilus lentigo
spindle cell n.
Spitz n.
stocking n.
strawberry n.
n. sudoriferous
Sutton n.
n. syringocystadenomatosus
  papilliferus
systematized n.
n. tardus
n. unius lateralis
n. unius lateris
n. vascularis
n. vasculosus
n. venosus

n. verrucosus
verrucous n.
Werther n.
white sponge n.
woolly-hair n.
nevus-cell nevus
New
N. Beginnings topical gel
sheeting
N. Decongestant
N. World leishmaniasis
N. Zealand mice
newborn
bullous impetigo of n.
hemolytic anemia of n.
hemolytic disease of n.
lamellar exfoliation of the n.
spontaneous gangrene of n.
subcutaneous fat necrosis of n.
Newcastle
N. disease (ND)
N. disease virus
newsprint
nexin-1
protease n.
nexine
Nezelof
N. syndrome
N. type of thymic
alymphoplasia
NGF
nerve growth factor
NGF antiserum
NGT topical
NHL
non-Hodgkin lymphoma
Niacels
niacin
n. deficiency
niacinamide
NIAMS
National Institute of Arthritis,
Musculoskeletal and Skin
Disorders
NiCad
nickel-cadmium

nickel
n. allergy
n. dermatitis
n. and dime lesion
n. sulfate
nickel-cadmium (NiCad)
Niclocide
niclosamide
Nicobid
Nicolar
Nicolle white mycetoma
nicotine
n. stomatitis
Nicotinex
Nico-Vert
NIDDM
non-insulin-dependent diabetes
mellitus
nidogen
Nidryl Oral
nidulans
Aspergillus n.
Nieden syndrome
Niemann-Pick disease
nifedipine
nifurtimox
niger
Aspergillus n.
Peptococcus n.
NightBird nasal CPAP
Nighttime
Arthritis Foundation N.
nigra
dermatosis papulosa n.
linea n.
pityriasis n.
seborrhea n.
tinea n.
nigricans
acanthosis n. (AN)
drug-induced acanthosis n.
keratosis n.
malignant acanthosis n.
pseudoacanthosis n.
Rhizopus n.
type A acanthosis n.

N

NOTES

nigricans *(continued)*
    type B acanthosis n.
    type C acanthosis n.
nigrities
    n. linguae
Nigrospora
NIH
    National Institute of Health
Nikolsky sign
Nilstat topical
nimitti midge
nimodipine
Nimotop
ninth-day erythema
NIP
    National Immunization Program
nit
nitazoxanide (NTZ)
nitidus
    lichen n.
nitrate
    econazole n.
    oxiconazole n.
    silver n.
    sulconazole n.
nitric oxide
nitritoid reaction
nitroblue
    n. tetrazolium
    n. tetrazolium test
nitrofurantoin
nitrofurazone
nitrogen (N)
    liquid n. (LN$_2$)
    n. mustard
nitrous oxide
Nivea moisturizer
Nix
    N. Creme Rinse
Nizoral
    N. Oral
    N. topical
NK
    natural killer
    NK cell
NKSF
    natural killer cell stimulating factor
NLE
    neonatal lupus erythematosus
NLF
    nasolabial fold
N-linked pattern

Nocardia
    N. asteroides
    N. brasiliensis
    N. caviae
    N. farcinica
    N. tenuis
    N. transvalensis
nocardiosis
nocturnal
    n. asthma
    n. hemoglobinuria
    n. myoclonus
    n. wheezing
nodal fever
node
    Bizzozero n.
    Bouchard n.
    Heberden n.
    juxta-articular n.
    lymph n.
    milkers' n.
    Osler n.
nodosa
    cutaneous polyarteritis n.
    dermatitis n.
    periarteritis n.
    polyarteritis n.
    systemic polyarteritis n.
    tinea n.
    trichomycosis n.
    trichomycosis axillaris n.
    trichorrhexis n.
nodose
nodositas
    n. crinium
nodosity
nodosum
    erythema n. (EN)
nodous
nodular
    n. amyloidosis
    n. basal cell carcinoma
    n. elastosis
    n. episcleritis
    n. fasciitis
    n. granulomatous vasculitis
    n. hidradenoma
    n. leprosy
    n. malignant melanoma
    n. melanoma
    n. migratory panniculitis
    n. myositis
    n. neurodermatitis

n. nonsuppurative panniculitis
n. non-X histiocytosis
n. panencephalitis
n. pattern
n. pulmonary amyloidosis
n. scabies
n. scleritis
n. subepidermal fibrosis
n. synovitis
n. syphilid
n. tuberculid
n. vasculitis
nodularis
    chondrodermatitis helicis n.
    prurigo n.
    trichomycosis axillaris n.
nodulation
nodule
    apple jelly n.
    athlete's n.
    Bohn n.
    cutaneous n.
    cutaneous-subcutaneous n.
    dark-staining n.
    Jeanselme n.
    juxta-articular n.
    lepromatous n.
    Lisch n.
    milkers' n.
    paraumbilical n.
    Picker n.
    picker's n.
    pulmonary necrobiotic n.
    red n.
    red papule and n.
    rheumatoid n.
    sharply circumscribed n.
    Sister Mary Joseph n.
    Stockman n.
    subcutaneous n.
    subcutaneous granulomatous n.
    subcutaneous rheumatoid n.
nodules, eosinophilia, rheumatism, dermatitis, and swelling (NERDS)
noduli (*pl. of* nodulus)
nodulocystic acne

nodulosis
    rheumatoid n.
nodulous
nodulus, pl. noduli
    n. cutaneus
noir
    talon n.
noire
    tache n.
Nolahist
Nolamine
Nolex LA
noma
nomenclature
    binary n.
    linnaean system of n.
non-A
    n.-A non-B (NANB)
    n.-A non-B hepatitis
    n.-A non-B hepatitis virus
nonacnegenic
nonarticular syndrome
non-B
    n.-B cell
    non-A n.-B (NANB)
nonblanchable
    n., abnormally colored lesion
nonbullous
    n. congenital erythrodermic ichthyosis
    n. congenital ichthyosiform erythroderma
    n. impetigo
noncaseating
    n. granuloma
noncatecholamine
noncavitary
noncomedogenic
nonconjugative plasmid
noncorticosteroid anti-inflammatory agent
non-cross-reactive drug
nondermatophyte fungal infection
Non-Drowsy
    Drixoral N.-D.
non-drug-related reaction
nongonococcal bacterial arthritis

N

NOTES

nonhemophiliac patient
non-Hodgkin lymphoma (NHL)
nonidentity
   reaction of n.
non-immediate-type immunologic
   drug reaction
nonimmune
   n. agglutination
   n. serum
nonimmunity
nonimmunologic
   n. basis
   n. complication
   n. drug reaction
noninflammatory
   n. edema
Nonin Onyx pulse oximeter
non-insulin-dependent diabetes
   mellitus (NIDDM)
nonirritating test substance
nonlinear IgA deposition
nonmeningeal
non-necrotizing angiitis
non-neoplastic disease
non-nucleoside reverse transcriptase
   inhibitor
nonoccluded virus
nonocclusive dressing
nonpalpable purpura
nonpathogenic fungus
nonpharmacologic measure of
   treatment
nonpoisonous
non-polio enterovirus
nonprecipitable antibody
nonprecipitating antibody
nonproductive cough
nonrapid eye movement (nonREM,
   NREM)
nonREM
   nonrapid eye movement
   nonREM sleep
nonresponder tolerance
nonrestorative sleep
nonrheumatoid
   n. episcleritis
   n. scleritis
nonscarring alopecia
nonsecretor
nonsedating antihistamine
nonsense triplet
nonshedding dog

nonspecific
   n. absorption
   n. anergy
   n. climatic change
   n. dermatitis
   n. protein
   n. therapy
nonsteroidal
   n. anti-inflammatory
   n. anti-inflammatory drug
   (NSAID)
nonstick gauze
nonsuction grasper
nonsyphilitic treponematosis
nonthrombocytopenic purpura
nontreponemal test
nontuberculous
   n. mycobacterial infection
nonvenereal syphilis
noon unit
No Pain-HP
Nordimmun
Norditropine
Nordryl
   N. injection
   N. Oral
norepinephrine bitartrate
norfloxacin
Norisodrine
normal
   n. animal
   n. antibody
   n. antitoxin
   n. cornification
   n. horse serum
   n. opsonin
   n. toxin
normocapnia
normocholesteremic xanthoma
normochromic
normocomplementemic
normocytic
normolipemic xanthomatosis
Noroxin Oral
Norpramin
Nor-tet Oral
North
   N. American blastomycosis
   N. American Contact
   Dermatitis Group (NACDG)
northern
   n. rat flea
   n. rat flea bite

Norvir
Norwalk
   N. agent
   N. virus
Norwalk-like agent
Norway itch
Norwegian scabies
nose
   saddle n.
Nosema
   N. connori
   N. corneum
   N. ocularum
nosematosis
nosocomial
   n. gangrene
   n. infection
   n. pneumonia (NP)
nosocomialis
   phagedena n.
Nosopsyllus
   N. fasciatus
   N. fasciatus bite
nosotoxic
nosotoxin
nostras
   elephantiasis n.
   piedra n.
Nostrilla
notalgia paresthetica
notatum
   Penicillium n.
Novacet
   N. topical
Novafed
Novahistine
Novocain
   N. injection
noxa, pl. noxae
NoxBOX monitor
noxythiolin
NP
   nosocomial pneumonia
NP-27
NPA
   nasopharyngeal aspirate

NR
   Tussi-Organidin N.
NREM
   nonrapid eye movement
NSAID
   nonsteroidal anti-inflammatory drug
      NSAID gastropathy
NSAIDs
N segments
Nt
   neutralizing
NTPPH
   nucleoside triphosphate
      pyrophosphohydrolase
NTZ
   nitazoxanide
      NTZ Long Acting Nasal
      solution
nuchae
   acne keloidalis n.
   cutis rhomboidalis n.
   erythema n.
   lichen n.
   ligamentum n.
   nevus flammeus n.
   sycosis n.
nuclear
   n. factor
   n. inclusion bodies
nucleatum
   Fusobacterium n.
nuclei (*pl. of* nucleus)
nucleic acid probe
nucleocapsid
nucleohistone
nucleoid
nucleolar staining
nucleoside
   n. triphosphate
      pyrophosphohydrolase
      (NTPPH)
nucleotidase
nucleotide
nucleotides
nucleotoxin
nucleus, pl. nuclei
   droplet n.

N

NOTES

Nucofed
nude mouse
Nu-Hope skin barrier strip
null
    n. cell
    n. cell leukemia
number
    chromosome n.
numbness
numerical taxonomy
nummular
    n. eczema
    n. lesion
    n. syphilid
nummulare
    eczema n.
nummularis
    psoriasis n.
Nuprin
Nursoy formula
nut
    Brazil n.
Nu-Tears
    N.-T. II solution
    N.-T. solution

Nutracort
Nu-Trake Weiss emergency airway
    system
Nutraplus topical
nutrient artery
nutritional disorder
Nutrotropin
NVAC
    National Vaccine Advisory
    Committee
Nydrazid injection
nylon
nystagmus
nystatin
    n. and triamcinolone
Nystat-Rx
Nystex topical
Nyst-Olone II topical
Nytol
    Maximum Strength N.

O
- O agglutinin
- O antigen

OA
- occupationally induced asthma
- osteoarthritis

OAF
- osteoclast-activating factor

oak
- Gambel o.
- live o.
- poison o.
- o. tree
- western poison o.
- white o.

oakridgensis
- *Legionella o.*

oat

oatmeal
- colloidal o.

obconica
- *Primula o.*

obesity
- protein-energy-related o.
- vitamin-related o.

objective synonym

obligate
- o. aerobe
- o. myiasis

obliterans
- arteriosclerosis o.
- balanitis xerotica o.

obliterative granulomatous fibrosis

obstruction
- episodic bronchial o.
- fixed airflow o.
- severe o.
- upper airway o.

obstructive sleep apnea (OSA)

obtusus
- lichen o.

obvious physical exhaustion

occidentalis
- *Dermacentor o.*

occipital
- o. forelock
- o. horn syndrome

occlude

occluded virus

Occlusal-HP
- O.-H. Liquid

occlusion
- portal o.

occlusive
- o. dressing
- o. moisturizer
- o. patch test
- o. therapy

occuloglandular syndrome

occult
- o. blood
- o. spina bifida

occupational
- o. acne
- o. allergen
- o. allergic alveolitis
- o. exposure
- o. therapy (OT)

occupationally induced asthma (OA)

occupation-related syndrome

Ochrobacterium anthropi

ochrodermia

ochronosis
- endogenous o.
- exogenous o.

ochronotic

Ockelbo disease

Octicair Otic

Octocaine
- O. injection

octreotide

octulosonic acid

OcuClear

OcuCoat
- O. Ophthalmic solution
- O. PF Ophthalmic solution

ocular
- o. adnexa
- o. albinism
- o. allergy
- o. atopic dermatitis
- o. hypertelorism
- o. larma migrans
- o. lesion
- o. lymphomatosis
- o. pemphigus
- o. toxicity

ocular-mucous membrane syndrome

O

ocularum
 Nosema o.
oculi
 orbicularis o.
oculocerebral syndrome of Cross and McKusick
oculocutaneous
 o. albinism
 o. telangiectasias
oculodermal melanosis
oculoglandular
Ocutricin
 O. HC Otic
 O. Topical Ointment
Ocu-Tropine Ophthalmic
odaxetic
ODD
 once-daily dosing
odds
 logarithm of o. (lod)
Odland body
odontoid process displacement
odor
 o. control
 volatile o.
odorans
 Alcaligenes o.
Oesophagostomum
oestruosa
 myiasis o.
OET
 open epicutaneous test
officinalis
 poxvirus o.
ofloxacin
Ofuji disease
Ohmeda hand-held oximeter
ohne Hauch
oidiomycin
"oid-oid" disease
oil
 o. of bergamot
 Cajuput o.
 citronella o.
 coal tar, lanolin, and mineral o.
 Derma Smoothe O.
 o. drop lesion
 fish o.
 o. gland
 o. immersion
 Jojoba o.
 mineral o.

 patchouli o.
 petitgrain o.
 silicone o.
 trypsin, balsam peru, and castor o.
 o. vaccine
 ylang-ylang o.
oil-based facial foundation
oiliness
oily granuloma
ointment
 A and D O.
 AK-Spore H.C. Ophthalmic O.
 AK-Spore Ophthalmic O.
 Cortisporin Ophthalmic O.
 Cortisporin Topical O.
 Medi-Quick Topical O.
 mupirocin o.
 Neosporin Ophthalmic O.
 Neosporin Topical O.
 Neotricin HC Ophthalmic O.
 Ocutricin Topical O.
 Panscol O.
 Salacid O.
 Septa Topical O.
 o. of tar
 Terak Ophthalmic O.
 Terramycin Ophthalmic O.
 Terramycin w/Polymyxin B Ophthalmic O.
 triamcinolone o. (TAO)
 Whitfield O.
Oka vaccine
OKT3
 Orthoclone O.
OKT cell
 Ortho-Kung T cell
olamine
 ciclopirox o.
old-man's pemphigus
Old World leishmaniasis
olecranon
 o. bursitis
 o. process
oleoresin
 plant o.
oleosa
 hyperhidrosis o.
 seborrhea o.
oleosus
Oligella
olighidria

oligoarthritis
asymmetric o.
seronegative o.
oligoarthropathy
asymmetric o.
oligoarticular seronegative
rheumatoid arthritis
oligocystic
oligodynamic
oligohidria
oligohidrosis
oligosaccharide
Lewis X o.
oligospermia
oligotrichia
oligotrichosis
O-linked pattern
olive
Russian o.
o. tree
Ollendorf syndrome
Olmstead, Olmsted
O. syndrome
olsalazine sodium
omega-3 fatty acid
omega-6 fatty acid
Omenn syndrome
Omnipen
Omnipen-N
omphalocele
Omsk
O. hemorrhagic fever
O. hemorrhagic fever virus
once-daily dosing (ODD)
Onchocerca
O. caecutiens
O. volvulus
onchocerciasis
onchocercosis
oncofetal antigen
oncogene
BNLF-1 o.
oncogenic virus
oncology
Onconase
oncornaviruses
Oncovirinae

oncovirus
oncus
Ondine curse, periodic breathing
one hand-two foot syndrome
ongles en raquette
onion
onset
insidious o.
ontogeny
onychalgia
o. nervosa
onychatrophia
onychatrophy
onychauxis
onychectomy
onychia
Candida o.
o. craquelé
o. lateralis
o. maligna
o. parasitica
o. periungualis
o. piannic
o. punctata
o. sicca
onychitis
onychoclasis
onychocryptosis
onychodystrophy
onychogenic
onychogryphosis, onychogryposis
onychoheterotopia
onychoid
onychology
onycholysis
onychoma
onychomadesis
onychomalacia
onychomycosis
onychonosus
onycho-osteodysplasia
onychopathic
onychopathology
onychopathy
onychophagia
onychophagy
onychophosis

O

NOTES

283

onychophyma
onychoptosis
onychorrhexis
onychoschizia
onychosis
onychotillomania
onychotomy
onychotrophy
Ony-Clear Nail
o'nyong-nyong
    o.-n. fever
    o.-n. virus
onyx
onyxis
onyxitis
oocysts
    Cryptosporidium o.
Oomycetes
oozing
    o. dermatitis
O&P
    ova and parasites
    test for O.
opacification
    amorphous parenchymal o.
    corneal o.
    ground-glass o.
opacities
    mottled o.
opaline patch
Opcon-A
open
    o. application test
    o. comedo
    o. epicutaneous test (OET)
    o. lung biopsy
    o. patch test
    o. reduction and internal
      fixation (ORIF)
    o. test
opera-glass deformity
opercula
opercularis
    Megalopyge o.
operculate
ophiasis
ophritis
ophryitis
ophryogenes
    ulerythema o.
Ophthacet Ophthalmic
Ophthalgan Ophthalmic

ophthalmia
    o. neonatorum
    spring o.
Ophthalmic
    Achromycin O.
    Acular O.
    AK-Chlor O.
    AK-Cide O.
    AK-Dex O.
    AK-Homatropine O.
    AK-Neo-Dex O.
    AK-Poly-Bac O.
    AK-Pred O.
    AK-Sulf O.
    AKTob O.
    AK-Tracin O.
    AK-Trol O.
    Alomide O.
    Atropair O.
    Atropine-Care O.
    Atropisol O.
    Betimol O.
    Bleph-10 O.
    Blephamide O.
    Cetamide O.
    Cetapred O.
    Chloroptic O.
    Chloroptic-P O.
    Ciloxan O.
    Dexacidin O.
    Dexasporin O.
    Econopred O.
    Econopred Plus O.
    Flarex O.
    Fluor-Op O.
    FML O.
    FML Forte O.
    Garamycin O.
    Genoptic O.
    Genoptic S.O.P. O.
    Gentacidin O.
    Gentak O.
    Herplex O.
    HMS Liquifilm O.
    Ilotycin O.
    Inflamase Forte O.
    Inflamase Mild O.
    Isopto Atropine O.
    Isopto Cetapred O.
    Isopto Homatropine O.
    Isopto Hyoscine O.
    I-Sulfacet O.
    I-Tropine O.

Livostin O.
Maxitrol O.
Metimyd O.
Metreton O.
Natacyn O.
NeoDecadron O.
Neo-Dexameth O.
Ocu-Tropine O.
Ophthacet O.
Ophthalgan O.
Ophthocort O.
Osmoglyn O.
Polysporin O.
Polytrim O.
Pred Forte O.
Pred-G O.
Pred Mild O.
Sodium Sulamyd O.
Sulf-10 O.
Sulfair O.
Timoptic O.
Timoptic-XE O.
TobraDex O.
Tobrex O. ·
Vasocidin O.
Vasosulf O.
Vira-A O.
Viroptic O.
ophthalmica
  zona o.
ophthalmicus
  herpes zoster o.
ophthalmomaxillaris
  nevus o.
  nevus fuscoceruleus o.
ophthalmomyiasis
Ophthocort
  O. Ophthalmic
opioid
oppilation
opportunistic
  o. infection
  o. organism
  o. pathogen
  o. systemic fungal infection
  o. systemic mycosis

OPSI
  overwhelming postsplenectomy
    infection
opsinogen
OpSite semipermeable dressing
opsogen
opsonic
  o. deficiency
opsonin
  common o.
  immune o.
  normal o.
  specific o.
  thermolabile o.
  thermostable o.
opsonization
opsonocytophagic
opsonometry
opsonophagocytic defect
opsonophilia
opsonophilic
optic
  o. atrophy
  o. glioma
  o. neuritis
Opticrom
Opti-Flex
OptiHaler
Optimine
optimum temperature
**Opti 1 portable pH/blood gas
  analyzer**
OPV
Orabase
  O. HCA
  Kenalog in O.
  O. with benzocaine
Oracit
oral
  Achromycin V O.
  Aller-Chlor O.
  o. allergy syndrome
  AllerMax O.
  Amino-Opti-E O.
  o. antihistamine
  o. aphthous ulcer
  Aquasol E O.

O

NOTES

285

oral *(continued)*
Asacol O.
Bactocill O.
Banophen O.
Beepen-VK O.
Belix O.
Benadryl O.
Betapen-VK O.
Bio-Tab O.
Blocadren O.
Brethine O.
Bricanyl O.
Calciferol O.
24Calm-X O.
o. candidiasis
Cataflam O.
o. cavity abnormality
CeeNU O.
Ceftin O.
o. challenge
Chlo-Amine O.
Chlorate O.
Chlor-Trimeton O.
Cipro O.
Coly-Mycin S O.
o. condyloma planus
Cortone Acetate O.
Cytoxan O.
Delta-Cortef O.
Deltasone O.
Diamine T.D. O.
Diflucan O.
Dimetabs O.
Dimetane O.
Dormin O.
Doryx O.
Doxy O.
Doxychel O.
Dramamine O.
Drisdol O.
Dynacin O.
E.E.S. O.
E-Mycin O.
o. epithelial nevus
o. (erosive) lichen planus
Eryc O.
EryPed O.
Ery-Tab O.
o. erythema multiforme
Erythrocin O.
o. erythromycin ethylsuccinate
Eryzole O.
Flagyl O.

o. florid papillomatosis
Floxin O.
Flumadine O.
Gantrisin O.
Gastrocrom O.
Genahist O.
o. hairy leukoplakia
o. hyposensitization
Ilosone O.
Imitrex O.
Indocin O.
Indocin SR O.
o. iron therapy
Kantrex O.
o. keratosis
Laniazid O.
Ledercillin VK O.
Liquid Pred O.
Marmine O.
Maxaquin O.
Meclomen O.
Medrol O.
o. melanoacanthoma
Mephyton O.
Meticorten O.
Minocin O.
Monodox O.
o. mucosa
Mycifradin Sulfate O.
Mycostatin O.
Neo-fradin O.
Neoral O.
Neo-Tabs O.
Nidryl O.
Nizoral O.
Nordryl O.
Noroxin O.
Nor-tet O.
Orasone O.
Oxsoralen-Ultra O.
Panmycin O.
PCE O.
PediaCare O.
Pediapred O.
Pediazole O.
Penetrex O.
Pentasa O.
Pen-Vee K O.
Pepcid O.
Phenameth O.
Phendry O.
Phenergan O.
Phenetron O.

poliovirus vaccine, live,
trivalent, o.
o. postinflammatory
hyperpigmentation
Prednicen-M O.
Prelone O.
Prostaphlin O.
Prothazine O.
Protostat O.
Retrovir O.
Rifadin O.
Rimactane O.
Robicillin VK O.
Robitet O.
Salagen O.
Sandimmune O.
Sleep-eze 3 O.
Sominex O.
Sporanox O.
Sterapred O.
Sumycin O.
o. tattoo
Tega-Vert O.
Telachlor O.
Teldrin O.
Teline O.
Terramycin O.
Tetracap O.
Tetralan O.
Tetram O.
o. thrush
Trisoralen O.
Twilite O.
o. ulceration
Unipen O.
Uri-Tet O.
Valium O.
Valrelease o.
Vancocin o.
V-Cillin K o.
Veetids o.
VePesid o.
Vibramycin o.
Videx o.
Vivotif Berna o.
Voltaren o.
Wellcovorin o.

Zantac o.
Zovirax o.
Oraminic II injection
orange
　　o. blossom
Orap
Orasone Oral
orbicular
　　o. eczema
orbiculare
　　Pityrosporum o.
orbicularis
　　o. oculi
　　psoriasis o.
orbital
　　o. inflammatory disease
　　o. myositis
　　o. pseudotumor
Orbivirus
orchard
　　o. grass
ordinal designation of the
　　exanthemata
Oregon ash
Orex
orf
　　human o. virus
　　o. virus
organ culture
Organidin
organism
　　calculated mean o. (CMO)
　　Cox o.
　　encapsulated o.
　　Gram-negative o.
　　Gram-positive o.
　　hypothetical mean o.
　　opportunistic o.
　　pleuro-pneumoniae-like o.
　　(PPLO)
　　prokaryotic extracellular o.
organization
　　health maintenance o. (HMO)
organoid nevus
organotaxis
organotropic
organotropism

O

NOTES

organotropy
organ-specific
    o.-s. antigen
Orgotein
Oriboca virus
oriental
    O. boil
    O. button
    o. rat flea
    o. rat flea bite
    O. ringworm
    O. sore
    O. ulcer
orientalis
    furunculosis o.
    Leishmania o.
ORIF
    open reduction and internal fixation
orifice
    follicular o.
orificial
orificialis
    tuberculosis cutis o.
origin
    antirabies serum, equine o.
    fever of unknown o. (FUO)
Orimune
Orinidyl
Orion
    O. device
    O. inhaler
oris
    cancrum o.
    leukokeratosis o.
Ormazine
Ornade
ornidazole
Ornidyl injection
Ornithodoros
ornithosis virus
oronasal
oropharyngeal candidiasis
oropharynx
orotic aciduria
orotidinuria
orphan
    chicken embryo lethal o.
    (CELO)
    o. disease
    o. drug
    enteric cytopathogenic
    bovine o. (ECBO)

    enteric cytopathogenic
      human o. (ECHO)
    enteric cytopathogenic
      monkey o. (ECMO)
    enteric cytopathogenic swine o.
    (ECSO)
    o. virus
orris root
Orthoclone OKT3
orthokeratinization
orthokeratosis
Ortho-Kung T cell (OKT cell)
orthomolecular therapy
Orthomyxoviridae
    O. virus
orthophosphate (P1)
orthopnea
Orthopoxvirus
    O. vaccinia
orthosis
    thoraco-lumbar-sacral o.
orthostatic hypotension
orthotic
Orudis
    O. KT
Oruvail
oryzae
    Aspergillus o.
    Rhizopus o.
orzihabitans
    Flavimonas o.
OSA
    obstructive sleep apnea
oscillation
    high frequency o.
oscillator
    Hayek o.
Osler
    O. disease
    O. hemangiomatosis
    O. node
    O. sign
Osler-Weber-Rendu
    O.-W.-R. disease
    O.-W.-R. syndrome
osmidrosis
Osmitrol injection
Osmoglyn Ophthalmic
osmolality
osmophil
osmotic shock

osseous
    o. heteroplasia
    o. lesion
ossicles
    intra-articular o.
ossificans
    myositis o.
ossification
    para-articular o.
ossium
    fibrogenesis imperfecta o.
osteitis
    o. fibrosa
    o. fibrosa cystica disseminata
osteoarthritis (OA)
    erosive o. (EOA)
    idiopathic hypertrophic o.
osteoarthropathy
    hypertrophic o.
osteoarticular candidiasis
osteocalcin
osteochondritis dissecans
osteochondrodysplasia
osteochondromatosis
osteoclast
osteoclast-activating factor (OAF)
osteocyte
    o. lacunae
osteodermatopoikilosis
osteodermatous
osteodermia
osteodystrophy
    Albright hereditary o.
osteogenesis
    o. imperfecta
    o. imperfecta tarda
OsteoGram bone density test
osteolytic bone lesion
osteoma cutis
osteomalacia
Osteomark urine-based test
osteomatosis
osteomyelitis
    Aspergillus o.
    blastomycotic o.
    Candida o.
    candidal o.

    coccidioidal o.
    pyogenic o.
osteon
osteonecrosis
osteonectin
osteo-onychodysplasia
osteopenia
osteopetrosis gallinarum
osteophyte
osteopoikilosis
osteopontin
osteoporosis
    age-related o.
    o. circumscripta
    juxta-articular o.
    periarticular o.
    type I o.
    type II o.
osteosis cutis
Osterballe precision needle
ostia
ostium
    pilosebaceous o.
ostracea
    parakeratosis o.
ostraceous
    o. scale
ostreacea
    psoriasis o.
OT
    occupational therapy
Ota
    nevus of O.
    O. nevus
Ot antigen
Otic
    Acetasol HC O.
    AK-Spore H.C. O.
    AntibiOtic O.
    Bacticort O.
    Cortatrigen O.
    Cortisporin O.
    O. Domeboro
    Drotic O.
    LazerSporin-C O.
    Octicair O.
    Ocutricin HC O.

O

NOTES

Otic *(continued)*
    Otobiotic O.
    Otocort O.
    Otomycin-HPN O.
    Otosporin O.
    PediOtic O.
    VoSol O.
    VoSol HC O.
oticus
    herpes zoster o.
otitis
    o. externa
    external o.
    o. media
Otobiotic Otic
Otocalm Ear
Otocort Otic
Otomycin-HPN Otic
otomycosis
otoscopy
    pneumatic o.
Otosporin Otic
ototoxicity
Ouchterlony
    O. method
    O. technique
    O. test
outer
    o. canthus
    o. root sheath
Outerbridge scale
output
    adequate urine o.
ovale
    Pityrosporum o.
    Plasmodium o.
ovalis
    Malassezia o.
ova and parasites (O&P)
overdosage
overdose
    drug o.
overlap
    o. disease
    o. myositis (OVLP)
    o. syndrome
overlay
    PAL pump for air mattress o.
overriding maxillary incisor
overuse syndrome
overwhelming postsplenectomy infection (OPSI)
overwintering

ovine progressive pneumonia
ovinia
oviposit
OVLP
    overlap myositis
ovomucoid
oxacillin
    o. disk diffusion test
    o. sodium
oxalate
    o. crystal
oxalosis
oxamniquine
Oxandrin
oxandrolone
oxaprozin
oxazepam
oxeye, ox-eye
    e. daisy
Oxford unit
oxiconazole
    o. nitrate
oxidase
    lysyl o.
    NADPH o.
    urate o.
oxidative burst
oxide
    ethylene o.
    mercuric o.
    nitric o.
    nitrous o.
oxidized cellulose
OxiFlow
oximeter
    Cricket recording pulse o.
    INVOS Cerebral O.
    Nellcor Symphony N-3000 pulse o.
    Nonin Onyx pulse o.
    Ohmeda hand-held o.
    Oxypleth pulse o.
    OxyTemp hand-held pulse o.
    SpotCheck+ handheld pulse o.
oxipurinol
Oxistat
    O. topical
Oxsoralen
    O. topical
    O.-Ultra Oral
oxtriphylline
Oxy-5
    O. Tinted

oxybenzone
methoxycinnamate and o.
Oxycel
oxychlorosene sodium
Oxyfil oxygen refilling system
oxygen
o. consumption per minute
(VO_2)
continuous low-flow o.
fraction of inspired o. (FIO_2)
o. free radical
humidified o.
hyperbaric o. (HBO)
o. metabolite
partial pressure of o. (PO_2)
partial pressure alveolar o.
(PAO_2)
partial pressure arterial o.
(PaO_2)
supplemental o.
oxygenation
extracorporeal membrane o.
(ECMO)

oxygenator
oxyhemoglobin (HbO_2)
oxymetazoline hydrochloride
oxymetholone
oxyphenbutazone
Oxypleth pulse oximeter
OxyTemp hand-held pulse oximeter
oxytetracycline
o. hydrochloride
o. and hydrocortisone
o. and polymyxin b
OxyTip
oxytoca
Klebsiella o.
Oxyuris vermicularis
oyster
o. mass of mucus
ozochrotia
ozone
ozzardi
Mansonella o.

NOTES

O

P

P antigen
P blood group antigen
P and PD

P1

orthophosphate

P450

cytochrome P.

p24

p. antigen
p. antigen testing

PA

polyarthritis

PABA

para-aminobenzoic acid

Pacheco parrot disease virus

pachyderma

p. lymphangiectatica
p. verrucosa
p. vesicae

pachydermatocele

pachydermatosis

pachydermatous

pachydermia

pachydermic

pachydermoperiostosis

pachyglossia

pachyhymenia

pachyhymenic

pachylosis

pachymenia

pachymenic

pachymeningitis

hypertrophic cervical p.
rheumatoid p.

pachyonychia

p. congenita

pachyotia

Pacific tick

pacificus

Ixodes p.

pacinian neurofibroma

packed red cell transfusion

paclitaxel

pad

herniated presacral fat p.
knuckle p.

Paecilomyces

Paederus

P. gemellus

P. gemellus sting
P. limnophilus
P. limnophilus sting

PAF

platelet-activating factor
platelet-aggregating factor

PAG

pregnancy alpha-2 glycoprotein

PAGE

polyacrylamide gel electrophoresis

Paget

P. cells
P. disease

pagetoid

p. cells
p. reticulosis

PAH

p-aminohippurate

pain

chronic p.
global rating of p.
limb p.
p. on motion
paranasal sinus p.
pleuritic chest p.

painful

p. adiposity
p. mouth
p. piezogenic pedal papule
p. tongue

painful-bruising syndrome

Pain-HP

No P.-H.

paint

Castellani p.

paired venom gland

Pak

Shingles Relief P.

PAL

powered air loss
PAL pump for air mattress
overlay

palatal papillomatosis

palate

hard p.
high-arched p.
itchy soft p.

palatinus

torus p.

pale color

P

palestinensis
  Acanthamoeba p.
palindromic rheumatism
palisade
  p. cell
  p. layer
palisaded encapsulated neuroma
palisading
  p. granuloma
  p. histiocyte
pallescense
pallesthesia
pallida
  Spirochaeta p.
pallidum
  microhemagglutination-
    Treponema p. (MHA-TP)
  Treponema p.
pallor
palm
  hyperlinear p.
  liver p.
  queen p.
  reddening of p.
  p. tree
  tripe p.
palmar
  p. aponeurosis
  p. crease
  p. erythema
  p. fascia
  p. fasciitis and polyarthritis
    syndrome
  p. syphilid
palmare
  erythema p.
  xanthoma striatum p.
palmaris
  pyosis p.
  xanthochromia striata p.
  xanthoma striata p.
palmellina
  trichomycosis p.
palmitate
  clofazimine p.
palmoplantar
  p. fibromatosis
  p. keratoderma (PPK)
palmoplantaris
  pustulosis p.
palm-sole involvement
palpable purpura
palpebral edema

palpebrarum
  pediculosis p.
  xanthelasma p.
  xanthoma p.
  p. xanthoma
palsy
  Bell p.
  facial nerve p.
  transitory p.
pamidronate
p-aminohippurate (PAH)
pamoate
  pyrantel p.
PAN
  polyacrylonitrile
  PAN membrane
Panadol
panagglutinable
panagglutinins
panama
  Salmonella p.
panaritium
Panasol II home phototherapy
  system
panatrophy of Gower
pancreatic
  p. disorder
  p. lobular panniculitis
pancreatitis
pancuronium bromide
pandemic
pandemicity
panel
  ABPA p.
  cellular immune p.
  humoral immunity status p.
  hypersensitivity pneumonitis p.
    (HSP)
  latex RIA p.
panencephalitis
  nodular p.
  subacute sclerosing p. (SSPE)
panhidrosis
panhypopituitarism
  autoimmune p.
  idiopathic p.
  secondary p.
panidrosis
panimmunity
panleukopenia
  p. virus of cats
Panmycin Oral
panniculitides

panniculitis
α_1 antitrypsin deficiency p.
chemical p.
cold p.
cytophagic histiocytic p.
cytophagic lobular p.
histiocytic cytophagic p.
idiopathic p.
idiopathic lobular p.
lobular p.
lupus erythematosus p.
nodular migratory p.
nodular nonsuppurative p.
pancreatic lobular p.
physical lobular p.
relapsing febrile nodular
nonsuppurative p.
scleroderma septal p.
septal p.
subacute migratory p.
subacute nodular migratory p.
pannus-cartilage junction
pannus cell
panophthalmitis
PanOxyl
PanOxyl-AQ
Panscol
P. Lotion
P. Ointment
panspermia
pan T-cell marker
pantothenic acid deficiency
pantropic virus
PAO₂
partial pressure alveolar oxygen
PaO₂
partial pressure arterial oxygen
pao ferro wood
papain
Papanicolaou test (Pap test)
papaverine
paper
Diazo p.
litmus p.
p. mulberry

p. mulberry tree
p. wasp
papilla, pl. papillae
anogenital vestibular p.
dermal p.
hypertrophy of tongue p.
vestibular p.
papillaris
pars p.
papillary
p. atrophy
p. dermis
p. ectasia
p. hidradenoma
p. necrosis
p. tumor
papilliferum
hidradenoma p.
syringocystadenoma p.
papilliferus
nevus
syringocystadenomatosus p.
papillitis
papilloadenocystoma
papillocarcinoma
papilloma
p. acuminatum
basal cell p.
canine oral p.
p. diffusum
p. durum
hard p.
p. inguinale tropicum
p. molle
Shope p.
soft p.
p. venereum
zymotic p.
papillomatosis
confluent and reticulate p.
florid cutaneous p. (FCP)
florid oral p.
p. of Gougerot-Carteaud
juvenile p.
laryngeal p.
malignant p.
oral florid p.

NOTES

P

papillomatosis *(continued)*
  palatal p.
  reticulated p.
papillomatosus
  lupus p.
  nevus p.
papillomatous
Papillomavirus
papillomavirus, papilloma virus
  human p. (HPV)
Papillon-Lèfevre syndrome
Papineau graft
Papovaviridae
papovavirus
pappataci
  p. fever
  p. fever virus
pappose
pappus
Pap test
papula
papular
  p. acne
  p. acrodermatitis
  p. acrodermatitis of childhood
  p. dermatitis of pregnancy
  p. fever
  p. fibroplasia
  p. mastocytosis
  p. mucinosis
  p. scrofuloderma
  p. stomatitis virus of cattle
  p. syphilid
  p. tuberculid
  p. urticaria
papulation
  granular p.
  perifollicular p.
papulatum
  erythema p.
papule
  Celsus p.
  discrete umbilicated p.
  fibrous p.
  follicular p.
  Gottron p.'s
  indolent p.
  indurated p.
  keratotic p.
  moist p.
  mucous p.
  painful piezogenic pedal p.
  penile pearly p.

  persistent pearly penile p.
  piezogenic pedal p.
  pruritic p.
  purple-red p.
  red p.
  split p.
papuliferous
papuloerythematous
papuloerythroderma
papulonecrotica
  tuberculosis p.
  tuberculosis cutis p.
papulonecrotic tuberculid
papulopustular
  p. lesion
papulopustule
papulosa
  acne p.
  p. nigra dermatosis
  stomatitis p.
  urticaria p.
papulose atrophicante maligne
papulosis
  atrophic p.
  p. atrophicans maligna
  bowenoid p.
  lymphomatoid p.
  malignant atrophic p.
papulosquamous
  p. dermatitis
  p. disorder
  p. lesion
  p. syphilid
papulosum
  eczema p.
papulovesicle
papulovesicular
  p. lesion
  p. rash
papyraceous
  p. scar
para-aminobenzoic acid (PABA)
para-aminosalicylate sodium
para-aminosalicylic acid
para-articular ossification
parachlorometaxylenol
parachlorophenylalanine
parachroma
parachromatosis
paracoccidioidal granuloma
Paracoccidioides brasiliensis
paracoccidioidin
  p. skin test

paracoccidioidomycosis
paracrine
paradox
    thoracoabdominal p.
paradoxical
    p. pulse
    p. sleep
paradoxus
    pulsus p.
paraffinoma
parafollicularis
    hyperkeratosis follicularis et p.
parafrenal abscess
paragonimiasis
Paragonimus
    P. kellicotti
    P. westermani
parahaemolyticus
    Haemophilus p.
parahidrosis
parainfluenza
    p. virus
parainfluenzae
    Haemophilus p.
parakeet feather
parakeratosis
    p. ostracea
    p. psoriasiformis
    p. pustulosa
    p. scutularis
    p. variegata
parallergic
paralysis
    acute atrophic p.
    acute flaccid p. (AFP)
    fowl p.
    immune p.
    immunological p.
    infectious bulbar p.
    myogenic p.
    phrenic nerve p.
    tick p.
parameter
paramethasone acetate
Paramyxoviridae
    P. virus

Paramyxovirus
paranasal
    p. sinus drainage
    p. sinus pain
paraneoplastic
    p. acrokeratosis
    p. syndrome
paraneoplastica
    acrokeratosis p.
parangi
Para-Pak Ultra Ecofix system
parapertussis
    Bordetella p.
paraphenylenediamine
    p. dermatitis
paraphimosis
parapneumonic effusion
Parapoxvirus
paraproteinemia
parapsilosis
    Candida p.
parapsoriasis
    p. acuta et varioliformis
    p. en gouttes
    p. en plaque
    p. guttata
    guttate p.
    large-plaque p.
    p. lichenoid
    p. lichenoides et varioliformis
        acuta
    poikilodermatous p.
    small plaque p.
    p. variegata
    p. varioliformis
pararama
parascarlatina
parasitaria
parasite
    metazoal p.
    ova and p.'s (O&P)
parasitic
    p. cyst
    p. disease
    p. granuloma
    p. melanoderma

NOTES

P

parasitica
    achromia p.
    onychia p.
parasiticum
    eczema p.
parasitosis
    delusion of p.
parasympathetic nerve fiber
parasyphilis
paratope
paratracheal region
paratrichosis
paratrimma
    erythema p.
paratripsis
paratriptic
paratyphi
    Salmonella p.
paraumbilical nodule
paraungual
paravaccinia
    p. virus
    p. virus infection
Paravespula
    P. sting
parchment skin
Par Decon
parenchyma
parenchymal
    p. amyloidosis
    p. fibrosis
parenteral
    p. absorption
    Coly-Mycin M P.
    p. corticosteroid
    p. diphenhydramine
    p. gold
paresis
paresthesia
paresthetica
    meralgia p.
    notalgia p.
paridrosis
Parinaud oculoglandular syndrome
Parker-Pearson needle
Parkes-Weber hemangiomatosis
Parkinson disease
Park-Williams bacillus
paromomycin
    p. sulfate
paronychia
    acute p.
    Candida p.

candidal p.
chronic p.
herpetic p.
paronychial
    p. wart
paronychomycosis
paronychosis
parotid gland
parotiditis
    epidemic p.
parotitis
paroxetine
    p. HCl
    p. hydrochloride
paroxysmal
    p. cold hemoglobinuria
    p. flushing
    p. nocturnal hemoglobinuria
    (PNH)
    p. sneezing
paroxysm of coughing
parrot
    p. feather
    p. virus
parrot-beak nail
Parry-Romberg syndrome
pars
    p. papillaris
    p. reticularis
parsley
parsnip
partial
    p. agglutinin
    p. antigen
    p. combined immunodeficiency
    disorder
    p. face-sparing lipodystrophy
    p. leukonychia
    p. lipodystrophy
    p. pressure alveolar oxygen
    (PAO$_2$)
    p. pressure arterial oxygen
    (PaO$_2$)
    p. pressure of carbon dioxide
    (PCO$_2$)
    p. pressure of oxygen (PO$_2$)
    p. thromboplastin time (PTT)
partialis
    hypertrichosis p.
partial-thickness burn
particle
    Dane p.
    defective interfering p.

DI p.
signal recognition p.
particulate matter
Partuss LA
parvilocular cyst
Parvoviridae
Parvovirus
parvovirus
human p. (HPV)
human p. B19
Parvovirus B 19
parvum bovine immunoglobulin concentrate
PAS
periodic acid-Schiff
PAS stain
PAS technique
P.A.S.
Sodium P.
Paschen bodies
Paser
Pasini epidermolysis bullosa
Pasini-Pierini idiopathic atrophoderma
passage
blind p.
percutaneous p.
serial p.
passant
en p.
passion purpura
passive
p. agglutination
p. anaphylaxis
p. cutaneous anaphylactic reaction
p. cutaneous anaphylaxis (PCA)
p. cutaneous anaphylaxis test
p. hemagglutination (PHA)
p. immunity
p. immunization
p. immunotherapy
p. motion
p. prophylaxis
p. range of motion exercise

p. transference
p. transfer test
Passy-Muir tracheostomy speaking valve
Paste
Triple P.
paste
baking soda p.
Camcreme ECG p.
Lassar p.
Pasteurella
P. aerogenes
P. multocida
P. pestis
P. tularensis
Pasteur vaccine
Pastia
P. line
P. sign
patagium
cervical p.
patch
butterfly p.
cotton-wool p.
eczematous p.
herald p.
moth p.
mucous p.
opaline p.
PediaPatch Transdermal P.
Peyer p.
pruritic erythematous p.
salmon p.
shagreen p.
soldier p.
p. stage
p. test
p. testing
p. test interpretation
Testoderm p.
p. test scarring
Transderm Scōp P.
Trans-Plantar Transdermal P.
Trans-Ver-Sal transdermal p.
Verukan solution
patchouli oil

NOTES

P

patchy
p. airspace consolidation
p. infiltrate
patellar tendinitis
patellofemoral
p. disease
p. joint
p. pain syndrome
pathergy
Pathocil
pathoclisis
pathogen
opportunistic p.
pathogenesis
pathogenetic
pathogenic blastomycetes
pathogenicity
pathognomic
pathognomonic
pathologically confirmed complete remission (PCR)
pathologic feature
pathology
bite p.
pathometric
pathometry
pathophysiology
pathway
effector p.
monooxygenase p.
Raper-Mason p.
patient
hemophiliac p.
nonhemophiliac p.
Patois virus
pattern
bimodal immunofluorescent p.
Christmas tree p.
p. of distribution
geographic p.
ground-glass p.
herringbone p.
livedo p.
netted p.
N-linked p.
nodular p.
O-linked p.
polycyclic p.
polygenic inheritance p.
restrictive ventilatory p.
reticular p.
rheumatoid p.
p. of staining

stellate p.
webbed p.
zosteriform p.
patterned
p. alopecia
p. leukoderma
pauciarticular
p. arthritis
p. juvenile rheumatoid arthritis
paucibacillary leprosy
pauci-inflammatory
Paul
P. reaction
P. test
paul
Salmonella st. p.
Paul-Bunnell test
paurometabolum
Tsukamurella p.
Pautrier
P. abscess
P. microabscess
Paxil
Paxton disease
PBMC
peripheral blood mononuclear cell
PBZ
pyribenzamine
PBZ-SR
PCA
passive cutaneous anaphylaxis
PCE Oral
PCNA
proliferating cell nuclear antigen
PCO$_2$
partial pressure of carbon dioxide
PCP
Pneumocystis carinii pneumonia
PCR
pathologically confirmed complete remission
polymerase chain reaction
arbitrary primed PCR (AP-PCR)
PCR assay
PCR for HIV DNA
mixed-linker PCR (ML-PCR)
repetitive PCR (Rep-PCR)
TB test by PCR
PCT
porphyria cutanea tarda
PD
P and P.

percussion and postural
drainage
PDGF
platelet-derived growth factor
PDL
pulsed dye laser
PE
Guiatuss P.
Halotussin P.
peach
peak
biclonal p.
p. expiratory flow (PEFR)
p. expiratory flow rate
p. flow meter
p. inspiratory ventilator
pressure
monoclonal p.
p. serum level
p. and trough
widow's p.
peanut
pear
pearls
Epstein p.
necklace of p.
Pearson chi square test
peas
peau
p. de chagrin
p. d'orange
pecan
p. tree
pectoris
pseudoangina p.
pectus excavatum
PediaCare
P. Oral
Pediacof
PediaPatch Transdermal Patch
Pediapred Oral
Pediatric
pediatric
American Academy of P.'s
(AAP)
Cleocin p.
Fedahist Expectorant p.

p. infectious disease
developmental screening test
(PIDDST)
p. scleroderma
Pediazole
P. Oral
pedicellaria
triple-jawed p.
Pedi-Cort V topical
pediculation
pediculicide
Pediculoides ventricosus
pediculosis
p. capitis
p. corporis
p. corporis vel vestimentorum
p. palpebrarum
p. pubis
p. vestimenti
pediculous
Pediculus
P. capitis
P. corporis
P. humanus
P. humanus capitis
P. humanus capitis infestation
Pedi-Dri
Pedinol
PediOtic Otic
Pedi-Pro topical
pedis
dermatomycosis p.
dysesthesia p.
malum perforans p.
spina p.
tinea p.
Pedituss
pedrosoi
Fonsecaea p.
Hormodendron p.
peduncle
pedunculated
peel
chemical p.
face p.
familial continuous skin p.
skin p.

NOTES

P

301

peeling-skin syndrome
PEEP
    positive end-expiratory pressure
pefloxacin
PEFR
    peak expiratory flow
peg
    rete p.
pegademase bovine
pelade
pelage
pelidnoma
pelioma
peliosis
pellagra
pellagra-associated dermatitis
pellagrin
pellagroid
    p. dermatitis
pellagrous
pelletieri
    Actinomadura p.
pellicle
    acquired p.
pellitory
    wall p.
pelt
peltation
pelvic inflammatory disease (PID)
pemphigoid
    benign mucosal p.
    bullous p. (BP)
    cicatricial p.
    lichen planus p.
    mucous-membrane p.
    p. syphilid
pemphigoides
pemphigosa
    variola p.
pemphigus
    p. acutus
    benign familial chronic p.
    Brazilian p.
    p. contagiosus
    p. erythematosus
    familial benign chronic p.
    foliaceous p.
    p. foliaceus
    p. gangrenosus
    p. leprosus
    p. neonatorum
    ocular p.
    old-man's p.

p. vegetans
p. vulgaris
pemphigus-like eruption
pen
    Pilot Spotlighter p.
penciclovir
pencil
    p. and cup deformity
    styptic p.
pendulum
    fibroma p.
Penecort
penetrans
    hyperkeratosis follicularis et
        parafollicularis in cutem p.
    Tunga p.
penetrant
Penetrex Oral
penicillamine
penicillin
    p. aqueous
    p. desensitization
    p. g benzathine
    p. g benzathine and procaine
        combined
    p. g procaine
    phenoxymethyl p.
    p. therapy
    unit of p.
    p. v potassium
    p. v suspension
penicillin G
penicillin-induced anaphylaxis
penicillin-penicilloyl human serum
    albumin (PPO-HSA)
penicillin-resistant *Streptococcus*
    pneumoniae **(PRSP)**
penicillin V
Penicillin VK
penicilliosis
Penicillium
    P. marneffei
    P. notatum
penicilloyl G
penicilloyl G/V
penicilloyl V
penile
    p. pearly papule
    p. sclerosing lymphangitis
penis
    Bowen disease of the glans p.
    glans p.

induratio p. plastica
median raphe cyst of the p.
Pentacarinat injection
Pentacef
Pentam-300 injection
pentamer
pentamidine
p. in aerosol form
p. isethionate
Pentasa Oral
Pentatrichomonas hominis
pentavalent gas gangrene antitoxin
penton
p. antigen
pentosan
sodium p.
pentoxifylline
Pentrax
Pen-Vee K Oral
pen VK
PEP
positive expiratory pressure
PEP mask
Pepcid
P. AC Acid Controller
P. I.V.
P. Oral
peplomer
peplos
pepper
black p.
green p.
peppertree
California p.
peptide
anaphylatoxin p.
anionic neutrophil activating p.
(ANAP)
p. antigen
chemotactic p.
connective tissue activating p.
(CTAP)
procollagen type III
aminoterminal p.
peptide-1
neutrophil-activating p.
Peptide T

peptidoglycan
Pepto-Bismol
Peptococcus niger
Peptostreptococcus
P. anaerobius
P. asaccharolyticus
P. magnus
P. prevotii
P. productus
P. saccharolyticus
peracute
perambulating ulcer
perch
perchlornaphthalin
Percogesic
percussion and postural drainage
(P and PD)
percutaneous
p. absorption
p. passage
p. test
peregrinum
Mycobacterium p.
perenne
Lolium p. (Lol p)
perennial
p. allergic rhinitis
p. rye
p. rye grass
perfloxacin
perforans
folliculitis nares p.
mal p.
malum p.
scleromalacia p.
perforant
mal p.
perforating
p. disease
p. folliculitis
p. granuloma annulare
p. ulcer of foot
perforin
perfrigeration
perfume
p. dermatitis
Periactin

NOTES

perianal
  p. pruritus
  p. streptococcal cellulitis
perianth
periaortitis
periapical
periarteritis nodosa
periarthritis
  calcific p.
  shoulder p.
periarticular
  p. disorder
  p. osteoporosis
  p. syndrome
periauricular
peribronchial desquamation
peribronchiolar lymphocyte
  infiltration
péribuccale
  erythrose pigmentaire p.
pericarditis
pericardium
perichondritis
  infectious p.
pericyte
periderm
perifollicular
  p. accentuation
  p. papulation
perifolliculitis
  p. abscedens et suffodiens
  p. capitis abscedens et
    suffodiens
  dissecting p.
  pustular p.
  superficial pustular p.
perihilar
perimyositis
perineural fibrosis
periocular area
period
  eclipse p.
  incubation p.
  induction p.
  latent p.
  prepatent p.
  refractory p.
periodic
  p. acid-Schiff (PAS)
  p. acid-Schiff stain
  p. acid-Schiff technique
  p. edema
  p. leg movement (PLM)

  p. peritonitis
  p. polyserositis
perionychia
perionyxis
perioral
  p. area
  p. dermatitis
periorbital
  p. area
  p. dermatitis
  p. purpura
periostosis
  idiopathic p.
peripheral
  p. airspace
  p. anergy
  p. arthritis
  p. blood count
  p. blood eosinophilia
  p. blood mononuclear cell
    (PBMC)
  p. fibrosis
  p. gangrene
  p. giant cell granuloma
  p. nerve
  p. nerve involvement
  p. nerve sheath tumor
  p. nervous system (PNS)
  p. neuritis
  p. neuromyopathy
  p. ossifying fibroma
  p. staining
  p. T-cell lymphoma
  p. type
periporate
periporitis
periporoma
peritendinitis crepitans
peritonitis
  acute p.
  benign paroxysmal p.
  feline infectious p.
  periodic p.
periungual
  p. erythema
  p. fibroma
  p. telangiectasia
  p. wart
periungualis
  onychia p.
perivascular infiltrate
perivasculitis
  retinal p.

perlecan
perlèche
Perles
    Tessalon P.
Permapen injection
permeability
    vascular p.
permethrin
permissive hypercapnia
perna disease
pernicious anemia
pernio
    p. cyanosis
    erythema p.
    lupus p.
perniosis
Pernox
peroneal
    p. nerve entrapment
    p. tendon
peroral intestinal biopsy
peroxidase
    eosinophil p.
peroxide
    benzoyl p.
    erythromycin and benzoyl p.
Peroxin
    P. A5
    P. A10
Persa-Gel
Persian Gulf syndrome
persistence
    microbial p.
persistent
    p. acantholytic dermatosis
    p. edema
    p. light reaction
    p. light reactor
    p. pearly penile papule
    p. pyoderma
persister
perspiration
    insensible p.
    sensible p.
perspire
perstans
    acrodermatitis p.

Dipetalonema p.
erythema p.
erythema dyschromicum p.
erythema figuratum p.
erythema gyratum p.
hyperkeratosis lenticularis p.
telangiectasia macularis
    eruptiva p. (TMEP)
urticaria p.
persulcatus
    Ixodes p.
persulfate salt
pertenue
    Treponema p.
pertrichosis
Pertussis
pertussis
    p. agglutination test
    Bordetella p.
    p. immune globulin
    p. immunoglobulin
    p. vaccine
Peru
    balsam of P.
peruana
    verruca p.
peruviana
    verruca p.
Peruvian wart
pes
    p. anserinus bursa
    p. febricitans
    p. planus
pest
    fowl p.
    swine p.
pestiferous
pestilence
pestilential
pestis
    Pasteurella p.
    Yersinia p.
Pestivirus
petechia, pl. petechiae
    calcaneal p.
    linear p.
    Tardieu p.

NOTES

P

petechial
    p. hemorrhage
petechiasis
petitgrain oil
Petriellidium boydii
petrolatum
    lanolin, cetyl alcohol, glycerin,
        and p.
    white p.
Pette-Döring disease
Peutz-Jeghers syndrome
Peyer patch
Peyronie disease
PF
    pulmonary function
Pfeiffer phenomenon
PFGE
    pulsed field gel electrophoresis
Pfizerpen
    P.-AS injection
    P. injection
PFS
    Folex P.
    Tarabine P.
PFT
    pulmonary function test
PG
    prostaglandin
P/G
    Fulvicin P.
PGD
    prostaglandin D
PGD2
    prostaglandin D2
PGE
    prostaglandin E
PGE1
    prostaglandin E1
PGE2
    prostaglandin E2
PGH2
    prostaglandin H2
pH
    blood p.
    low urine p.
PHA
    passive hemagglutination
    phytohemagglutinin
phacoanaphylactic uveitis
phacoanaphylaxis
phacomatosis
phaeohyphomycosis

phage
    β p.
    defective p.
phagedena
    p. gangrenosa
    p. nosocomialis
    sloughing p.
    p. tropica
    tropical sloughing p.
phagedenic
    p. ulcer
phagocyte
    p. dysfunction
    p. oxidative burst
phagocytic
    p. deficiency
    p. dysfunction disorders
        immunodeficiency
    p. dysfunction
        immunodeficiency
    p. function
    p. index
phagocytin
phagocytize
phagocytoblast
phagocytolysis
phagocytolytic
phagocytosable debris
phagocytose
phagocytosis
    induced p.
    spontaneous p.
phagolysis
phagolysosome
phagolytic
phagosome
phagotype
phakomatosis
phalange
    proximal p.
phaneroscope
phanerozoite
phantom tumor
Pharmacia lancet
pharmacokinetic
    Dapsone P.'s
pharmacologic
    p. mediators of anaphylaxis
    p. therapy
pharyngeal pouch syndrome
pharyngitis
    arcanobacterial p.

herpangina p.
streptococcal p.
pharyngoconjunctival
   p. fever
   p. fever virus
phase
   p. I rheumatoid arthritis
   p. II rheumatoid arthritis
   anagen p.
   catagen p.
   eclipse p.
   growth p.
   horizontal growth p.
   lag p.
   logarithmic p.
   negative p.
   positive p.
   presensitization p.
   resting p.
   stationary p.
   telogen p.
   vertical growth p.
Phazet lancet
Phenameth Oral
Phenazine injection
phenazopyridine
   sulfisoxazole and p.
Phendry Oral
Phenerbel-S
Phenergan
   P. injection
   P. Oral
Phenetron Oral
phenindamine tartrate
pheniramine, phenylpropanolamine,
  and pyrilamine
phenobarbital
   theophylline, ephedrine, and p.
phenol
   camphor and p.
   camphor, menthol and p.
phenolated disinfectant
phenolformaldehyde
phenology
phenol-preserved extract
phenomenon, pl. phenomena
   adhesion p.

Arthus p.
autoimmune p.
Bordet-Gengou p.
Danysz p.
Debré p.
Denys-Leclef p.
d'Herelle p.
Ehrlich p.
erythrocyte adherence p.
generalized Shwartzman p.
Gengou p.
Gordon p.
hunting p.
immune adherence p.
isomorphic p.
Köbner p.
Koch p.
LE p.
Lucio leprosy p.
Pfeiffer p.
quellung p.
Raynaud p.
red cell adherence p.
Sanarelli p.
Sanarelli-Shwartzman p.
Schultz-Charlton p.
Shwartzman p.
Splendore-Hoeppli p.
spreading p.
Theobald Smith p.
Twort p.
Twort-d'Herelle p.
phenothiazine
phenotype
   Fairbanks arthritis p.
   Ribbing arthritis p.
   VanA p.
phenotypic
   p. mixing
phenoxybenzamine hydrochloride
phenoxymethyl penicillin
phenylalanine metabolism
phenylbutazone
phenylephrine
   brompheniramine and p.
   chlorpheniramine,

NOTES

P

phenylephrine *(continued)*
    phenyltoloxamine,
    phenylpropanolamine and p.
    guaifenesin,
    phenylpropanolamine, and p.
    p. hydrochloride
    isoproterenol and p.
    sodium sulfacetamide and p.
Phenylfenesin L.A.
phenylketonuria
phenylpropanolamine
    brompheniramine and p.
    chlorpheniramine, phenylephrine,
      and p.
    chlorpheniramine, pyrilamine,
      phenylephrine, and p.
    clemastine and p.
    guaifenesin and p.
    p. hydrochloride
phenyltoloxamine
    acetaminophen and p.
    chlorpheniramine, phenylephrine,
      and p.
    p., phenylpropanolamine, and
      acetaminophen
phenytoin
pheochromocytoma
pheomelanin
Phialophora
    P. richardsiae
    P. verrucosa
phimosis
pHisoHex
phlebectasia
    congenital generalized p.
Phlebotomus
    P. fever
    P. fever virus
Phlebovirus
phlegmasia
    p. alba
    p. alba dolens
    p. malabarica
phlegmon
    diffuse p.
phlegmonous
    p. cellulitis
    p. erysipelas
    p. ulcer
phlei
    Mycobacterium p.
phlogosin
phlogotherapy

phlyctena
phlyctenar
phlyctenoid
phlyctenosis
phlyctenous
phlyctenular
phlyctenule
PHN
    postherpetic neuralgia
Phoma
    P. betae
    P. fungus
    P. species
phorbol ester
Phormia
phosphatase
phosphate
    Aralen P.
    Aralen Phosphate With
      Primaquine P.
    basic calcium p. (BCP)
    chloroquine p.
    Cleocin P.
    Decadron P.
    dexamethasone sodium p.
    Hexadrol P.
    histamine p.
    Hydrocortone P.
    primaquine p.
phosphatidylinositol
phosphodiesterase
    p. inhibitor
    p. isoenzyme inhibitor
phospholipase A
phospholipase A2
phospholipase C
phospholipid
phosphonoformate
phosphorhidrosis
phosphoribosyltransferase
    hypoxanthine-guanine p.
      (HGPRT)
phosphoridrosis
phosphorus
phosphorylation
phosphorylatoin
photo
    p. aging
    p. protection
photoallergen
photoallergic
    p. contact dermatitis
    p. drug reaction

p. reaction
p. sensitivity
photoallergy
photobiologic reaction
photobiology
photochemical
p. reaction
p. smog
photochemistry
photochemotherapy
extracorporeal p.
photocontact
p. dermatitis
photodermatitis
photodermatosis
photodistribution
photodrug
p. reaction
photodynamic
p. sensitization
photoerythema
PhotoGenica laser system
photoinactivation
photoingestant dermatitis
photology
photometry
reflectance p.
photomicrography
photon absorptiometry
photoncia
photonosus
photo-onycholysis
photo-patch, photopatch
p.-p. test
photopathy
photopheresis
photophobia
photophoresis
extracorporeal p.
photophytodermatitis
photoplethysmography (ppg)
photosensitive
p. nonscarring dermatitis
photosensitivity
p. dermatitis
drug-induced bullous p.

p., ichthyosis, brittle hair,
intellectual impairment
p., ichthyosis, brittle hair,
intellectual impairment,
decreased fertility, and short
stature (PIBIDS)
p. reaction
photosensitization
contact p.
phototherapy
photothermolysis
selective p.
phototoxic
p. contact dermatitis
p. drug reaction
p. sensitivity
phototoxicity
phototoxis
PHP
pseudohypoparathyroidism
phragmospore
phrenic
p. nerve
p. nerve paralysis
phrynoderma
phthalic anhydride
phthiriasis
Phthirus
phycomycosis
subcutaneous p.
phylacagogic
phylaxis
Phyllocontin Tablet
phylogenetic atavism
phyma
phymatosis
physical
p. allergy
p. barrier
p. lobular panniculitis
p. stimulus
p. sunscreen
p. urticaria
physiological
p. dead space
p. dead space ventilation per
minute

NOTES

P

physiologic test
physiology
   sleep p.
phytanic
   p. acid
   p. acid storage
   p. acid storage disease
phytoagglutinin
phytodermatitis
phytohemagglutinin (PHA)
phytomitogen
phytonadione
phytophlyctodermatitis
phytophotodermatitis
phytotoxic
phytotoxin
pian
   p. bois
   hemorrhagic p.
piannic
   onychia p.
PIBIDS
   photosensitivity, ichthyosis, brittle
    hair, intellectual impairment,
    decreased fertility, and short
    stature
   P. syndrome
Picker nodule
picker's
   p. acne
   p. nodule
Pick and Go monitor
Picornaviridae
   P. virus
picornavirus
PID
   pelvic inflammatory disease
PIDDST
   pediatric infectious disease
    developmental screening test
PIE
   pulmonary infiltrate with
    eosinophilia
   PIE syndrome
piebaldism
piebaldness
piebald skin
piece
   Fab p.
   Fc p.
piechaudii
   Alcaligenes p.

piedra
   black p.
   p. nostras
   white p.
Piedraia
   P. hortae
pied rond rheumatism
Pierini
   atrophoderma of Pasini and P.
   idiopathic atrophoderma of
    Pasini and P.
piesesthesia, piezesthesia
piezogenic pedal papule
pig
   guinea p.
   p. skin
pigeon
   p. breeder's disease
   p. droppings
   p. feather
   p. serum protein (PSP)
pigment
   abnutzung p.
   p. cell transplantation
   p. change
   incontinence of p.
   minimal p. (MP)
pigmentary
   p. abnormality
   p. atopic dermatitis
   p. demarcation line
   p. syphilid
pigmentation
   amiodarone p.
   arsenic p.
   exogenous p.
pigmented
   p. basal cell carcinoma
   p. hair epidermal nevus
   p. purpura
   p. purpuric lichenoid dermatitis
   p. purpuric lichenoid dermatitis
    of Gougerot
   p. purpuric lichenoid
    dermatosis
   p. villonodular synovitis
    (PVNS)
pigmenti
   incontinentia p.
pigmentolysin
pigmentosa
pigmentosum
   morphea p.

urticaria p.
xeroderma p.
pigmentosus
nevus p.
pigs
mycoplasma pneumonia of p.
virus pneumonia of p.
pigweed
redroot p.
spiny p.
pilar
p. sheath acanthoma
p. tumor of scalp
pilaris
juvenile pityriasis rubra p.
keratosis p.
lichen p.
pityriasis rubra p.
pilary
pileous
pili (*pl. of* pilus)
p. annulatus
p. incarnati
p. multigemini
p. torti
piliferous
p. cyst
piliform
pilocarpine
p. iontophoresis sweat test
piloerection
piloid
piloleiomyoma
pilomatricoma
pilomatrixoma
p. carcinoma
pilomotor reflex
pilonidal
p. cyst
p. fistula
p. sinus
pilorum
p. agenesis
arrectores p.
scissura p.
pilose

pilosebaceous
p. apparatus
p. follicle
p. ostium
p. structure
p. unit
pilosis
pilosus
nevus p.
nevus pigmentosus et p.
Pilot Spotlighter pen
pilus, pl. **pili**
arrector p.
p. bifurcatus
F p.
I p.
R p.
p. tortus
Pima
pimozide
pimple
pincer
p. jaw
p. nail
pine
Australian p.
loblolly p.
lodgepole p.
ponderosa p.
p. resin
p. resin-colophony
slash p.
white p.
pineapple
pinhead-sized milia
pink
p. disease
p. salmon
pinkeye
pinkus
Pinkus tumor
pinna
pinocyte
pinocytosis
active p.
pinosome
pinpoint electrocoagulation

NOTES

P

311

pinpoint-sized milia
Pin-Rid
pinta
pintids
pintoid
pintos
    mal de los p.
pinworm
Pin-X
PIP
    positive inspiratory pressure
    proximal interphalangeal
piperacillin
    p. sodium
    p. sodium and tazobactam
      sodium
piperazine
    p. citrate
piperonal butoxide
Pipracil
pirbuterol
    p. acetate
piriformis syndrome
piritrexim isethionate
piroxicam
Pirquet
    P. reaction
    P. test
pistachio
pistillate
pit
    discrete p.
    ear p.
    Mantoux p.
    nail p.
    tooth p.
    p. viper bite
    p. viper snake
pitch wart
pitted
    p. keratolysis
    p. nail
pitting
    p. edema
    nail p.
    p. of nail
pituitary disorder
pityriasic
pityriasis
    p. alba
    p. alba atrophicans
    p. amiantacea
    p. capitis

    p. circinata
    p. folliculorum
    p. lichenoid
    lichenoid acute p.
    p. lichenoides chronica
    p. lichenoides et varioliformis
      acuta (PLEVA)
    p. linguae
    p. maculata
    p. nigra
    p. rosea
    p. rosea-like eruption
    p. rubra
    p. rubra pilaris
    p. sicca
    p. versicolor
pityriasis-type scale
pityrodes
    alopecia p.
pityroid
Pityrosporum
    P. folliculitis
    P. orbiculare
    P. ovale
pivalate
    clocortolone p.
Pixy321
P-K
    P.-K. antibodies
    P.-K. test
placebo
placenta-eluted gamma globulin
placental
    p. sulfatase deficiency
    p. sulfatase deficiency
      syndrome
pladaroma
plague
    bubonic p.
    cattle p.
    duck p.
    fowl p.
    rabbit p.
    p. vaccine
    vector of p.
Plain
    Citanest P.
plakins
plana
    verruca p.
planci
    Acanthaster p.

plane
diffuse p.
Frankfort horizontal p.
p. wart
planing
planopilaris
lichen p.
plant
p. agglutinin
p. antitoxin
arum p.
p. dermatitis
p. oleoresin
p. toxin
p. virus
planta, pl. plantae
verruca p.
plantain
English p.
plantar
p. dermatitis
p. desquamation
p. fascia
p. maceration
p. nerve syndrome
p. syphilid
p. wart
plantaris
epidermolytic keratosis palmaris
et p.
ichthyosis palmaris et p.
keratoderma palmaris et p.
keratosis palmaris et p.
pustulosis palmaris et p.
tylosis palmaris et p.
verruca p.
planum
xanthoma p.
planus
annular lichen p.
atrophic lichen p.
bullous lichen p.
condyloma p.
erosive lichen p.
follicular lichen p.
genital erosive lichen p.
hypertrophic lichen p.

lichen p.
lichen ruber p.
linear lichen p.
oral condyloma p.
oral (erosive) lichen p.
pes p.
ulcerative lichen p.
plaque
annular erythematous p.
atrophic p.
attachment p.
bacterial p.
cytoplasmic p.
degenerative collagenous p.
dental p.
disseminées parapsoriasis
en p.'s
eczematoid pruritic p.'s
erythematous p.
inflammatory p.
lichenified p.
mucous p.
parapsoriasis en p.
p. psoriasis
psoriatic p.
red-purple p.
p. stage
submucosal p.
ulcero-vegetating p.
urticarial p.
violaceous p.
warty keratotic p.'s
plaque-like cutaneous mucinosis
Plaquenil
plaque-type psoriasis
plasma
p. cell
p. cell balanitis
p. cell dyscrasia with
polyneuropathy, organomegaly,
endocrinopathy, monoclonal
protein
p. cell mucositis
p. cell myeloma
p. cell neoplasm
p. cell pneumonia
p. cellularis

NOTES

P

plasma *(continued)*
  p. cell vulvitis
  p. fibronectin
  fresh frozen p.
  frozen p.
  p. kallikrein
  p. membrane
  p. protein
  p. protein autoantibody
  p. therapy
  zoster immune p. (ZIP)
plasmacyte
plasmacytoapheresis
plasmacytoma
plasmapheresis
  exchange p.
plasmid
  bacteriocinogenic p.
  conjugative p.
  F p.
  infectious p.
  nonconjugative p.
  R p.
  resistance p.
  transmissible p.
plasmin
plasminogen
  p. activator
plasmodia
Plasmodium
  chloroquine-resistant *P.*
    falciparum (CRPF)
  P. falciparum
  P. malariae
  P. ovale
  P. vivax
Plaster
  Mediplast P.
  Sal-Acid P.
plastic
  p. adhesive dressing
  p. iritis
plastica
  induratio penis p.
plastid
Plastizote shoe
plate
  nail p.
platelet
  p. basic protein
  p. concentrate
  p. factor-4

hemolysis, elevated liver
  enzymes, low p. (HELLP)
p. neutralization procedure
p. neutralization test
platelet-activating factor (PAF)
platelet-aggregating factor (PAF)
**platelet-derived growth factor
  (PDGF)**
platelets
  washed maternal p.
plate-like crystal
plates
  lamellar p.
Platinol
Platinol-AQ
platinum
  salt of p.
platybasia
platyonychia
platypnea
platysma
platyspondylia
pleocytosis
pleomorphic lipoma
Plesiomonas shigelloides
plethysmograph
plethysmography
pleura
pleural
  p. abrasion
  p. amyloidosis
  p. friction rub
  p. tag
pleurectomy
pleurisy
  benign dry p.
  diaphragmatic p.
  epidemic benign dry p.
  epidemic diaphragmatic p.
  rheumatoid p.
  tuberculous p.
pleuritic chest pain
pleuritis
pleurodesis
  doxycycline p.
  mechanical p.
pleurodynia
  epidemic p.
pleuropericarditis
**pleuro-pneumoniae-like organism
  (PPLO)**

PLEVA
   pityriasis lichenoides et varioliformis
   acuta
plexiform
   p. neurofibroma
   p. neuroma
plexus
   Kiesselbach p.
plica
   p. polonica
   p. syndrome
plicata
   lingua p.
plicatic acid
PLM
   periodic leg movement
plombage
plug
   follicular p.
   laminated epithelial p.
   mucous p.
plugging
   mucous p.
plum
Plummer-Vinson syndrome
pluriorificialis
   ectodermosis erosiva p.
pluripotent
pluriresistant
plus
   Cold-Eezer P.
   Sustacal P.
plus strand
PM, P.M.
   Excedrin P.
   Midol P.
PML
   polymorphonuclear leukocyte
   progressive multifocal
   leukoencephalopathy
PMLE
   polymorphous light eruption
   eczematous PMLE
   familial PMLE
PMN
   polymorphonuclear neutrophil
PM-Scl antigen

PncCRM vaccine
PND
   postnasal drip
pneumatic otoscopy
pneumococcal
   p. antigenuria
   p. C-polysaccharide (CPS)
   p. infection
   p. otitis média
   p. pneumolysin
   p. pneumonia
   p. polysaccharide
   p. polysaccharide/protein
    conjugate vaccine
   p. polysaccharide vaccine
   p. stain
   p. vaccine
pneumococcidal
pneumococcolysis
Pneumococcus
pneumoconiosis
Pneumocystis
   P. carinii
   P. carinii pneumonia (PCP)
pneumocystosis
   extrapulmonary p.
pneumocyte
   hydropic change in p.
   type II p.
pneumolysin
   pneumococcal p.
pneumomediastinum
pneumonia
   atypical p.
   bacterial pneumococcal p.
   bronchiolitis obliterans with
    organizing p. (BOOP)
   chronic eosinophilic p. (CEP)
   community-acquired p. (CAP)
   desquamative interstitial p.
    (DIP)
   Eaton agent p.
   eosinophilic p.
   Friedländer p.
   idiopathic acute eosinophilic p.
   lipoid p.
   mycoplasmal p.

NOTES

P

pneumonia *(continued)*
 nosocomial p. (NP)
 ovine progressive p.
 plasma cell p.
 pneumococcal p.
 Pneumocystis carinii p. (PCP)
 polymicrobial p.
 primary atypical p.
 progressive p.
 recurrent bacterial p.
 recurrent viral p.
 usual interstitial p. (UIP)
 ventilator-associated p.
 viral p.
 p. virus of mice (PVM)
pneumoniae
 Chlamydia p.
 Klebsiella p.
 Mycoplasma p.
pneumonitis
 acute hypersensitivity p.
 acute lupus p.
 acute radiation p.
 chronic hypersensitivity p.
 desquamative interstitial p.
 hypersensitivity p. (HP)
 lymphocytic interstitial p. (LIP)
 radiation p.
 uremic p.
Pneumopent
pneumoperitoneum
pneumophila
 Legionella p.
pneumothorax, pl. **pneumothoraces**
 iatrogenic p.
Pneumovax 23
Pneumovirus
PNH
 paroxysmal nocturnal
  hemoglobinuria
PNS
 peripheral nervous system
PNU
 protein nitrogen unit
Pnu-Imune 23
PO$_2$
 partial pressure of oxygen
pock
pocket
 necrotic p.
Pockethaler
 Vancenase P.
Pocketpeak peak flow meter

Pocket SPO$_2$T
pockmark
podagra
Pod-Ben-25
podobromidrosis
Podocon-25
Podofilox
podofilox
Podofin
podophyllum resin
PodoSpray nail drill system
Podoviridae
POEMS
 polyneuropathy, organomegaly,
  endocrinopathy, monoclonal
  gammopathy, and skin changes
 POEMS syndrome
poikiloderma
 p. atrophicans and cataract
 p. atrophicans vasculare
 Civatte p.
 p. of Civatte
 p. congenitale
 reticulated pigmented p.
 p. vasculare atrophicans
 p. vascularis atrophicans
poikilodermatomyositis
poikilodermatous parapsoriasis
point
 Castellani p.
 fibromyalgia trigger p.
 p. mutation
pointed
 p. condyloma
 p. wart
pointing
poison
 p. ivy
 p. ivy dermatitis
 p. oak
 p. oak dermatitis
 p. sumac
 p. sumac dermatitis
poisoning
 ciguatera p.
 lead p.
 mercury p.
 silver p.
 strychnine p.
 systemic p.
poisonous
Poisson-Pearson formula
pokeweed mitogen (PWM)

Poladex
Polaramine
polio
polioencephalitis infectiva
poliomyelitis
    acute anterior p.
    acute bulbar p.
    chronic anterior p.
    p. immune globulin (human)
    p. immunoglobulin
    mouse p.
    p. vaccine
    p. virus
poliosis
    p. circumscripta
poliovirus
    p. hominis
    p. vaccine
    p. vaccine, inactivated
    p. vaccine, live, trivalent, oral
polish
    nail p.
Polistes
    P. sting
polka fever
pollen
    p. antigen
    p. extract
    grass p.
    windborne p.
pollen-induced allergic rhinitis
pollenosis
pollination
pollinosis
    Cupressaceae p.
pollution
    air p.
Polocaine injection
polonica
    plica p.
poloxamer 331
polyacrylamide gel electrophoresis
    (PAGE)
polyacrylonitrile (PAN)
polyad
polyangiitis
    microscopic p.

polyarteritis
    p. in childhood
    p. nodosa
polyarthralgia
polyarthritis (PA)
    asymmetric p.
    epidemic p.
    erosive p.
    juvenile chronic p.
polyarticular
    p. arthritis
    p. gonococcal arthritis
    p. juvenile rheumatoid arthritis
polychemotherapy
polychondritis
    relapsing p.
polychromatic
Polycillin
Polycillin-N
Polycillin-PRB
polyclonal
    p. activator
    p. antibody
    p. B cell
    p. gammopathy
polycyclic pattern
polycythemia vera
polydactylia
polyene
Polygam S/D
polygenic inheritance pattern
polygonal
polyhedral body
polyhidrosis
Poly-Histine C
Poly-Histine DM
polyidrosis
polyleptic fever
polymastia
polymer
    collagen p.
    p. film dressing
    p. foam dressing
polymerase
    p. chain reaction (PCR)

NOTES

P

polymerase *(continued)*
  p. chain reaction-based
    detection of hepatitis G virus
    RNA p.
polymerization
polymerized antigen
polymethyl methacrylate
polymicrobial
  p. arthritis
  p. bacteremia
  p. pneumonia
polymicrobic
polymorphe
  erythema p.
polymorphic
  p. reticulosis
polymorphism
  lipoprotein p.
  restriction fragment length p.
    (RFLP)
polymorphonuclear
  p. cell
  p. leukocyte (PML)
  p. leukocyte collagenase
  p. leukocyte-dependent tissue
    destruction
  p. leukocyte elastase
  p. neutrophil (PMN)
polymorphous
  p. exanthema
  p. light eruption (PMLE)
Polymox
polymyalgia
  p. rheumatica
polymyositis
  juvenile dermato/p. (JDMS/PM)
polymyxa
  Bacillus p.
polymyxin
  p. b and hydrocortisone
  p. b sulfate
polynesic
polyneuritiformis
  heredopathia atactica p.
polyneuritis
  acute idiopathic p.
  infectious p.
polyneuropathic amyloidosis
polyneuropathy
  familial amyloidotic p.
    syndrome
  p., organomegaly,
    endocrinopathy, monoclonal

gammopathy, and skin
    changes (POEMS)
polynucleotide antibody
Polyomavirus
polyonychia
polyostotic fibrous dysplasia
polyp
  fibroepithelial p.
  intestinal p.
  nasal p.
polypapilloma
polypectomy
polypeptide
  CD4, human truncated-365
    AA p.
  p. chain
  p. hormone
  p. inhibitor
polyphaga
  Acanthamoeba p.
polypi
polypoid lesion
polypophyrin
polyposis
Poly-Pred
  P.-P. Ophthalmic suspension
polypus
polyradiculoneuropathy
polyradiculopathy
polysaccharide
  p. antigen
  pneumococcal p.
  specific soluble p.
polyserositis
  familial paroxysmal p.
  familial recurrent p.
  periodic p.
polysomnograph
polysomnography (PSG)
Polysporin
  P. Ophthalmic
  P. topical
polystichia
Polytar
Polytec PI LaseAway
polythelia
polytrichia
polytrichosis
Polytrim Ophthalmic
polyunguia
polyvalent
  p. allergy
  p. antiserum

antivenin (crotalidae) p.
p. serum
p. vaccine
polyvinyl chloride (PVC)
POM
pulse oximetry monitoring
pomade
p. acne
pompholyx
pomphus
Poncet disease
ponderosa
p. pine
p. pine tree
Ponstel
Pontocaine
P. injection
P. topical
poona
Salmonella p.
poorly reversible asthma
poor marrow function
Popeye sign
poplar
Lombardy p. tree
p. tree
white p. tree
popliteal
p. cyst
p. fossa
popliteal-arcuate complex
population-based testing
porate
porcine
p. hemagglutinating
encephalomyelitis virus
p. transmissible gastroenteritis
porcupine
p. disease
p. skin
pore   *pore of*
dilated p.   *Winer*
Kohn p.
Porges-Meier test
pork
PORN
progressive outer retinal necrosis

porocarcinoma
poroid hidradenoma
porokeratosis
actinic p.
disseminated superficial
actinic p.
linear p.
Mibelli p.
p. of Mibelli
p. punctata
poroma
eccrine p.
follicular p.
porphobilinogen
porphyria
acute intermittent p.
ALA dehydratase deficiency p.
(ADP)
congenital erythropoietic p.
p. cutanea tarda (PCT)
erythropoietic p.
hepatic p.
hepatoerythropoietic p.
symptomatic p.
variegate p. (VP)
porphyric
porrigo
p. decalvans
p. favosa
p. furfurans
p. larvalis
p. lupinosa
p. scutulata
portal
p. occlusion
Portuguese
P. jellyfish
P. man-of-war
P. man-of-war sting
port-wine
p.-w. mark
p.-w. stain
positive
p. anergy
p. end-expiratory pressure
(PEEP)
p. expiratory pressure (PEP)

NOTES

P

positive *(continued)*
    Gram p.
    p. inspiratory pressure (PIP)
    p. phase
    p. reaction
    p. rheumatoid factor
possible
    minimal dose p.
posterior
    p. interosseous nerve syndrome
    p. interosseous neuropathy
    p. scleritis
    p. synechia formation
posteriores
    limbi palpebrales p.
postexertional microtrauma
postherpetic
    p. erythema multiforme
    p. neuralgia (PHN)
posthitis
post hoc analysis
postinfection lipoatrophy
postinfectious steatorrhea
postinflammatory
    p. hyperpigmentation
    p. hypopigmentation
post-kala azar dermal leishmanoid
postmortem
    p. pustule
    p. tubercle
    p. wart
postnasal drip (PND)
postnatal therapy
postpartum alopecia
postphlebitic syndrome
postprimary tuberculosis
poststreptococcal glomerulonephritis
postsynaptic terminal
post-thrombotic disease
post-traumatic
    p.-t. arthritis
    p.-t. pustular eruption
postulate
    Ehrlich p.
    Henle-Koch p.
    Koch p.
postulates
postural drainage
postvaccinal
    p. encephalitis
postvenereal reactive arthritis
potassium
    p. chloride stain (KOH)

    p. hydroxide (KOH)
    p. hydroxide preparation
    p. iodide
    penicillin v p.
Potassium Iodide Enseals
potato
    sweet p.
potential
    stress-generated electric p.
    zoonotic p.
potion
    Donizetti p.
    Wagner p.
Pott
    P. gangrene
    P. puffy tumor
poultice
poultry handler's disease
poultryman's itch
poverty weed
povidone-iodine
Powassan
    P. encephalitis
    P. virus
powder
    facial p.
    full-coverage facial p.
    Lotrimin AF P.
    Lotrimin AF Spray P.
    transparent facial p.
    Zeasorb-AF P.
powered air loss (PAL)
pox
    chicken p.
    Kaffir p.
Poxviridae
poxvirus
    p. officinalis
PPD
    purified protein derivative of
    tuberculin
ppg
    photoplethysmography
PPH
    primary pulmonary hypertension
PPHP
    pseudo-pseudohypoparathyroidism
PPi
    pyrophosphate
PPK
    palmoplantar keratoderma
PPLO
    pleuro-pneumoniae-like organism

PPL skin test
PPO-HSA
    penicillin-penicilloyl human serum
      albumin
PP-ribose-P
Practice
    Advisory Committee on
      Immunization P. (ACIP)
Prader-Willi syndrome
praecox
    icterus p.
prairie itch
PrameGel
Pramosone
    P. cream
pramoxine
    p. HCl
    p. hydrochloride
pratensis
Prausnitz-Küstner
    P.-K. antibody
    P.-K. reaction
    P.-K. test
pravastatin
Prax
praziquantel
prazosin hydrochloride
PRCA
    pure red cell aplasia
preauricular
    p. cyst
    p. sinus
precancer
precancerosa
    melanosis circumscripta p.
precancerous
    p. lesion
precipitate
    p. in gel
    p. in solution
precipitating antibody
precipitation
    double antibody p.
    hapten inhibition of p.
    immune p.
    p. test

precipitin
    p. assay
    p. reaction
    rheumatoid arthritis p. (RAP)
    serum p.
    p. test
precipitinogen
precipitinogenoid
precipitogen
precipitoid
precipitophore
precocious puberty
Pred
    P. Forte Ophthalmic
    P. Mild Ophthalmic
Predaject injection
Predalone injection
Predcor injection
Pred-G Ophthalmic
Predicort-50 injection
predictive
    p. patch test
    p. testing
predispose
predisposition
prednicarbate
Prednicen-M Oral
prednisolone
    chloramphenicol and p.
    p. and gentamicin
    neomycin, polymyxin b,
      and p.
    sodium sulfacetamide and p.
    p. tebutate
Prednisol TBA injection
prednisone
    p. burst
    p. pulse
    p. taper
predominant
    p. DIP joint involvement
    p. spondylitis
preeruptive
pre-existing antibody
**preformed granule-associated mast
cell**
Prefrin Ophthalmic solution

NOTES

P

Pregestimil
pregnancy
 p. alpha-2 glycoprotein (PAG)
 mask of p.
 papular dermatitis of p.
 pruritic urticarial papules and
  plaques of p. (PUPPP)
pregnancy-associated glycoprotein
Preiser disease
Prelone
 P. Oral
premalignant
 p. tumor
prematura
 alopecia p.
premature
 p. aging
 p. alopecia
premenstrual acne
Premier H. pylori assay
premorbid
premunition
premunitive
premycotic
prenatal therapy
preoperative anesthetic
preosteoblast
preosteoclast
preparation
 alum-precipitated p.
 hyperimmune gamma
  globulin p.
 KOH p.
 leukocyte-poor p.
 potassium hydroxide p.
 scabies p.
 tar p.
 Tzanck p.
prepatellar bursitis
prepatent period
Pre-Pen
prepolypoid
prepuce
preputiale
 sebum p.
presenile spontaneous gangrene
presenilis
 alopecia p.
presensitization phase
presenting clinical manifestation
preservative
pressure
 p. alopecia

bi-level positive airway p.
 (BiPAP)
p. blister
blood p.
p. bulla
continuous positive airway p.
 (CPAP)
expiratory positive airway p.
 (EPAP)
p. gangrene
inspiratory positive airway p.
 (IPAP)
peak inspiratory ventilator p.
positive end-expiratory p.
 (PEEP)
positive expiratory p. (PEP)
positive inspiratory p. (PIP)
pulmonary artery p.
p. sore
p. support ventilation (PSV)
p. urticaria
zero end-expiratory p. (ZEEP)
pressure-controlled inverse ratio
 ventilation
pressure-regulated volume control
 ventilation
PreSun
 P. lotion and gel
presynaptic terminal
pretibial
 p. fever
 p. myxedema
Prevention
 Centers for Disease Control
  and P. (CDC)
preventive
 p. treatment
Prevotella melaninogenica
prevotii
 Peptostreptococcus p.
prezone
prick
 p. puncture test
 p. test
 p. test concentration
 p. testing
Pricker needle
prickle
 p. cell
 p. cell layer
prickle-cell
 p.-c. carcinoma
 p.-c. epithelioma

prickly heat
prick-prick test
prick-test method
prilocaine
primaquine
    chloroquine and p.
    p. phosphate
primary
    p. adrenocortical failure
    p. amyloid
    p. amyloidotic arthropathy
    p. atrophy
    p. atypical pneumonia
    p. bubo
    p. cell-mediated deficiency
    p. complex
    p. cutaneous B-cell
      lymphocytic leukemia
    p. cutaneous B-cell lymphoma
    p. cutaneous T-cell lymphoma
    p. epithelial germ
    p. genital herpes simplex virus
    p. herpes simplex infection
    p. herpetic stomatitis
    p. hyperhidrosis
    p. hypogammaglobulinemia
    p. idiopathic macular atrophy
    p. immune response
    p. infection
    p. irritant
    p. irritant dermatitis
    p. lesion
    p. lymphedema
    p. macular atrophy of skin
    p. neuroendocrine carcinoma of
      the skin
    p. neuroendocrine tumor
    p. pulmonary hypertension
      (PPH)
    p. pulmonary parenchymal
      disease
    p. pyoderma
    p. reaction
    p. rejection
    p. Sjögren syndrome
    p. syphilis
    p. systemic amyloidosis

    p. telangiectasia
    p. tuberculosis
Primatene Mist
Primaxin
priming renal dialysis unit
Primula obconica
Principen
principle
    Castaneda p.
    diagnostic p.
Pringle disease
print
    scent p.
    tentacle p.
prion
    p. protein
    p. protein-origin amyloid
      deposit
prior drug exposure
priority
    law of p.
private antigen
privet
    p. tree
proactivator
    C3 p.
Pro-Air
proalpha-chain
Proampacin
probacteriophage
    defective p.
Probalan
probe
    Acradinium-ester-labeled nucleic
      acid p.
    cDNA p.
    IntraDop p.
    nucleic acid p.
    radioactive p.
    viral p.
Proben-C
probenecid
    ampicillin and p.
    colchicine and p.
probiosis
probiotic

NOTES

P

problem-oriented
  p.-o. algorithm
  p.-o. diagnosis
procainamide
procaine
  p. hydrochloride
  penicillin g p.
procapsid
Procaryotae (*var. of* Prokaryotae)
procaryote (*var. of* prokaryote)
procaryotic (*var. of* prokaryotic)
procaterol
procedure
  Caldwell-Luc p.
  elimination p.
  fluorometric p.
  Microsporidia diagnostic p.
  platelet neutralization p.
  Z-plasty p.
process
  airspace p.
  exocrinopathic p.
  host-immune p.
  olecranon p.
procollagen
  p. suicide
  p. type II
  p. type III aminoterminal
    peptide
Procort
Procrit
proctitis
proctocolitis
  ulcerative p.
Proctocort
Pro-Depo injection
prodromal
  p. stage
  p. symptom
Prodrox injection
product
  Exact skin p.
  home cleaning p.
production
  cytokine p.
  p. of lymphokine
  purulent sputum p.
productus
  Peptostreptococcus p.
Proetz maneuver
Profen
  P. II
  P. LA

Profeta law
profile
  angioedema p.
  Western blot vaccine p.
profunda
  miliaria p.
  tinea p.
profundus
  lupus p.
  lupus erythematosus p.
profundus/panniculitis
  lupus p.
profusa
  lentiginosis p.
progenitalis
  herpes p.
progeria
  Hutchinson-Gilford p.
  true p.
progesterone
prognosis, pl. **prognoses**
prognostic
progonoma
  melanotic p.
Prograf
Program
  National Asthma Education P.
    (NAEP)
  National Immunization P.
    (NIP)
progression
  malignant p.
progressiva
  granulomatosis disciformis
    et p.
progressive
  p. acinar consolidation
  p. azotemia
  p. bacterial synergistic
    gangrene
  p. facial hemiatrophy
  p. idiopathic atrophoderma
  p. interstitial fibrosis
  p. multifocal
    leukoencephalopathy (PML)
  p. outer retinal necrosis
    (PORN)
  p. pigmentary dermatosis
  p. pneumonia
  p. pneumonia virus
  p. symptom sclerosis (PSS)
  p. systemic sclerosis
  p. vaccinia

proguanil
prohormone
Prokaryotae, Procaryotae
prokaryote, procaryote
prokaryotic, procaryotic
    p. extracellular organism
prolactin
prolapse
    mitral valve p.
Prolastin
proleukin
prolidase deficiency
proliferating
    p. cell nuclear antigen (PCNA)
    p. pilar cyst
    p. systematized
        angioendotheliomatosis
    p. trichilemmal cyst
proliferation
    acanthotic epidermal p.
    endothelial cell p.
    gliomatous p.
    intravascular endothelial p.
    Masson intravascular
        endothelial p.
proliferative
    p. cell
    p. dermatitis
    p. glomerulonephritis
    p. inflammatory disease
    p. lesion
    p. synovitis
    p. synovium
ProLine endoscopic instrument
prolixus
    Rhodnius p.
prolongation
    p. of expiration
    expiratory p.
prolonged
    p. diarrhea
    p. pulmonary eosinophilia
Proloprim
prolyl
Prometa

promethazine
    p. HCl
    p. hydrochloride
Prometh injection
Promit
pronator teres syndrome
Propadrine
Propagest
properdin
    p. factor A
    p. factor B
    p. factor D
    p. factor E
    p. system
prophage
    defective p.
prophylactic
    p. antibody
    p. treatment
prophylaxis
    active p.
    p. agent
    chemical p.
    malaria p.
    passive p.
Prophyllin
propionate
    clobetasol p.
    fluticasone p.
    halobetasol p.
Propionibacterium
    P. acnes
    P. propionicus
propionicus
    Propionibacterium p.
proportional assist ventilation
propranolol hydrochloride
propria
    atrophia pilorum p.
    lamina p.
proptosis
propylene glycol
proquazone
Prorex injection
prosector's
    p. tubercle
    p. wart

NOTES

P

ProSobee
prosodemic
prostacyclin
   p. I3
prostaglandin (PG)
   p. D (PGD)
   p. D2 (PGD2)
   p. E (PGE)
   p. E1 (PGE1)
   p. E2 (PGE2)
   p. H2 (PGH2)
   p. synthesis inhibition
Prostaphlin
   P. injection
   P. Oral
prostatitis
prosthesis, pl. prostheses
   silicone rubber p.
prosthetic
protease
   p. inhibitor
   neutral p.
   p. nexin-1
protease-antiprotease imbalance
protection
   photo p.
   p. test
protective protein
protector
   Heelbo decubitus p.
protein
   acetylation of cellular p.
   acetylation of serum p.
   actin-binding p.
   acute phase p.
   adhesion p.
   AL p.
     immunoglobulin light chain-
      origin amyloid deposit
   amyloid A p.
   antibiotic p.
   p. antigen
   antiviral p. (AVP)
   Australian parrot p.
   azurophil granule p.
   bactericidal/permeability-
     increasing p.
   Bence Jones p.
   BvgS p.
   p. C
   cartilage matrix p.
   p. C deficiency
   cell adhesion p.

   p. C1 esterase inhibitor
   complement p.
   p. contact dermatitis
   control p.'s C1s–C3s
     (C1s–C3s)
   C-reactive p. (CRP)
   eosinophil cationic p.
   p. fever
   foreign p.
   freeze-dried p.
   heat shock p. (HSP)
   heterologous p.
   immune p.
   220-kD p.
   45-kilodalton p.
   M p.
   MacMARCKS p.
   macrophage inflammatory p.
     (MIP)
   major basic p.
   monoclonal p.
   mouse serum p. (MSP)
   mouse urine p. (MUP)
   myeloblastic p.
   neutrophil activating p. (NAP)
   p. nitrogen unit (PNU)
   nonspecific p.
   p. origin amyloid deposit
   pigeon serum p. (PSP)
   plasma p.
   plasma cell dyscrasia with
     polyneuropathy, organomegaly,
     endocrinopathy, monoclonal p.
   platelet basic p.
   prion p.
   protective p.
   rat serum p. (RSP)
   rat urine p. (RUP)
   rhoGDI p.
   p. S
   secretory leukoprotease
     inhibitor p.
   p. shock
   p. shock therapy
   Tamm-Horsfall p.
   ToxR p.
protein-1
   human monocyte
     chemoattractant p.
   monocyte chemoattractant p.
     (MCP-1)
proteinase
   aspartic p.

connective tissue p.
cysteine p.
α_1 p. deficiency
ECM-degrading p.
lysosomal p.
mast cell p.
neutral p.
serine p.
proteinase-inhibitor
protein-energy-related obesity
protein-losing enteropathy
proteinosis
lipoid p.
proteinuria
proteoglycan
proteolysis
proteolytic enzyme
Proteus
P. mirabilis
P. vulgaris
Prothazine
P. injection
P. Oral
protist
protistologist
protistology
protobe
protobiology
Protoctista
proto-oncogene
Fos p.-o.
Jun p.-o.
protopianoma
protoplast
protoporphyria
erythropoietic p.
protoporphyrin
Protostat Oral
Prototheca
protothecosis
Protovir
Protox
Protozoa
protozoal parasitic disease
protracta
Triatoma p.
Protropin II

protrusio acetabuli
protuberans
dermatofibrosarcoma p.
proud flesh
Provatene
Pro-Vent arterial blood sampling kit
Proventil
P. HFA (hydrofluoroalkane-134a)
P. Repetabs
provirus
provocation
bronchial p.
p. typhoid
provocative
p. dose testing
p. use test (PUT)
Provocholine
Prowazek bodies
Prowazek-Greeff bodies
prowazekii
Rickettsia p.
proxetil
cefpodoxime p.
proximal
p. bronchiectasis
p. interphalangeal (PIP)
p. nail matrix
p. phalange
Prozac
prozone
p. reaction
PRSP
penicillin-resistant Streptococcus pneumoniae
pruinosum
Chrysosporium p.
prune
pruriginosus
strophulus p.
pruriginous
prurigo
actinic p.
p. agria
Besnier p.
p. of Besnier

NOTES

P

prurigo *(continued)*
  p. estivalis
  p. ferox
  p. gestationis
  Hebra p.
  p. hiemalis
  Hutchinson summer p.
  p. infantilis
  p. mitis
  p. nodularis
  p. simplex
  p. simplex subacuta
  summer p.
pruritic
  p. dermatosis
  p. erythematous patch
  p. lesion
  p. papule
  p. urticarial papules and
   plaques of pregnancy
   (PUPPP)
pruritogenic
pruritus
  p. ani
  aquagenic p.
  p. balnea
  bath p.
  central p.
  essential p.
  p. estivalis
  genital p.
  p. hiemalis
  perianal p.
  psychogenic p.
  p. scroti
  senile p.
  p. senilis
  symptomatic p.
  p. vulva
PSE
  Guaifenex P.
Pseudallescheria boydii
pseudarthrosis
  Girdlestone p.
pseudoacanthosis nigricans
pseudoagglutination
pseudo-ainhum
pseudoallergic reaction
pseudo-alopecia areata
pseudoanaphylactic
  p. shock
pseudoanaphylaxis

pseudoaneurysm
  ventricular p. (PVA)
pseudoangina pectoris
pseudoangiosarcoma
  Masson p.
pseudoarthrosis
pseudobacteremia
pseudobacteriuria
pseudocavitation
pseudochancre
pseudochromidrosis
pseudocolloid
  p. of lips
pseudocowpox
  p. virus
pseudocyst
pseudocystic rheumatoid arthritis
pseudodiphtheria
pseudodiphtheriticum
  Bacillus p.
pseudodysentery
pseudoedema
pseudoephedrine
  acetaminophen,
   chlorpheniramine, and p.
  brompheniramine and p.
  carbinoxamine and p.
  chlorpheniramine and p.
  p. and dextromethorphan
  guaifenesin and p.
  p. HCl
  p. and ibuprofen
  loratadine and p.
  terfenadine and p.
  triprolidine and p.
pseudoepitheliomatous
  p. hyperplasia
pseudoerysipelas
pseudoexfoliation
pseudofolliculitis
  p. barbae
pseudofracture
Pseudo-Gest Plus Tablet
pseudogout
pseudohypoparathyroidism (PHP)
pseudoicterus
pseudoinfection
pseudojaundice
pseudolepromatous leishmaniasis
pseudolymphocytic choriomeningitis
  virus
pseudolymphoma
  B-cell p.

Spiegler-Fendt p.
T-cell p.
pseudolysogenic
   p. strain
pseudolysogeny
pseudomalignant lymphoma
pseudomallei
   Malleomyces p.
   Pseudomonas p.
pseudomembrane
pseudomembranous
   p. colitis
pseudomeningitis
pseudomilium
   colloid p.
Pseudomonas
   P. aeruginosa
   P. aeruginosa bacteremia
   P. elastase
   P. pseudomallei
pseudomonilethrix
pseudonit
pseudopelade
   p. of Brocq
pseudophlegmon
   Hamilton p.
pseudopilus, pl. pseudopili
   p. annulatus
pseudopneumonia
pseudopodagra
pseudoporphyria
pseudoproteinuria
pseudo-pseudohypoparathyroidism (PPHP)
pseudo-pseudothrombophlebitis
pseudorabies
   p. virus
pseudoradicular syndrome
pseudoreaction
pseudoreplica
pseudorheumatism
pseudorheumatoid
pseudorubella
pseudosarcomatous fasciitis
pseudoscar
   spontaneous p.
   stellate p.

pseudoscarlatina
pseudoseptic
pseudosmallpox
pseudosyndactyly
pseudothrombophlebitis
pseudotrichinosis
pseudotuberculosis
   Yersinia p.
pseudotumor
   p. cerebri
   orbital p.
pseudotumoral mediastinal amyloidosis
pseudo-Turner syndrome
pseudovariola
pseudoxanthoma elasticum
PSG
   polysomnography
psilate
psilosis
psilothin
psilotic
psittaci
   Chlamydia p.
psittacosis
   p. inclusion bodies
   p. virus
psoas
psora
psoralen
   p. ultraviolet A-range (PUVA)
Psorcon
   P. topical
   P. topical steroid
psorelcosis
psoriasic
psoriasiform
   p. dermatitis
   p. eruption
psoriasiformis
   parakeratosis p.
psoriasis
   p. annularis
   p. arthropica
   p. circinata
   p. diffusa
   p. discoidea

NOTES

P

psoriasis *(continued)*
    drop-like p.
    erythrodermic p.
    exfoliative p.
    generalized pustular p.
    genital p.
    p. geographica
    p. guttata
    guttate p.
    p. gyrata
    intertriginous p.
    intraepidermal microabscess
      of p.
    p. inveterata
    localized pustular p.
    microabscess of p.
    p. nummularis
    p. orbicularis
    p. ostreacea
    plaque p.
    plaque-type p.
    p. punctata
    pustular p.
    p. rupioides
    p. spondylitica
    p. universalis
    von Zumbusch pustular p.
psoriatic
    p. arthritis
    p. arthritis mutilans
    p. arthritis with spinal
      involvement
    p. arthropathy
    p. plaque
    p. sacroiliitis
    p. spondylitis
psoriatica
    arthropathia p.
psoriatic-type scale
psoriaticum
    erythroderma p.
psoric
psoriGel
Psorion Cream
psoroid
psoroptic acariasis
psorous
PSP
    pigeon serum protein
PSS
    progressive symptom sclerosis
P&S Shampoo

PSV
    pressure support ventilation
    Quantum PSV
psychocutaneous disease
Psychodidae
psychogalvanic
psychogalvanometer
psychogenic
    p. factor
    p. pain syndrome
    p. pruritus
    p. purpura
    p. reaction
psychological stimuli
psycho-neuro-immuno-endocrine axis
psychophysiologic disorder
psychosis
psychotropic
    p. agent
    p. agent therapy
psyllium
    p. seed
pteronyssinus
    Dermatophagoides p.
pterygium
    p. colli
    p. unguis
pthiriasis
    p. capitis
    p. corporis
    p. pubis
Pthirus
    P. pubis
    P. pubis infestation
ptosis
PTT
    partial thromboplastin time
puberty
    precocious p.
pubes
pubescence
pubic
    p. baldness
    p. lice
    p. louse
pubis
    pediculosis p.
    pthiriasis p.
    Pthirus p.
public antigen
pubomadesis
pudenda (*pl. of* pudendum)
pudendal ulcer

pudendi
  granuloma p.
pudendum, pl. pudenda
  ulcerating granuloma of p.
pudoris
  erythema p.
puerorum
  hydroa p.
puerperal fever
puerperium
Pulex irritans
pulicans
  purpura p.
pulicide
pulicosis
pulling boat hand
pullulans
  Aureobasidium p.
Pullularia
Pulmanex
Pulmicort
Pulmo-Aide
  P.-A. nebulizer
  P.-A. Traveler
pulmonale
  cor p.
pulmonary
  p. adenomatosis of sheep
  p. agenesis
  p. amyloidosis
  p. artery pressure
  p. disease anemia syndrome
  p. embolism
  p. function (PF)
  p. function test (PFT)
  p. hemorrhage
  p. hemosiderosis
  p. hypertension
  p. infiltrate with eosinophilia (PIE)
  p. lesion
  p. lymphoma
  p. mycosis
  p. necrobiotic nodule
  p. sling syndrome
  p. surfactant

  p. toilet
  p. vascular resistance (PVR)
pulmonic valve closure sound
PulmoSonic
pulmowrap
Pulmozyme
pulse
  p. methylprednisolone
  p. oximetry device
  p. oximetry monitoring (POM)
  paradoxical p.
  prednisone p.
  p. rate
  spin-echo p.
  steroid p.
  p. test
pulsed
  p. dye laser (PDL)
  p. field gel electrophoresis (PFGE)
PulseDose oxygen delivery technology
pulsus paradoxus
Pulvules
  Cinobac P.
  Co-Pyronil 2 P.
  Seromycin P.
pumilus
  Bacillus p.
pump
  elastomeric p.
pump-1
pumpkin
punch
  p. biopsy
  Dyonics suction p.
  skin p.
  upcurved p.
punctata
  acne p.
  chondrodysplasia p.
  keratosis p.
  keratosis palmoplantaris p.
  onychia p.
  porokeratosis p.
  psoriasis p.

NOTES

punctate
    erythema p.
    p. hemorrhage
    p. keratoderma
    p. porokeratotic keratoderma
punctated metalloproteinase
punctatum
    keratoderma p.
punctum
puncture
    p. wound
pupate
pupil
    Argyll Robertson p.
PUPPP
    pruritic urticarial papules and
    plaques of pregnancy
Puralube Tears solution
pure red cell aplasia (PRCA)
purging
    tumor cell p.
purified
    p. protein derivative
    p. protein derivative of
      tuberculin (PPD)
purine
    p. analogue
    p. nucleoside phosphorylase
      deficiency
    p. nucleotide cycle
    p. nucleotides adenosine
      triphosphate
    p. ribonucleotide
    p. ring
purple-red papule
purpura
    actinic p.
    acute idiopathic
      thrombocytopenic p.
    acute vascular p.
    allergic p.
    allergic nonthrombocytopenic p.
    anaphylactoid p.
    p. angioneurotica
    p. annularis telangiectodes
    p. annularis telangiectodes of
      Majocchi
    autoimmune p.
    chronic idiopathic
      thrombocytopenic p.
    cutaneous p.
    drug-induced p.
    essential thrombocytopenic p.

    factitious p.
    fibrinolytic p.
    p. fulminans
    Gardner-Diamond p.
    p. hemorrhagica
    Henoch p.
    Henoch-Schönlein p. (HSP)
    hypergammaglobulinemic p.
    hyperglobulinemic p.
    idiopathic thrombocytopenic p.
      (ITP)
    p. iodica
    macular p.
    Majocchi p.
    p. nervosa
    nonpalpable p.
    nonthrombocytopenic p.
    palpable p.
    passion p.
    periorbital p.
    pigmented p.
    psychogenic p.
    p. pulicans
    p. rheumatica
    Schamberg p.
    Schönlein p.
    senile p.
    p. senilis
    p. simplex
    skin p.
    solar p.
    p. symptomatica
    thrombocytopenic p.
    thrombotic thrombocytopenic p.
      (TTP)
    traumatic p.
    p. urticans
    Waldenström p.
    Werlhof p.
purpurascens
    Epicoccum p.
purpureum
    Trichophyton p.
purpuric
    p. eruption
    p. halo
    p. lesion
pursed lips breathing
purulent
    p. sputum
    p. sputum production
pus

puss
    p. caterpillar
    p. caterpillar sting
pustulant
pustular
    p. acne
    p. acrodermatitis
    p. bacterid
    p. dermatosis
    p. eruption
    p. folliculitis
    p. lesion
    p. melanosis
    p. miliaria
    p. patch-test reaction
    p. perifolliculitis
    p. psoriasis
    p. syphilid
pustulation
pustule
    follicular p.
    Kogoj p.
    malignant p.
    postmortem p.
    spongiform p.
    sterile p.
pustuliform
pustulocrustaceous
pustulosa
    acne p.
    acrodermatitis p.
    miliaria p.
    parakeratosis p.
    trichomycosis p.
pustulosis
    p. palmaris et plantaris
    p. palmoplantaris
    p. vacciniformis acuta
pustulosum
    eczema p.
    erysipelas p.
PUT
    provocative use test
putrescentiae
    Tyrophagus p.
PUVA
    psoralen ultraviolet A-range

    foil bath PUVA
    topical PUVA
PUVA-induced
    P.-i. lentigo
PVA
    ventricular pseudoaneurysm
PVC
    polyvinyl chloride
PVM
    pneumonia virus of mice
    PVM virus
PVNS
    pigmented villonodular synovitis
PVR
    pulmonary vascular resistance
PWM
    pokeweed mitogen
pycnidia
pycnidium
pyemia
pyemic
Pyemotes ventricosus
pyknosis
pyknotic cell
pylori
    Campylobacter p.
    Helicobacter p.
Pym fever
Pyocidin-Otic
pyocin
pyocyanine
pyocyanolysin
pyoderma
    blastomycosis-like p.
    chancriform p.
    p. faciale
    p. gangrenosum
    granulomatous p.
    intractable p.
    malignant p.
    persistent p.
    primary p.
    secondary p.
    superficial follicular p.
    superficial granulomatous p.
    p. vegetans
pyodermatitis

NOTES

P

333

pyodermatosis
pyodermatous
    p. infection
    p. skin lesion
pyodermia
    p. facialis
    p. gangrenosa
pyogenes
    Streptococcus p.
pyogenic
    p. arthritis
    p. bacterium
    p. fever
    p. granuloma
    p. infection
    p. osteomyelitis
    p. sacroiliitis
pyogenicum
    granuloma p.
pyohemia
pyomyositis
pyosis
    Manson p.
    p. palmaris
    p. tropica
pyostomatitis
    p. vegetans
pyrantel
    p. pamoate
pyrazinamide (PZA)
    rifampin, isoniazid, and p.
pyrethrins
pyrethroid
    synthetic p.

pyrethrum
pyrexia
    tick p.
pyribenzamine (PBZ)
pyridoxine
    p. deficiency
pyridoxol
    p. deficiency
pyrilamine
    pheniramine,
       phenylpropanolamine, and p.
pyrimethamine
    sulfadoxine and p.
Pyrinate
    A-200 P.
Pyrinyl II
pyrithione
    zinc p.
Pyrobombus
    P. sting
pyrogen
pyroglobulins
pyroglyphid mite
pyrophosphate (PPi)
    alkaline phosphatase and p.
    p. arthropathy
pyrophosphohydrolase
    nucleoside triphosphate p.
    (NTPPH)
pyrotoxin
pyruvate kinase deficiency
PZA
    pyrazinamide

Q
      Q fever
QIE
      quantitative immunoelectrophoresis
Q-switched Nd:YAG laser
Quadra-Hist
Quadrinal
quail bronchitis virus
Quant broth
Quantikine ELISA kit
quantitation of B cell
quantitative
      q. complement assay
      q. HCV RNA
      q. immunoassay for urine
        myoglobin
      q. immunoelectrophoresis (QIE)
      q. immunoglobulin analysis
Quantum PSV
Quaranfil virus
quarantine
quarter
      lamb's q.
quarter-evil
quarter-ill
quartz lamp
quaternary
      q. ammonium
      q. syphilis
quaternium-15
queen
      q. palm
      q. palm tree

Queensland tick typhus
quellung
      q. phenomenon
      q. reaction
      q. test
quenching
      fluorescence q.
Quest
      Tranquility Q.
Queyrat
      erythroplasia of Q.
Quibron
      Q.-T
      Q.-T/SR
QuickVue One-Step Allergen Screen
Quiess
quinacrine
Quincke
      Q. disease
      Q. edema
quinidine
quinine sulfate
quinolones
Quinquaud disease
Quinsana Plus topical
quintana
      Bartonella q.
quinti
      adductor digiti q.
quinupristin/dalfopristin

R
R antigen
R factor
R pilus
R plasmid
r24 antibody
RA
rheumatoid arthritis
rabbit
r. bush
r. epithelium
r. fibroma
fibromatosis virus of r.
r. fibroma virus
r. myxoma virus
r. plague
virus III of r.
rabbitpox
r. virus
rabid
rabies
r. immune globulin, human
r. immune globulin (human)
r. immunoglobulin
r. vaccine
r. vaccine, Flury strain egg-
passage
r. virus
r. virus, Flury strain
r. virus, Kelev strain
r. virus vaccine
raccoon eyes
racemosa
livedo r.
racemosus
Mucor r.
Racet topical
racial melanoderma
racket nail
rad
radial
r. immunodiffusion (RID)
r. scar
radiation
r. burn
r. dermatitis
r. dermatosis
electromagnetic r.
ionizing r.

r. pneumonitis
ultraviolet r.
radical
free r.
r. mastectomy
oxygen free r.
radicans
Rhus r.
Toxicodendron r.
radicular nerve root
radiculitis
radiculoganglionitis
radiculopathy
radioactive probe
radioallergosorbent test (RAST)
radioassay
C1qR r.
radiobacter
Agrobacterium r.
radiodermatitis
chronic r.
radioepidermitis
radioepithelitis
radiographic contrast media (RCM)
radioimmunoassay (RIA)
Raji cell r.
radioimmunodiffusion
radioimmunoelectrophoresis
radioimmunoprecipitation
radioimmunosorbent test (RIST)
radiolabeled iodine
radiolunate
radiometry
BACTEC r.
radionuclide
r. ventriculography
radioreceptor assay
radiosensitivity
radiotherapy
radish
RADS
reactive airways dysfunction
syndrome
RAEB
refractory anemia with excess blasts
ragweed
canyon r.
r. dermatitis
desert r.
false r.

R

ragweed *(continued)*
    giant r.
    short r.
    slender r.
    Western r.
ragwort
rail
    Railguard bed r.
Railguard bed rail
Rainbow vacuum
rain splash
raised border
raisin
Raji
    R. cell
    R. cell radioimmune assay
    R. cell radioimmunoassay
rale
    coarse r.
ram horn nail
Ramsay Hunt syndrome
Ranawat triangle method
Ranikhet disease
ranitidine hydrochloride
RANTES
ranula
RAP
    rheumatoid arthritis precipitin
Rapamune
rapamycin
Raper-Mason pathway
rapid
    r. canities
    r. cooling
    r. eye movement (REM)
    r. plasma reagin (RPR)
Rappaport classification
raquette
    ongles en r.
rare
    r. mycosis
    r. system reaction
rarefaction
    mottled r.
rash
    ammonia r.
    antitoxin r.
    astacoid r.
    atopic dermatitis r.
    black currant r.
    brown-tail r.
    butterfly r.
    cable r.

    caterpillar r.
    crystal r.
    diaper r.
    drug r.
    ecchymotic r.
    generalized maculopapular r.
    gum r.
    heat r.
    heliotrope r.
    hemorrhagic r.
    hydatid r.
    JRA r.
    lupus erythematous-like r.
    macular r.
    maculopapular r.
    malar r. (MR)
    malar butterfly r.
    mulberry r.
    Murray Valley r.
    napkin r.
    nettle r.
    papulovesicular r.
    red r.
    rose r.
    serum r.
    skin r.
    "slapped cheek" r.
    summer r.
    sunburn-like r.
    tooth r.
    wandering r.
    wildfire r.
raspberry tongue
RAST
    radioallergosorbent test
    RAST test
rat
    r. flea bite
    r. mite dermatitis
    r. serum protein (RSP)
    r. urine protein (RUP)
rat-bite fever
rate
    erythrocyte sedimentation r.
    (ESR)
    glomerular filtration r. (GFR)
    low flow r.
    moisture vapor transmission r.
    (MVTR)
    peak expiratory flow r.
    pulse r.
    respiratory r.
    Westergren sedimentation r.

R

ratio
    carpal to metacarpal r.
    CD4/CD8 r.
    dead space:tidal volume r.
    inspiratory to expiratory r.
      (I:E)
    International Normalization R.
      (INR)
    residual volume to total lung
      capacity r. (RV/TLC)
    risk r. (RR)
    therapeutic r.
    ventilation-perfusion r.
rats
    Wistar r.
rattlesnake
    r. bite
Rauscher
    R. leukemia virus
    R. virus
rauwolfia drug
RAV
    Rous-associated virus
Raynaud
    R. disease
    R. phenomenon
    R. syndrome
rays
    grenz r.
RBC
    RBC surface
rCD4
    CD4, human recombinant
      soluble r.
RCM
    radiographic contrast media
RCR
    replication-competent retrovirus
    RCR assay
    RCR testing
RD
    rhabdomyosarcoma
    human RD
RDS
    respiratory distress syndrome
reactants
    acute phase r.

Reactine
reaction
    accelerated r.
    acute anaphylactic r.
    acute phase r.
    acute pulmonary r.
    acute transfusion r.
    adverse drug r.
    allergic r.
    anamnestic r.
    anaphylactic r.
    anaphylactic hypersensitivity r.
    anaphylactoid r.
    angry back r.
    antigen-antibody r.
    Arthus r.
    arthus-type r.
    Ascoli r.
    associative r.
    autoimmune type of r.
    autologous mixed leukocyte r.
    capsular precipitation r.
    cell-mediated r.
    cell-mediated drug r.
    cell-mediated immunologic
      drug r.
    Chantemesse r.
    cholera-red r.
    cocarde r.
    complement-fixation r.
    constitutional r.
    cross r.
    cutaneous r.
    cutaneous graft versus host r.
    cytotoxic r.
    cytotoxic immunologic drug r.
    Dale r.
    delayed r.
    delayed hypersensitivity r.
    delayed-hypersensitivity
      immunologic drug r.
    delayed systemic r.
    delayed transfusion r.
    demarcated r.
    depot r.
    dermatophytid r.
    dermotuberculin r.

NOTES

reaction *(continued)*
    diffuse histiocytic r.
    dopa r.
    drug r.
    early r.
    eczematous r.
    epicutaneous r.
    false-negative r.
    false-positive r.
    Fernandez r.
    fixation r.
    fixed drug r.
    flocculation r.
    focal r.
    foreign-body r.
    Forssman antigen-antibody r.
    Frei-Hoffmann r.
    fungal id r.
    gel diffusion r.
    Gell and Coombs r.
    graft versus host r. (GVHR)
    granulomatous inflammatory r.
    group r.
    Gruber r.
    Gruber-Widal r.
    Haber-Weiss r.
    Hapten-type r.
    hematologic r.
    Herxheimer r.
    homocytotropic r.
    homograft r.
    hunting r.
    hypersensitivity r.
    hypersensitivity r.
    hysterical r.
    id r.
    r. of identity
    idiosyncratic drug r.
    IgE-dependent immunologic
        drug r.
    immediate hypersensitivity r.
    immediate transfusion r.
    immune complex immunologic
        drug r.
    immune complex-mediated
        drug r.
    immunologic drug r.
    incompatible blood
        transfusion r.
    inflammation r.
    insulin r.
    intracutaneous r.
    intradermal r.

    irritant patch-test r.
    Jarisch-Herxheimer r.
    Köbner r.
    late r.
    late phase allergic r.
    latex fixation r.
    lepromatous r.
    lepromin r.
    local r.
    Loewenthal r.
    marked localized r.
    Mazzotti r.
    miostagmin r.
    miscellaneous r.
    Mitsuda r.
    mixed agglutination r.
    mixed lymphocyte culture r.
    negative r.
    Neufeld r.
    neutrophil antibody and
        transfusion r.
    nitritoid r.
    non-drug-related r.
    r. of nonidentity
    non-immediate-type
        immunologic drug r.
    nonimmunologic drug r.
    r. of partial identity
    passive cutaneous
        anaphylactic r.
    Paul r.
    persistent light r.
    photoallergic r.
    photoallergic drug r.
    photobiologic r.
    photochemical r.
    photodrug r.
    photosensitivity r.
    phototoxic drug r.
    Pirquet r.
    polymerase chain r. (PCR)
    positive r.
    Prausnitz-Küstner r.
    precipitin r.
    primary r.
    prozone r.
    pseudoallergic r.
    psychogenic r.
    pustular patch-test r.
    quellung r.
    rare system r.
    reversed Prausnitz-Küstner r.
    Schultz-Charlton r.

Schultz-Dale r.
self-limited allergic r.
serum r.
severe acute allergic r.
severe immediate r.
severe systemic r.
Shwartzman r.
skin r.
specific r.
suprasternal r.
symptomatic r.
systemic r.
toxic systemic r.
transfusion r.
Treponema pallidum
  immobilization r.
two-stage r.
type I–III hypersensitivity r.
type III immune complex
  drug r.
type I–IV immunologic drug r.
type IV delayed
  hypersensitivity r.
vaccinoid r.
vascular r.
vasomotor r.
vasovagal r.
in vivo r.
Wassermann r. (W.r.)
Weil-Felix r.
Weinberg r.
well-demarcated skin r.
wheal-and-erythema r.
wheal-and-flare r.
whitegraft r.
Widal r.
zonal type r.
reactions
reactivate
reactivation
  sunburn r.
reactive
  r. airways disease
  r. airways dysfunction
    syndrome (RADS)
  r. angioendotheliomatosis

  r. arthritis
  r. perforating collagenosis
  r. postinfectious synovitis
  r. salpingitis
reactivity
  immediate skin r.
  specific alteration in
    immunologic r.
reactor
  persistent light r.
reading
  delayed patch test r.
reading-frame-shift mutation
reagent
  Melzer r.
reagin
  atopic r.
  rapid plasma r. (RPR)
reaginic
  r. antibody
  r. hypersensitivity
Rea-Lo
Reatine
rebound dermatitis
recall
  ultraviolet r.
Receptin
receptor
  B-cell antigen r.
  brush border r.
  C4B r.
  C3b r.
  C5b-9 r.
  C3bBb r.
  C3/C4 r.
  C3dg r.
  complement r. (1–4) (CR
    (1–4))
  Fc r.
  fibronectin r.
  homing r.
  lymphocyte homing r.
  r. site
  surface r.
  T-cell r.
  T-cell antigen r.

NOTES

recessive
 autosomal r.
 r. X-linked ichthyosis
recidivans
 leishmaniasis r.
recidive
 chancre r.
reciprocal transfusion
Recklinghausen
 R. disease
 R. disease type I
reclusa
 Loxosceles r.
recognition factor
recoil
 elastic r.
recombinant
 R. HIV-1 latex agglutination
 test
 r. human interleukin-1 receptor
 antagonist
 r. immunoblot assay (RIBA)
 r. strain
 r. vector
recombinase activating gene
recombination
 genetic r.
 high frequency of r. (Hfr,
 HFR)
Recombivax HB
recorder
 SNAP r.
 SNAP sleep r.
recovery
 short tau inversion r. (STIR)
recrudescent
 r. typhus
 r. typhus fever
recruitment
 host-generated neutrophils r.
rectal
 Rowasa R.
 r. ulceration
rectus abdominis syndrome
recurrens
 herpes simplex r.
recurrent
 r. aspiration
 r. bacterial pneumonia
 r. cutaneous abscess
 r. genital herpes simplex virus
 r. infection
 r. infundibulofolliculitis

 r. intraoral herpes simplex
 virus
 r. labial herpes simplex virus
 r. ulcer
 r. urticaria
 r. viral pneumonia
recurrentis
 Borrelia r.
red
 r. albinism
 r. alder
 r. alder tree
 r. ant
 r. birch
 r. blood cell
 r. bug bite
 r. cedar
 r. cedar tree
 r. cell adherence phenomenon
 r. cell adherence test
 r. cell antigen
 r. cell membrane alteration
 r. eye
 r. granulation
 r. half-moon
 r. halo
 r. imported fire ant
 r. imported fire ant sting
 r. maple
 r. maple tree
 r. mulberry
 r. mulberry tree
 r. neuralgia
 r. nodule
 r. papule
 r. papule and nodule
 r. rash
 r. sweat
 r. top
reddening
 r. of oropharyngeal mucosa
 r. of palm
 r. of soles of feet
"red man" syndrome
redox stress
red-purple plaque
redroot pigweed
redtop
 r. A grass
 r. grass
reduced joint survey (RJS)
reducing substance

reductase
    5 alpha r.
reduction
    leukotriene r.
Redutemp
Reduviidae
rédux
    chancre r.
redwood
    r. tree
reed
    r. canary
    common r.
reedy nail
re-enameling
reepithelialization
Reese's Pinworm Medicine
reflectance photometry
reflex
    r. cough
    pilomotor r.
    stretch r.
    submersion r.
    r. sympathetic dystrophy (RSD)
    r. sympathetic dystrophy
        syndrome (RSD syndrome)
reflux
    gastroesophageal r. (GER)
refractory
    r. anemia with excess blasts
        (RAEB)
    r. period
Refresh
    R. Ophthalmic solution
    R. Plus Ophthalmic solution
Refsum
    R. disease
    R. syndrome
region
    complementarity determining r.
    constant r.
    hypervariable r.
    I r.
    intertriginous r.
    paratracheal r.
    ringworm of genitocrural r.

    switch r.
    variable r.
regional granulomatous
    lymphadenitis
Regranex
regressing atypical histiocytosis
regression
    spontaneous r.
Regular
    Iodex R.
regulation
    leukotriene r.
regulator
    cystic fibrosis
        transmembrane r.
regulon
    BvgAS r.
reinfection
    r. tuberculosis
reinoculation
Reiter
    R. disease
    R. syndrome
    R. test
rejection
    accelerated r.
    acute cellular r.
    allograft r.
    chronic allograft r.
    first-set r.
    hyperacute r.
    primary r.
    second set r.
Relafen
relapsing
    r. febrile nodular
        nonsuppurative panniculitis
    r. fever
    r. polychondritis
relationship
    temporal r.
relative
    r. immunity
    immunochemical r.
    r. risk
relaxation
    smooth muscle r.

R

NOTES

343

relaxin
release
    allergen-induced mediator r.
    delayed anagen r.
    delayed telogen r.
    immediate antigen r.
    immediate telogen r.
    leukocyte histamine r.
    myoglobin r.
    sustained r.
releaser
    direct histamine r.
releasing factor (RF)
relevant sting history
Relief
    Mini Thin Asthma R.
    R. Ophthalmic solution
    Vicks DayQuil Sinus Pressure
      & Congestion R.
Reliever
    Arthritis Foundation Pain R.
REM
    rapid eye movement
    reticular erythematous mucinosis
    REM sleep
    REM sleep-related hypoxemia
    REM syndrome
remission
    pathologically confirmed
      complete r. (PCR)
remitting seronegative symmetrical
synovitis
remodeling
    extracellular matrix r.
    tissue r.
removal
    excisional r.
Remune
renal
    r. biopsy
    r. cyst
    r. failure
    r. involvement
Rendu-Osler-Weber
    R.-O.-W. disease
    R.-O.-W. syndrome
Renova
Reoviridae
REO virus
Reovirus
reovirus-like agent
repair
    abnormal DNA r.

DNA r.
    staged abdominal r. (STAR)
    tissue r.
repeated
    r. exposure
    r. respiratory infection
repeat open reaction application
test
repeats
    variable numbers of tandem r.
      (VNTR)
repellent
repens
    dermatitis r.
    erythema gyratum r.
Repetabs
    Proventil R.
repetitive PCR (Rep-PCR)
replacement
    enzyme r.
    r. therapy
replica
replicase
replicate
replication
replication-competent
    r.-c. retrovirus (RCR)
    r.-c. retrovirus assay
replicative form (RF)
replicator
Rep-PCR
    repetitive PCR
requirement
    immunization r.
RES
    reticuloendothelial system
Rescriptor
Resectisol Irrigation solution
reserve
    breathing r. (BR)
    heart rate r. (HRR)
reservoir
    r. host
    r. of infection
residual
    r. volume
    r. volume to total lung
      capacity ratio (RV/TLC)
resin
    epoxy r.
    formaldehyde r.
    pine r.

podophyllum r.
thermosetting r.
resin-colophony
pine r.-c.
resistance
airway r.
bacteriophage r.
r. factor
insulin r.
r. plasmid
pulmonary vascular r. (PVR)
resistance-inducing factor
resistance-transfer factor
resistance-transferring episome
resistant
resorptive arthropathy
Respaire
R.-120 SR
R.-60 SR
Respa-1st
Respbid
RespiGam
Respihaler
Decadron Phosphate R.
Respinol-G
respiration
Cheyne-Stokes r.
respirator
BABYbird r.
respiratory
r. acidosis
r. burst
r. changes
r. distress
r. distress syndrome (RDS)
r. enteric orphan virus
r. failure
r. rate
r. syncytial virus (RSV)
r. syncytial virus IV immune
globulin
Respirgard II nebulizer
Respitrace machine
response
anamnestic r.
antigen-specific immune r.

biphasic r.
booster r.
cholinergic r.
early-phase r.
histiocytic r.
host r.
IgE-mediated r.
immune r.
immunologic r.
irritant patch-test r.
isomeric r.
isomorphic r.
late-phase r.
primary immune r.
secondary immune r.
seroconversion r.
somatosensory evoked r.
triple r.
in vitro proliferative
lymphocyte r.
white line r.
responsiveness
airway r.
rest hypoxemia
rest, ice, compresses, elevation
(RICE)
resting phase
restitope
Reston subtype
restorative sleep
restriction
r. fragment length
r. fragment length
polymorphism (RFLP)
MHC r.
restrictive
r. cardiomyopathy
r. functional impairment
r. lung disease
r. ventilatory pattern
restrictus
Aspergillus r.
resuscitation
cardiopulmonary r.
retardation
growth r.

NOTES

rete
    r. peg
    r. ridges
retention
    r. cyst
    r. triad
reticular
    r. degeneration
    r. dermis
    r. dysgenesis
    r. erythematous mucinosis
      (REM)
    r. lesion
    r. pattern
reticularis
    angiitis livedo r.
    dermatopathia pigmentosa r.
    idiopathic livedo r.
    livedo r.
    pars r.
reticulata
    folliculitis ulerythema r.
    folliculitis ulerythematosa r.
reticulate
    r. array
    r. pigmented anomaly
reticulated
    r. papillomatosis
    r. pigmented poikiloderma
reticulin fiber
reticulocyte count
reticuloendothelial
    r. cell
    r. system (RES)
reticuloendothelioma
reticuloendotheliosis
reticuloendotheliosis
    avian r.
    familial r.
reticuloendothelium
reticulogranuloma
reticulohistiocytic granuloma
reticulohistiocytoma
reticulohistiocytosis
    congenital self-healing r.
    multicentric r. (MR)
    self-healing r.
reticuloid
    actinic r.
reticulosis
    benign inoculation r.
    disseminated pagetoid r.
    lipomelanic r.

    localized pagetoid r.
    pagetoid r.
    polymorphic r.
reticulum
    r. fiber
reticulum-cell sarcoma
retiform
Retin-A
    R.-A. topical
retina
retinacula of ankle
retinal
    r. examination
    r. exudate
    r. hemorrhage
    r. perivasculitis
    r. thrombophlebitis
retinitis
    cytomegalovirus r.
    VZV r.
retinoic acid
retinoid
    r. therapy
retractions
retroperitoneal fibrosis
retropharyngeal
Retrovir
    R. injection
    R. Oral
Retroviridae
retrovirus
    r.-associated lymphoma
    r. group
    replication-competent r. (RCR)
revaccination
reverse
    r. passive hemagglutination
    r. transcriptase
reversed
    r. anaphylaxis
    r. passive anaphylaxis
    r. passive latex agglutination
    r. Prausnitz-Küstner reaction
reversion
revertant
revulsion
Reye syndrome
Rezine
RF
    releasing factor
    replicative form
    rheumatoid factor
    IgG RF

immunoglobulin G
rheumatoid factor
IgM RF
immunoglobulin M
rheumatoid factor
RF test
RFLP
restriction fragment length
polymorphism
R-Gel
RH
rheumatoid
Rh
R. antigen
R. blocking test
R. immune globulin
intravenous (RhIGIV)
rhabdomyolysis
rhabdomyoma
rhabdomyosarcoma (RD)
Rhabdoviridae
rhabdovirus
rhagades
rhagadiform
rhagas
RH$_o$(D)
R. immune globulin
R. immunoglobulin
rheophoresis
rhesus rotavirus (RRV)
Rheumatex
R. test
R. test for rheumatoid factor
rheumatic
r. fever
rheumatica
polymyalgia r.
purpura r.
scarlatina r.
rheumaticum
erythema annulare r.
rheumatism
palindromic r.
pied rond r.
tuberculous r.
rheumatocelis
rheumatoid (RH)

r. arthritis (RA)
r. arthritis precipitin (RAP)
r. clawing
r. disease
r. episcleritis
r. factor (RF)
r. nodule
r. nodulosis
r. pachymeningitis
r. pattern
r. pleurisy
r. rheumatic vasculitis
r. scleritis
r. synovial cell
r. synovial macrophage-
like/dendritic cell
r. vasculitis
rheumatologist
rheumatology
American College of R.
(ACR)
Rheumaton
R. test
R. test for rheumatoid factor
Rheumatrex
RhIGIV
Rh immune globulin intravenous
rhinitis
acute r.
allergic r.
endocrine r.
foreign body r.
granulomatosis r.
gustatory r.
infectious r.
r. medicamentosa
r. nervosa
perennial allergic r.
pollen-induced allergic r.
seasonal allergic r.
vasomotor r. (VMR)
rhinocerebral infection
Rhinocladiella aquaspersa
rhinoconjunctivitis
allergic r.
Rhinocort
rhinomanometry

R

NOTES

rhinophyma
rhinopneumonitis
    equine r.
Rhinoprobe
rhinorrhea
    cerebrospinal r.
rhinoscleroma
rhinoscleromatis
    Klebsiella r.
rhinoscopy
rhinosinusitis
rhinosporidiosis
Rhinosporidium seeberi
Rhinosyn
    R. Liquid
    R.-PD Liquid
rhinotracheitis
    feline viral r.
    infectious bovine r. (IBR)
Rhinovirus
rhinovirus
    bovine r.'s
    r. challenge test
    equine r.'s
Rhizopus
    R. nigricans
    R. oryzae
Rhodnius prolixus
Rhodococcus
    R. equi
    R. erythropolis
Rhodotorula rubra
rhoGDI protein
rhomboid
    r. glossitis
    r. swelling
rhonchi
rhopheocytosis
rhubarb
Rhus
    R. diversiloba
    R. radicans
    R. toxicodendron
    R. toxicodendron antigen
    R. venenata
    R. venenata antigen
    R. vernix
rhus
    r. dermatitis
rhusiopathiae
    Erysipelothrix r.
rhyparia

rhysodes
    Acanthamoeba r.
rhytidectomy
rhytidoplasty
RIA
    radioimmunoassay
RIBA
    recombinant immunoblot assay
    HCV by RIBA
    RIBA HCV
Ribas-Torres disease
ribavirin
Ribbing arthritis phenotype
riboflavin deficiency
ribonucleic acid (RNA)
ribonucleoprotein (RNP)
    small nuclear r. (snRNP)
ribonucleotide
    purine r.
ribosomal
ribosome
ribovirus
RICE
    rest, ice, compresses, elevation
rice
    r. bodies
    r. itch
richardsiae
    Phialophora r.
Richner-Hanhart syndrome
richteria
    Solenopsis saevissima r.
Richter syndrome
ricin
    anti-B4 blocked r.
    B4 blocked r.
ricinus
    Ixodes r.
rickets
rickettsia
    R. akari
    R. australis
    R. conorii
    R. prowazekii
    R. rickettsii
    R. typhi
    r. vaccine, attenuated
rickettsial infection
rickettsialpox
rickettsii
    Rickettsia r.
rickettsiosis
    eastern tick-borne r.

rickettsiostatic
Ricobid
RID
    radial immunodiffusion
Ridaura
Rida virus
Ridenol
ridge
ridges
    interpapillary r.
    rete r.
RIE
    rocket immunoelectrophoresis
Riedel struma
Riehl
    R. melanoderma
    R. melanosis
rifabutin
Rifadin
    R. injection
    R. Oral
Rifamate
rifampin
    r. and isoniazid
rifampin, isoniazid, and
  pyrazinamide
rifampin-isoniazid-streptomycin-
  ethambutol (RISE)
rifamycin
rifapentine
Rifater
rifaximin
Rift
    R. Valley fever
    R. Valley fever virus
Right
    Breathe R.
rigid thoracoscope
rigor
Riley-Day syndrome
Rilutek
riluzole
Rimactane Oral
rimantadine
    r. hydrochloride
rimexolone

rinderpest
    r. virus
ring
    Kayser-Fleischer r.
    r. precipitin test
    purine r.
    r. shadow
    r. ulcer
    Wessely r.
    Woronoff r.
ringed hair
ringworm
    r. of beard
    black-dot r.
    r. of body
    crusted r.
    r. of foot
    r. of genitocrural region
    honeycomb r.
    r. of nail
    Oriental r.
    r. of scalp
    scaly r.
    Tokelau r.
    r. yaws
Rinkel serial endpoint titration
Rinkle testing
Rinne test
Rinse
    Nix Creme R.
Rio rosewood
RISE
    rifampin-isoniazid-streptomycin-
      ethambutol
risedronate
RISE-resistant tuberculosis
risk
    r. ratio (RR)
    relative r.
RIST
    radioimmunosorbent test
Ritchie articular index
ritonavir
Ritter disease
river
    r. birch
    r. blindness

NOTES

RJS
    reduced joint survey
RNA
    ribonucleic acid
        RNA glycosidase toxin
        HAV RNA
        HCV RNA
        RNA polymerase
        quantitative HCV RNA
        RNA tumor virus
        RNA virus
Rnase P
RNP
    ribonucleoprotein
    RNP antigen
road burn
Ro antigen
Robaxin
Robicillin VK Oral
Robinson disease
Robinul
    R. Forte
Robitet Oral
Robitussin
    R.-PE
    R. Severe Congestion Liqui-
      Gels
Robomol
robustus
    arthritis r.
Rocaltrol
Rocephin
Rochalimaea henselae
Rocha-Lima inclusion
rocket immunoelectrophoresis (RIE)
Rocky
    R. Mountain spotted fever
    R. Mountain spotted fever
      vaccine
    R. Mountain tick
rod
    Gram-negative r.
    Gram-positive r.
rodent ulcer
rodhaini
    Babesia r.
rodonalgia
roentgen
roetheln
RoEzIt skin moisturizer
Roferon-A
Rogaine
Rokitansky-Aschoff sinus

rolled shoulder lesion
Romana sign
Romberg
    R. hemiatrophy
    R. syndrome
Römer test
Rondec
    R. Drops
    R. Filmtab
    R. Syrup
    R.-TR
Rondo inhaler
ronds
    corps r.
room temperature
root
    nail r.
    orris r.
    radicular nerve r.
rope burn
roquinimex
rosacea
    acne r.
    corticosteroid r.
    granulomatous r.
    hypertrophic r.
    tuberculoid r.
rosaceaform dermatitis
rosacea-like
    r.-l. tuberculid
    r.-l. tuberculid of Lewandowski
Rosai-Dorfman
    R.-D. disease
    R.-D. syndrome
rose
    r. cold
    r. fever
    r. rash
    r. spot
rosea
    atypical pityriasis r.
    pityriasis r.
Rosenbach disease
Rosenthal-French dosimeter
roseola
    epidemic r.
    idiopathic r.
    r. infantilis
    r. infantum
    syphilitic r.
roseola-like illness
roseolous

rosette
- E r.
- EAC r.
- T-cell r.
- r. test

rosette-forming cell
Rose-Waaler test
rosewood
- Rio r.

rosin
Ross
- R. River fever
- R. River virus

rot
- Barcoo r.
- jungle r.

Rotacaps
- Ventolin R.

Rotahaler inhaler
rotating
- r. air impactor
- r. arm impactor

rotation
- timed intermittent r.

rotator cuff
rotavirus
- group C r.
- rhesus r. (RRV)

röteln
Rothia dentocariosa
Rothmann-Makai syndrome
Rothmund syndrome
Rothmund-Thomson syndrome
Roth spot
Rotorod sampler
rotoslide
rouge
- homme r.
- l'homme r.

rough marsh elder
round body
roundworm
Rous
- R. sarcoma
- R. sarcoma virus (RSV)
- R. sarcoma virus immune globulin intravenous (RSV-IGIV)
- R. tumor

Rous-associated virus (RAV)
Roux spatula
Rowasa Rectal
roxithromycin
Royl-Derm wound hydrogel dressing
RPR
- rapid plasma reagin

RR
- risk ratio

RRV
- rhesus rotavirus

RSD
- reflex sympathetic dystrophy
- RSD syndrome

RSP
- rat serum protein

RSV
- respiratory syncytial virus
- Rous sarcoma virus

RSV-IGIV
- Rous sarcoma virus immune globulin intravenous

Rs virus
rub
- pleural friction r.
- r. test

Rubarth
- R. disease
- R. disease virus

rubber
- r. additive dermatitis
- Brazilian r.
- r. man syndrome

rubedo
rubefacient
rubefaction
rubella
- congenital r.
- r. HI test
- r. IgG ELISA test
- r. and mumps vaccines, combined
- r. vaccine virus

NOTES

R

rubella *(continued)*
r. virus
r. virus vaccine, live
rubeola
r. virus
rubeosis
ruber
lichen r.
Rubivirus
rubor
skin r.
rubra
miliaria r.
pityriasis r.
Rhodotorula r.
stria r.
rubrifacient
rubrum
eczema r.
Trichophyton r.
ruby
r. laser
r. spot
Rud syndrome
rufous
r. albinism
r. oculocutaneous albinism
ruga, pl. **rugae**
Rugger-jersey spine
rugose
rugous
Rumalon
ruminantium
Cowdria r.
Rumpel-Leede
R.-L. sign
R.-L. test
runaround
runt disease
runting syndrome
Runyon classification
RUP
rat urine protein

rupia
r. escharotica
rupial
r. syphilid
rupioid
rupioides
psoriasis r.
rural cutaneous leishmaniasis
Russell
R. bodies
R. viper venom time
Russian
R. autumn encephalitis
R. autumn encephalitis virus
R. olive
R. olive tree
R. spring-summer encephalitis (Eastern subtype)
R. spring-summer encephalitis virus
R. spring-summer encephalitis (Western subtype)
R. thistle
R. tick-borne encephalitis
Ru-Tuss
R.-T. DE
Ruvalcaba-Myhre-Smith syndrome
Ru-Vert-M
RV/TLC
residual volume to total lung capacity ratio
rye
r. meal
perennial r.
wild r.
Rymed
Rymed-TR
Ryna Liquid
Rynatan
Rynatuss

S
    S antigen
    S unit of streptomycin
SA
    salicylic acid
SAARD
    slow-acting antirheumatic drug
saber shin
Sabin-Feldman dye test
Sabin vaccine
Sabouraud
    S. agar
    S. medium
sabre
    coup de s.
    en coup de s.
sacbrood
saccharolyticus
    Peptostreptococcus s.
Saccharomyces neoformans
sacer ignis
Sachs-Georgi test
sacroiliitis
    psoriatic s.
    pyogenic s.
sacrospinalis muscle
Sactimed-I-Sinald disinfectant
saddle
    s. back caterpillar
    s. back caterpillar sting
    s. nose
    s. nose deformity
Saenger macula
Saf-Clens wound cleanser
Safe Tussin
sage
    coast s.
sagebrush
sailor's skin
Saint
    S. Anthony's fire
    S. Ignatius itch
Saizen
Salacid Ointment
Sal-Acid Plaster
Salagen Oral
Salazopyrin
salbutamol
Saleto-200
Saleto-400

Saleto CF
Salflex
Salgesic
salicylate
    choline s.
salicylic
    s. acid (SA)
    s. acid collodion
    s. acid and lactic acid
    s. acid and propylene glycol
salicylism
saligna
    eucalyptus s.
salina
    Artemisia s.
saline
    s. agglutinin
    Broncho S.
    s. isohemagglutinin
Salisbury common cold virus
saliva
    enzymatic s.
    s. substitute
Salivart
salivary
    s. gland
    s. gland virus
    s. gland virus disease
    s. virus
Salk vaccine
salmeterol
    s. xinafoate
salmincola
    Nanophyetus s.
salmon
    s. calcitonin
    s. patch
    pink s.
Salmonella
    S. arizonae
    S. arthritis
    S. bredeney
    S. choleraesuis
    S. enteritidis
    S. montevideo
    S. panama
    S. paratyphi
    S. poona
    S. st. paul

S

Salmonella *(continued)*
   S. typhi
   S. typhimurium
salmonellosis
salmonicolor
   Sporobolomyces s.
salpingitis
   reactive s.
salsalate
Salsitab
salt
   s. cedar
   s. cedar tree
   Epsom s.'s
   gold s.'s
   s. grass
   persulfate s.
   s. of platinum
   s. sensitivity
   silver s.'s
   sodium s.
   theophylline s.
   s. water boil
saltbush
saltwater catfish
saltwort
salute
   allergic s.
salvage therapy
sampler
   inertial suction s.
   Rotorod s.
   Sartorious air s.
San
   S. Joaquin fever
   S. Miguel sea lion virus
Sanarelli phenomenon
Sanarelli-Shwartzman phenomenon
sand
   s. flea
   s. flea bite
sandal
   keratodermic s.
   s. strap dermatitis
sandfly
   s. bite
   s. fever
   s. fever virus
Sandimmune
   S. injection
   S. Oral
Sandoglobulin
sandworm disease

Sanfilippo
   S. mucopolysaccharidosis
   S. syndrome
sanguineus
   Allodermanyssus s.
   nevus s.
   sudor s.
sanguisuga
   Triatoma s.
Sansert
Santyl
saphenous nerve entrapment
saprophytic
   s. disease
   s. flora
saquinavir
   s. mesylate
sarcoid
   s. arthritis
   Boeck s.
   Darier-Roussy s.
   Spiegler-Fendt s.
sarcoidal
sarcoidosis
   cutaneous s.
   extrapulmonary s.
sarcolemma
sarcoma
   African-variety Kaposi s.
   avian s.
   epithelioid s.
   Kaposi s. (KS)
   multiple idiopathic
     hemorrhagic s.
   reticulum-cell s.
   Rous s.
sarcomatous
sarcomere
Sarcophaga
sarcophagi fly
Sarcopsylla
Sarcoptes
   S. hominis
   S. scabiei
sarcoptic
   s. acariasis
   s. mange
sardine
sargassum
   Japanese s.
Sarna
Sartorious air sampler

SAS
  statistical analysis system
Sastid Plain Therapeutic Shampoo
  and Acne Wash
satellite
  s. cell
  s. lesion
satellitosis
saturated solution of potassium
  iodide (SSKI)
saturation analysis
Saunders-Zwilling hypothesis
sauriasis
sauriderma
sauriosis
sauroderma
sausage
  s. digit
  s. finger
  s. toe
savitum
  Helminthosporium s.
saxitoxin
SBE
  subacute bacterial endocarditis
sc
  subcutaneous
scab
scabby mouth
Scabene
  S. Lotion
  S. shampoo
scabetic
scabicidal
scabicide
scabiei
  Sarcoptes s.
scabies
  animal s.
  Boeck s.
  crusted s.
  environmental s.
  hair follicle mite s.
  s. incognito
  nodular s.
  Norwegian s.
  s. preparation

scabietic
  s. mite
scabieticide
scabious
scabrities
  s. unguium
scalded skin syndrome
scale
  Borg s.
  branny s.
  carpet-tack s.
  lamellar s.
  lichen-type s.
  micaceous s.
  ostraceous s.
  Outerbridge s.
  pityriasis-type s.
  psoriatic-type s.
  Sessing pressure ulcer
    assessment s.
  Shea pressure ulcer
    assessment s.
  Shea s. (stages I-IV)
  silver-white s.
  silvery s.
  visual analogue s. (VAS)
scalene
scaling
  s. lesion
  s. skin-colored lesion
scall
  milk s.
scalp
  dissecting cellulitis of s.
  dissection cellulitis of s.
  s. infection
  s. louse
  pilar tumor of s.
  ringworm of s.
  seborrheic dermatitis of the s.
Scalpicin
scaly
  s. ringworm
  s. tetter
scan
  HRCT s.
  indium chloride s.

S

NOTES

scan *(continued)*
  SPECT s.
  Tc polyphosphate s.
  technetium s.
  ventilation-perfusion lung s.
  ventilation/perfusion lung s.
    (V/Q lung scan)
  V/Q lung s.
    ventilation/perfusion lung scan
Scanner
  SilkTouch C02 Flash S.
scanning
  indium-labeled s.
Scanpor
  S. acrylate adhesive
  S. tape
scapularis
  Ixodes s.
scapulocostal syndrome
scapulothoracic syndrome
scar
  atrophic white s.
  s. formation
  hypertrophic s.
  ice-pick type s.
  keloidal type s.
  papyraceous s.
  radial s.
  shilling s.
  white s.
scarf nevus
scarification
  s. test
scarificator
scarifier
  Berkeley s.
scarify
scarlatina
  anginose s.
  s. hemorrhagica
  s. latens
  s. maligna
  s. rheumatica
  s. simplex
scarlatinal
  s. nephritis
scarlatinella
scarlatiniform
  s. eruption
  erythema s.
  s. erythema
scarlatinoid

scarlet
  s. fever
  s. fever antitoxin
  s. fever erythrogenic toxin
scarring
  s. alopecia
  cigarette-paper s.
  keloidal s.
  patch test s.
scavenger cell
SCC
  squamous cell carcinoma
SCD
  sickle cell disease
Scedosporium apiospermum
scent print
Schamberg
  S. comedo extractor
  S. dermatitis
  S. disease
  S. progressive pigmented
    purpuric dermatosis
  S. purpura
Schaumann body
Scheie
  S. mucopolysaccharidosis
  S. syndrome
Schenck disease
schenckii
  Sporothrix s.
  Sporotrichum s.
Schick
  S. method
  S. test
  S. test toxin
Schiff
  periodic acid-S. (PAS)
Schirmer test
Schistosoma
  S. haematobium
  S. japonicum
  S. mansoni
  S. mekongi
schistosomal dermatitis
schistosome granuloma
schistosomiasis
  ectopic cutaneous s.
schizonychia
schizotrichia
Schober test
schoenleinii
  Achorion s.
  Trichophyton s.

Schönlein
    S. disease
    S. purpura
Schönlein-Henoch syndrome
Schridde cancer hair
Schuco 2000 nebulizer
Schultz-Charlton
    S.-C. phenomenon
    S.-C. reaction
Schultz-Dale reaction
Schwann cell
schwannoma
Schweninger-Buzzi
    anetoderma of S.-B.
    S.-B. anetoderma
sciatic nerve entrapment
SCID
    severe combined immunodeficiency
    severe combined immunodeficiency
        disorder
    SCID mice
scintigraphy
scintiscan
scissors
    Gradle s.
    iris s.
    serrated iris s.
scissura pilorum
Scl-70
SCLE
    subacute cutaneous lupus
        erythematosus
sclera
    donor s.
scleral defect
scleredema
    s. adultorum
    Buschke s.
    s. diutinum
    s. neonatorum
sclerema
    s. adiposum
    s. neonatorum
scleriasis
scleritis
    diffuse s.
    nodular s.

    nonrheumatoid s.
    posterior s.
    rheumatoid s.
scleroatrophy, sclerotylosis
    anetoderma s.
    atrophoderma s.
    lichen sclerosus s.
    striae s.
sclerodactylia
sclerodactyly
scleroderma
    diffuse s.
    environmental s.
    linear s.
    localized s.
    pediatric s.
    s. septal panniculitis
scleroderma-like
    s.-l. eruption
    s.-l. skin thickening
sclerodermatitis
sclerodermatous
scleroderma
sclerodermoid
ScleroLASER
scleromalacia
    s. perforans
scleromyxedema
scleronychia
sclerosed
sclerosing
    s. agent
    s. cholangitis
    s. hemangioma
    s. lymphangitis
sclerosis
    amyotrophic lateral s. (ALS)
    s. corii
    s. cutanea
    diffuse progressive systemic s.
    drug-induced progressive
        symptom s.
    environment progressive
        symptom s.
    limited progressive systemic s.
    linear progressive systemic s.

S

NOTES

357

sclerosis *(continued)*
    localized progressive
      systemic s.
    multiple s.
    progressive symptom s. (PSS)
    progressive systemic s.
    systemic s.
    tuberous s.
sclerosus
    genital lichen s.
    lichen s.
    s. lichen
sclerotherapy
sclerothrix
sclerotic
sclerotrichia
sclerotylosis *(var. of* scleroatrophy)
scoliosis
Scolopendra
    S. heres
    S. heres bite
scopolamine
Scopulariopsis brevicaulis
scorbutic
score
    APACHE II s.
    Brasfield chest radiograph s.
    Shwachman clinical s.
    t s.
    z s.
scorpion
    bark s.
    common striped s.
    s. fish
    s. sting
Scotch Tape test
scrapie
scraping
    fungal s.
    nasal s.
scratch
    s. chamber test
    s. test
    s. testing
Screen
    QuickVue One-Step
      Allergen S.
screening
    s. audiometry
    spirometric s.
Screening Patch Test Kit
screen test
screw-worm fly

scrofula
scrofuloderma, scrofulodermia
    s. gummosa
    papular s.
    verrucous s.
scrofulosorum
    acne s.
    lichen s.
scrofulous
    lichen s.
scrotalis
    lingua s.
scrotal tongue
scroti
    pruritus s.
scrub
    Exidine S.
    Techni-Care surgical s.
    s. typhus
scruff
sculpturatus
    Centruroides s.
scurf
scurvy
scutular
scutularis
    parakeratosis s.
scutulata
    ichthyosis s.
    porrigo s.
scutulum
Scytalidium
    S. dimidiatum
    S. hyalinum
SD
    standard deviation
    WinRho SD
S/D
    Gammagard S.
    Polygam S.
SEA
    seronegativity, enthesopathy,
    arthropathy
sea
    s. anemone
    s. anemone sting
    s. boot foot
    s. cucumber
    s. cucumber sting
    s. snake
    s. snake bite
    s. urchin

s. urchin granuloma
s. urchin sting
seabather's eruption
seal finger
season
growing s.
seasonal
s. allergic rhinitis
s. allergy
sebacea
ichthyosis s.
sebaceous, sebaceus
s. adenoma
s. carcinoma
s. cyst
s. gland
s. horn
s. hyperplasia
lupus s.
nevus s.
s. trichofolliculoma
s. tubercle
s. tumor
sebaceum
adenoma s.
molluscum s.
tuberculum s.
sebolith
sebopsoriasis
seborrhea
s. adiposa
s. capitis
s. cerea
concrete s.
s. corporis
eczematoid s.
s. faciei
s. furfuracea
s. nigra
s. oleosa
s. sicca
s. squamosa neonatorum
seborrheic
s. dermatitis
s. dermatitis-like condition
s. dermatitis of the scalp

s. dermatosis
s. eczema
s. keratosis
s. verruca
s. wart
seborrheica
corona s.
dermatitis s.
seborrhiasis
Sebulex
Sebulon
sebum
s. cutaneum
s. preputiale
second
s. degree burn
forced expiratory volume in
1 s. (FEV$_1$)
s. set rejection
secondary
s. adrenocortical failure
s. agammaglobulinemia
s. amyloid
s. antibody deficiency
s. cataract
s. cutaneous B-cell
lymphocytic leukemia
s. cutaneous B-cell lymphoma
s. disease
s. effect
s. encephalitis
s. hyperparathyroidism
s. hypogammaglobulinemia
s. immune response
s. immunodeficiency
s. infection
s. lesion
s. lymphedema
s. panhypopituitarism
s. psychiatric disorder
s. pyoderma
s. Sjögren syndrome
s. smoke
s. syphilid
s. syphilis
s. systemic amyloidosis

S

NOTES

secondary *(continued)*
  s. telangiectasia
  s. tuberculosis
second-line drug (SLD)
Secrétan syndrome
secrete
secretion
  excessive s.
secretor
  s. factor
secretory
  s. antibody study
  s. coil
  s. component
  s. component deficiency
  s. immunoglobulin
  s. leukoprotease inhibitor
  s. leukoprotease inhibitor
    protein
  s. otitis media
secretory immunoglobulin A
section
  horizontal s.
  vertical s.
SED
  spondyloepiphyseal dysplasia
sedative
  s. therapy
Sedi-Stain
seeberi
  Rhinosporidium s.
seed
  s. corn
  millet s.
  psyllium s.
  sesame s.
  s. tick
  s. wart
seglycin CS/DS
segment
  apicoposterior s.
segmental
  s. hyalinizing vasculitis
  s. neurofibromatosis
  s. vitiligo
Segond fracture
seizure
Seldane
  S.-D
selectins
selection
  tumor cell negative s.
selective photothermolysis

selenium
  s. deficiency
  s. sulfide
Selestoject
"self" antigen
self-healing reticulohistiocytosis
self-infection
self-injecting epinephrine
self-limited allergic reaction
self-nonself discrimination
Selsun
  S. Blue
  S. Gold
  S. Gold for Women
selvagem
  fogo s.
semelincident
semicircular
  s. lipoatrophy
  s. lipotrophy
semi-impermeable membrane
semimembranosus complex
semipermeable dressing
semiquantitative
semisynthetic analog
Semliki Forest virus
Semple vaccine
Semprex
Semprex-D
Sendai virus
Senear-Usher
  S.-U. disease
  S.-U. syndrome
seneca snakeroot
senile
  s. angioma
  s. atrophoderma
  s. ectasia
  s. elastosis
  s. fibroma
  s. gangrene
  s. hemangioma
  s. keratoderma
  s. keratoma
  s. keratosis
  s. lentigo
  s. melanoderma
  s. pruritus
  s. purpura
  s. sebaceous hyperplasia
  s. skin
  s. wart

senilis
  alopecia s.
  keratosis s.
  lentigo s.
  pruritus s.
  purpura s.
  verruca s.
  verruca plana s.
senior synonym
sennetsu
  Ehrlichia s.
sensible perspiration
sensitiva
  trichosis s.
sensitive
  temperature s. (TS)
sensitivity
  acquired s.
  allergic s.
  animal dander s.
  antibiotic s.
  aspirin s.
  atopic s.
  autoerythrocyte s.
  idiosyncratic s.
  induced s.
  multiple chemical s.
  photoallergic s.
  phototoxic s.
  salt s.
sensitization
  active s.
  autoerythrocyte s.
  cross s.
  photodynamic s.
sensitize
sensitized
  s. antigen
  s. cell
  s. lymphocyte
sensitizer
sensitizing
  s. dose
  s. injection
  s. substance
sensor
  ClipTip reusable s.

  Cross Top replacement
    oxygen s.
  Infinity s.
  SpiroSense flow s.
Sensorcaine
  S.-MPF
sensory ganglion
sensu stricto
sentinel
  s. animal
  s. tag
seositis
seotonin
Sephadex beads
Seprafilm bioresorbable membrane
sepsis
sepsis-induced
  s.-i. disseminated intravascular
    coagulation
  s.-i. thrombocytopenia
septa
  interlobular s.
septal
  s. embolus
  s. panniculitis
Septa Topical Ointment
septic
  s. arthritis
  s. dactylitis
  s. embolus
  s. shock
septicemia
  Aeromonas s.
  bacterial s.
  Candida s.
  DF2 s.
  gonococcal s.
  streptococcal s.
  typhoid s.
Septisol
Septra
  S. DS
sequela of influenza
sequence
  chi s.
sequences
  long terminal repeat s. (LTR)

S

NOTES

sequestration
 s. cyst
 s. dermoid
sequestrum
sera (*pl. of* serum)
Serax
Serevent
Sergent white line
serial
 s. dilutional intradermal skin
  test
 s. passage
serine
 s. esterase
 s. proteinase
serivumalb
sermorelin acetate
seroconversion
 s. response
serodiagnosis
seroepidemiology
serofast
serologic
 s. test for syphilis (S.T.S.)
serology
Seromycin Pulvules
seronegative
 s. oligoarthritis
 s. spondyloarthropathy
seronegativity, enthesopathy, arthropathy (SEA)
seropositive
 s. rheumatoid arthritis
seropurulent
serosanguineous
serotaxis
serotherapy
serotonin
serotype
 heterologous s.
 homologous s.
serotyping
serovaccination
serovar
serpentine
serpiginosa
 elastosis perforans s.
 zona s.
serpiginosum angioma
serpiginosus
 lupus s.

serpiginous
 s. ulcer
serpigo
serpin
serrated iris scissors
Serratia marcescens
sertraline
 s. HCl
 s. hydrochloride
serum, pl. sera
 s. accident
 s. agglutinin
 s. alpha-antitrypsin
 anticomplementary s.
 antiepithelial s.
 s. anti-glomerular-basement-
  membrane antibody
 antilymphocyte s. (ALS)
 antirabies s.
 antireticular cytotoxic s.
 antitoxic s.
 bacteriolytic s.
 blood s.
 s. C3
 s. C4
 s. complement C1–C9 (C1–C9)
 s. complement level
 convalescent s.
 Coombs s.
 s. disease
 dried human s.
 s. eruption
 foreign s.
 s. hepatitis (SH)
 s. hepatitis virus
 horse s.
 human s.
 human measles immune s.
 human pertussis immune s.
 human scarlet fever immune s.
 hyperimmune s.
 s. IgA
 s. IgM
 immune s.
 inactivated s.
 liquid human s.
 measles convalescent s.
 mouse s.
 s. nephritis
 s. neutralization
 nonimmune s.
 normal horse s.
 polyvalent s.

s. precipitin
s. protein electrophoresis
s. protein electrophoretic
   finding
s. rash
s. reaction
s. shock
s. sickness
specific s.
s. therapy
thyrotoxic s.
serumal
serum-fast
sesame seed
sessile
Sessing pressure ulcer assessment
   scale
seta, pl. **setae**
set of idiotopes
setosa
trichosis s.
severe
s. acute allergic reaction
s. anemia
s. chronic allergic condition
s. combined immunodeficiency
   (SCID)
s. combined immunodeficiency
   disorder (SCID)
s. combined immunodeficient
   mice
s. deforming osteogenesis
   imperfecta
s. immediate reaction
s. obstruction
s. respiratory failure
s. systemic reaction
severity of allergy symptom
sewer fly
sex factor
sexine
sexually transmitted disease (STD)
Sézary
S. cell
S. erythroderma
S. syndrome

SF
stimulating factor
synovial fluid
SH
serum hepatitis
shadow
ring s.
shaft
hair s.
shagbark
s. hickory
s. hickory tree
shaggy thick wall
shagreen
s. patch
s. skin
Sham
S. TENS
shampoo
G-well S.
Head and Shoulders s.
Kwell S.
P&S S.
Scabene s.
T/SAL S.
Zincon S.
sharp
s. dissection
s. spoon
sharply circumscribed nodule
shave
s. biopsy
s. technique
shawl distribution
Shea
S. pressure ulcer assessment
   scale
S. scale (stages I-IV)
sheath
s. cell
cuticle of inner root s.
fibrous s.
inner root s.
nerve s.
outer root s.
tendon s.

S

NOTES

shedding
    virus s.
Sheehan syndrome
sheep
    contagious ecthyma (pustular
      dermatitis) virus of s.
    s. epithelium
    pulmonary adenomatosis of s.
    s. sorrel
    s. wool
sheep-pox
    s.-p. virus
sheet
    keratinous s.
    Silk Skin s.
sheeting
    DermaSof s.
    New Beginnings topical gel s.
sheets of nevus cells
shellfish
shell nail
shelter foot
shift
    antigenic s.
Shiga-like toxin
Shigella
    S. dysenteriae
    S. flexneri
    S. flexneri dysenteriae
    S. infection
    S. sonnei
shigelloides
    Aeromonas s.
    Plesiomonas s.
shigellosis
Shiley tracheostomy tube
shilling scar
shimamushi disease
shin
    saber s.
    s. splint
    s. spot
    toasted s.
shiner
    allergic s.
shingles
Shingles Relief Pak
ship fever
shipping
    s. fever
    s. fever virus
shock
    anaphylactic s.

    anaphylactoid s.
    s. antigen
    endotoxin s.
    histamine s.
    osmotic s.
    protein s.
    pseudoanaphylactic s.
    septic s.
    serum s.
shocking dose
shoe
    Plastizote s.
Shope
    S. fibroma
    S. fibroma virus
    S. papilloma
    S. papilloma virus
short
    s. anagen telogen effluvium
    s. incubation hepatitis
    s. ragweed
    s. tau inversion recovery
      (STIR)
short-chain
    s.-c. type collagen
    s.-c. type X collagen
short-haired breed
shoulder
    frozen s.
    Head & S.'s
    s. periarthritis
shoulder-hand syndrome
shrimp
shrinking lung syndrome
Shuco-Myst nebulizer
Shulman syndrome
shunt
    arteriovenous s.
    ventriculoperitoneal s. (VP)
shunting
    venoarterial s.
Shwachman clinical score
Shwartzman
    S. phenomenon
    S. reaction
SI
    syncytium-inhibiting
sialadenitis
sialidase
sialidosis
sialometaplasia
    necrotizing s.
sialomucin

Sibine
>S. *stimulea*
>S. *stimulea* sting

sicca
>cholera s.
>keratoconjunctivitis s.
>onychia s.
>pityriasis s.
>seborrhea s.
>s. syndrome

sick building syndrome
sickle
>s. cell anemia
>s. cell disease (SCD)
>s. cell trait
>s. cell ulcer

sickness
>African horse s.
>motion s.
>serum s.
>spotted s.

side-chain theory
side effect
sideroderma
sign
>Auspitz s.
>bandage s.
>Bunnell s.
>Buschke-Ollendorf s.
>butterfly s.
>Comby s.
>Crowe s.
>Cullen s.
>cutaneous s.
>Darier s.
>Dawbarn s.
>daylight s.
>Dennie-Morgan s.
>dimple s.
>Ewart s.
>Faget s.
>flag s.
>Gottron s.
>Grisolle s.
>groove s.
>hair collar s.
>Hertoghe s.

>Hoover s.
>Hutchinson s.
>impingement s.
>Leser-Trélat s.
>Lovibond profile s.
>McMurray s.
>melanoma warning s.
>Mirchamp s.
>Muerhrcke s.
>Nikolsky s.
>Osler s.
>Pastia s.
>Popeye s.
>Romana s.
>Rumpel-Leede s.
>tail s.
>Thomson s.
>Vierra s.
>Walker-Murdoch s.
>Yergason supination s.

signal
>s. recognition particle
>s. transduction

signet ring lymphoma
significance
>McNemar test of s.

Silafed Syrup
Silaminic Expectorant
Silastic tubing
Sildicon-E
silencer
"silent" chest
silent lupus nephritis
Silfedrine
>Children's S.

silica granuloma
silicone
>s. deposition
>s. grease
>s. oil
>s. rubber prosthesis
>s. synovitis

silicosis
silk
Silk Skin sheet
SilkTouch C02 Flash Scanner

S

NOTES

Sillence
S. type II–IV osteogenesis
imperfecta
Siloskin dressing
Silvadene
silver
s. nitrate
s. poisoning
s. protein, mild
s. salts
s. stain (IFA)
s. sulfadiazine
silver-methenamine stain
silver-white scale
silvery scale
Simbu virus
simian vacuolating virus No. 40
(SV40)
simian virus 40
simian virus (SV)
Simmond syndrome
Simplastin EXCEL
simple
s. drug
s. lentigo
s. pulmonary eosinophilia
simplex
acne s.
angioma s.
dermatitis s.
disseminated herpes s.
EB s.
epidermolysis s.
epidermolysis bullosa s.
erythema s.
herpes s.
hidroacanthoma s.
ichthyosis s.
lentigo s.
lichen chronicus s.
lymphangioma superficium s.
prurigo s.
purpura s.
scarlatina s.
toxoplasmosis, other infections,
rubella, cytomegalovirus
infection, and herpes s.
(TORCH)
s. variant
verruca s.
Simulium
simvastatin

Sinarest 12 Hour Nasal solution
Sindbis
S. fever
S. virus
Sine-Aid
S.-A. IB
Sinequan
Singh index
single
s. (gel) diffusion precipitin test
in one dimension
s. immunodiffusion
s. photon emission computed
tomography (SPECT)
s. radial immunodiffusion
(SRID)
s. spike
single-breath nitrogen washout test
single-peak pork insulin
single-stranded
s.-s. anti-DNA antibody
s.-s. DNA
sinobronchial
sinopulmonary disease
Sinubid
Sinufed Timecelles
Sinulin
sinus
barber's pilonidal s.
cutaneous s.
dental s.
s. histiocytosis
Motrin IB S.
pilonidal s.
preauricular s.
Rokitansky-Aschoff s.
s. tract
transillumination of s.
sinusitis
acute paranasal s.
chronic paranasal s.
ethmoid s.
sinusoid
cavernous s.
Sinutab Tablet
sinuvertebral nerve
Siphonaptera
Siphoviridae
sippy diet
siro
Acarus s.
Tyroglyphus s.

SIRS
systemic inflammatory response
syndrome
sisal
Sister Mary Joseph nodule
site
antibody combining s.
antigen-binding s.
antigen-combining s.
combining s.
immunologically privileged s.
receptor s.
sitophila
Neurospora s.
situ
carcinoma in s.
in s.
malignant melanoma in s.
sixth
s. disease
s. venereal disease
size
lesion s.
Sjögren
S. disease
S. syndrome (SS)
Sjögren-Larsson syndrome
skeletal abnormality
skin
alligator s.
s. atrophy
blistering s.
bronzed s.
s. cancer
combination s.
deciduous s.
diamond s.
s. disease syndrome
s. dissemination
dry s.
elastic s.
s. eruption
farmer's s.
Favre-Racouchot s.
fish s.
glabrous s.
glossy s.

golfer s.
golfer's s.
granulomatous slack s.
hanging s.
hidden nail s.
hyperirritable s.
India-rubber s.
infantile acute hemorrhagic
edema of the s.
s. involvement
leopard s.
s. lesion
loose s.
s. lubrication
s. lubrication therapy
lymphocytic infiltration of
the s.
marble s.
mixed tumor of s.
monoclonal protein, s.
parchment s.
s. peel
piebald s.
pig s.
porcupine s.
primary macular atrophy of s.
primary neuroendocrine
carcinoma of the s.
s. punch
s. purpura
s. rash
s. reaction
s. rubor
sailor's s.
senile s.
shagreen s.
slack s.
s. stones
striate atrophy of s.
s. tag
s. test
s. testing
thickened s.
toad s.
s. trephine
true s.
s. type

S

NOTES

skin *(continued)*
    s. ulcer
    volar s.
    s. wheal
    s. window technique
    s. writing
    yellow s.
skinbound disease
skin-colored
    s.-c. lesion
skin-limited histiocytosis
skin-puncture test
Skin-So-Soft
    Avon S.-S.-S.
SkinTech medical tattooing device
Sklowsky symptom
SK-SD
    streptokinase-streptodornase
sky-blue spot
slack skin
slapped
    "s. cheek" appearance
    "s. cheek" rash
    "s. face" appearance
slash
    s. pine
    s. pine tree
SLC
    synovial lining cell
SLD
    second-line drug
SLE
    systemic lupus erythematosus
sleep
    alpha-NREM s.
    s. anomaly
    s. apnea
    s. apnea/hypopnea syndrome
    s. apnea syndrome
    delta s.
    desynchronized s.
    s. efficiency
    nonREM s.
    nonrestorative s.
    paradoxical s.
    s. physiology
    REM s.
    restorative s.
    slow wave s.
    stage 1 s.
    stage 4 s.
    s. study
sleep-disordered breathing

Sleep-eze 3 Oral
Sleepinal
SLE-like syndrome
slender ragweed
Sleuth
    CO S.
    ETO S.
    HBT S.
slim disease
slippery
    s. elm
    s. elm tree
Slo-bid
Slo-Niacin
slope shouldered lesion
Slo-Phyllin
    S.-P. GG
slough
sloughed bronchial epithelium
sloughing
    s. phagedena
    s. ulcer
slow
    s. fever
    s. virus
    s. virus disease
    s. vital capacity (SVC)
    s. wave sleep
slow-acting antirheumatic drug (SAARD)
slow-reacting
    s.-r. factor of anaphylaxis (SRF-A)
    s.-r. substance (SRS)
    s.-r. substance of anaphylaxis (SRS-A)
slurry
    talc s.
Sly
    S. mucopolysaccharidosis
    S. syndrome
small
    s. nuclear ribonucleoprotein (snRNP)
    s. plaque parapsoriasis
    s. tonsil
    s. vessel vasculitis
small airways dysfunction
smallpox
    fulminating s.
    hemorrhagic s.
    malignant s.
    modified s.

S

s. vaccine
s. virus
West Indian s.
Sm antigen
Smart Trigger
smear
nasal s.
Tzanck s.
wet s.
Ziehl-Neelsen s.
smegmatis
Mycobacterium s.
Smith-Riley syndrome
smog
industrial s.
photochemical s.
smoke
cigarette s.
s. inhalation
secondary s.
tobacco s.
smooth
s. leprosy
s. lesion
s. muscle relaxation
s. skin-colored lesion
s. stinger
smotherweed
smut
Bermuda s.
corn s.
cultivated barley s.
cultivated corn s.
cultivated oat s.
cultivated rye s.
cultivated wheat s.
Johnson s.
snake
Arizona coral s.
s. bite
copperhead s.
coral s.
cottonmouth s.
Eastern coral s.
pit viper s.
sea s.
terrestrial s.

Texas coral s.
s. venom
venomous s.
water moccasin s.
snakebite
snakeroot
seneca s.
SNAP
S. recorder
S. sleep recorder
Snaplets
S.-EX
S.-FR granule
snapping
s. finger
s. hip
Sneddon syndrome
Sneddon-Wilkinson disease
sneezeweed
sneezing
paroxysmal s.
snowshoe hare virus
snRNP
small nuclear ribonucleoprotein
U3 s.
SO₂
sulfur dioxide
soak therapy
soap
Ayndet moisturizing s.
Baby Magic s.
Derma S.
Derm-Vi S.
sobria
Aeromonas s.
sodium
alendronate s.
aminosalicylate s.
s. bicarbonate
carboxymethylcellulose s.
cefazolin s.
cefmetazole s.
cefonicid s.
cefoperazone s.
cefotaxime s.
cefoxitin s.
ceftizoxime s.

NOTES

369

sodium *(continued)*
  ceftriaxone s.
  cephalothin s.
  cephapirin s.
  s. citrate and citric acid
  cloxacillin s.
  colistimethate s.
  cromolyn s.
  diclofenac s.
  dicloxacillin s.
  Diphenylan S.
  s. etidronate
  foscarnet s.
  s. hypochlorite solution
  meclofenamate s.
  2-mercaptoethane sulphonate s.
    (mesna)
  methicillin s.
  mezlocillin s.
  nafcillin s.
  naproxen s.
  nedocromil s.
  olsalazine s.
  oxacillin s.
  oxychlorosene s.
  para-aminosalicylate s.
  S. P.A.S.
  s. pentosan
  piperacillin s.
  piperacillin sodium and
    tazobactam s.
  s. salt
  stibogluconate s.
  S. Sulamyd Ophthalmic
  s. sulfacetamide
  s. sulfacetamide and
    fluorometholone
  s. sulfacetamide and
    phenylephrine
  s. sulfacetamide and
    prednisolone
  s. thiosulfate
  tolmetin s.
  s. versenate solution
  warfarin s.
sodium-PCA
  lactic acid and s.-P.
Sof-Cil
soft
  s. chancre
  s. corn
  s. keratin
  s. lesion

  s. papilloma
  s. sore
  s. tick
  s. tissue
  s. tissue calcification
  s. ulcer
  s. wart
Softech endotracheal tube
solani
  Stemphylium s.
solar
  s. cheilitis
  s. dermatitis
  s. elastosis
  s. fever
  s. keratosis
  s. lentigo
  s. purpura
  s. urticaria
solare
  erythema s.
solaris
  s. urticaria
Solatene
soldering
  s. flux
  s. fumes
soldier patch
sole
  s. dyshidrosis
Solenopsis
  S. geminata
  S. invecta
  S. invecta sting
  S. richteri sting
  S. saevissima richteria
Solganal
solid
  s. carbon dioxide
  s. hidradenoma
  s. phase immunoassay
solid-phase C1q-binding assay
solid-tumor marker
solitary
  s. keratoacanthoma
  s. simple lymphangioma
soluble
  s. antigen
  s. specific substance (SSS)
Soluble T4
Solu-Cortef
Solu-Medrol
  S.-M. injection

Solurex
    S. L.A.
Soluspan
    Celestone S.
solution
    Adsorbotear Ophthalmic s.
    Afrin Nasal s.
    AK-Dilate Ophthalmic s.
    AK-Nefrin Ophthalmic s.
    Akwa Tears s.
    Allerest 12 Hour Nasal s.
    AquaSite Ophthalmic s.
    aqueous s.
    Atrovent Inhalation s.
    Bion Tears s.
    Burow s.
    carbol-fuchsin s.
    Chlorphed-LA Nasal s.
    Comfort Tears s.
    Crolom Ophthalmic s.
    Dakrina Ophthalmic s.
    Dey-Drop Ophthalmic s.
    Dristan Long Lasting Nasal s.
    Dry Eyes s.
    Dry Eye Therapy s.
    Duofilm s.
    Duration Nasal s.
    Dwelle Ophthalmic s.
    Eye-Lube-A s.
    flunisolide nasal s.
    Freezone s.
    Fungoid Topical s.
    HypoTears s.
    HypoTears PF s.
    hypotonic s.
    Intal Nebulizer s.
    I-Phrine Ophthalmic s.
    Isopto Frin Ophthalmic s.
    Isopto Plain s.
    Isopto Tears s.
    Just Tears s.
    Lacril Ophthalmic s.
    Liquifilm Forte s.
    Liquifilm Tears s.
    Lotrimin AF s.
    LubriTears s.
    Monsel s.
    Murine s.
    Murocel Ophthalmic s.
    Mydfrin Ophthalmic s.
    Nasalcrom Nasal s.
    Nature's Tears s.
    Neosporin Ophthalmic s.
    Neo-Synephrine Ophthalmic s.
    NTZ Long Acting Nasal s.
    Nu-Tears s.
    Nu-Tears II s.
    OcuCoat Ophthalmic s.
    OcuCoat PF Ophthalmic s.
    precipitate in s.
    Prefrin Ophthalmic s.
    Puralube Tears s.
    Refresh Ophthalmic s.
    Refresh Plus Ophthalmic s.
    Relief Ophthalmic s.
    Resectisol Irrigation s.
    Sinarest 12 Hour Nasal s.
    sodium hypochlorite s.
    sodium versenate s.
    Tear Drop s.
    TearGard Ophthalmic s.
    Teargen Ophthalmic s.
    Tearisol s.
    Tears Naturale s.
    Tears Naturale Free s.
    Tears Naturale II s.
    Tears Plus s.
    Tears Renewed s.
    Trans-Ver-Sal transdermal patch
     Verukan s.
    trivalent oral poliovirus s.
    Ultra Tears s.
    Vicks Sinex Long-Acting
     Nasal s.
    Viva-Drops s.
    4-Way Long Acting Nasal s.
solvent-based mascara
somaliensis
    Streptomyces s.
somatic
    s. agglutinin
    s. antigen
somatomedin C

S

NOTES

somatosensory
> s. evoked response

somatropin
Sominex Oral
SomnoStar apnea testing device
sonnei
> *Shigella s.*

Sony VHS HQ Digital Picture video
soot wart
Sorbsan alginate dressing
sordes
sore
> bay s.
> bed s.
> canker s.
> cold s.
> desert s.
> fever s.
> fungating s.
> hard s.
> s. mouth
> Naga s.
> Oriental s.
> pressure s.
> soft s.
> summer s.
> tropical s.
> veldt s.
> venereal s.
> water s.

soremouth
> s. virus

soremuzzle
soreness
sorghum
> s. grass

sorivudine
sorrel
> sheep s.

sorter
> fluorescence-activated cell s. (FACS)

Soto syndrome
souffle
sound
> coarse breath s.
> diminished breath s.
> pulmonic valve closure s.

source
> monochromatic light s.

South American blastomycosis
Southern blot

sowdah
Soyalac
soybean
> s. flour
> s. grain dust mite
> s. meal

soy milk
SP-10 spirometer
SpA
> spondyloarthropathy

space
> intercellular s.
> physiological dead s.
> Tenon s.

spacer
> Ellipse compact s.

spade finger
Spanish
> S. fly
> S. fly sting
> S. influenza

sparfloxacin
sparing
> island of s.

SPART analyzer
spasm
> epidemic transient diaphragmatic s.

spasmogen
spatula
> Roux s.

SPE
> streptococcal pyrogenic exotoxin

specialized transduction
special lesion
species
> Phoma s.

species-specific
> s.-s. antigen

specific
> s. active immunity
> s. alteration in immunologic reactivity
> s. anergy
> s. antigen
> s. antiserum
> s. bactericide
> s. capsular substance
> s. disease
> s. hemolysin
> s. IgE antibody level
> s. immune globulin (human)
> s. opsonin

s. passive immunity
s. reaction
s. serum
s. soluble polysaccharide
s. soluble sugar
s. transduction
specificity
speck finger
speckled
s. lentiginous nevus
s. staining
speckled-pattern ANA
SPECT
single photon emission computed
tomography
SPECT scan
Spectam injection
Spectazole
S. topical
spectinomycin hydrochloride
spectra
spectral
s. analysis
Spectrobid
spectroscopy
flame emission s. (FES)
spectrum
antimicrobial s.
broad s., broad-spectrum
S. ruby laser
toxin s.
wide s.
spermatolysin
spermatolysis
spermatolytic
spermatoxin
spermine
spermolysis
spermotoxin
Spexil
SPF
sun protection factor
sphacelation
sphaceloderma
sphaericus
Bacillus s.
sphenoethmoidectomy

sphenoid dysplasia
spherocytosis
hereditary s.
Sphingobacterium
sphingolipidosis
sphingomyelinase-D
SPI
Standards for Pediatric
Immunization
spica cast
spider
s. angioma
antivenin, black widow s.
arterial s.
s. bite
black widow s.
brown recluse s.
fiddle-back s.
s. hemangioma
s. mole
s. nevus
s. telangiectasia
s. telangiectasis
s. venom
violin-back s.
spider-burst
Spiegler-Fendt
S.-F. pseudolymphoma
S.-F. sarcoid
spike
single s.
spiloma
spiloplaxia
spilus
nevus s.
spinach
spinale
tache s.
spina pedis
spindle
s. cell
s. cell carcinoma
s. cell hemangioendothelioma
s. cell lipoma
s. cell nevus
spine
horny s.

S

NOTES

spine *(continued)*
 Rugger-jersey s.
 venom-bearing s.
spin-echo pulse
Spinhaler inhaler
spinipalpis
 Ixodes s.
spinosa
 ichthyosis s.
spinosum
 stratum s.
spinulosa
 trichostasis s.
spinulosus
 lichen s.
 lichen pilaris seu s.
spiny
 s. pigweed
 s. structure
spiradenitis
spiradenoma
 eccrine s.
spiralis
 Trichina s.
 Trichinella s.
spirals
 Curschmann s.
spiramycin
Spirillum minus
spirit
Spirochaeta pallida
spirochete
 corkscrew s.
 s. infection
spirochetemia
spirochetolysis
spirochetosis
spirogram
 forced expiratory s. (FES)
spirometer
 Flash portable s.
 Micro Plus s.
 SP-10 s.
 Spirovit SP-1 portable s.
spirometric screening
spirometry
 incentive s.
spironolactone
Spiroplasma apis
SpiroSense flow sensor
Spirovit SP-1 portable spirometer
spiruroid larva migrans
Spitz nevus

splash
 rain s.
 wave s.
splendens
 lamina s.
Splendore-Hoeppli phenomenon
splenectomy
splenic index
splenomegaly
splenotoxin
splint
 hindfoot s.
 shin s.
splinter hemorrhage
split
 s. papule
 s. tolerance
splitting nail
split-virus vaccine
spodogenous
spodophorous
Spondweni virus
spondylitica
 psoriasis s.
spondylitis
 ankylosing s. (AS)
 s. ossificans ligamentosa
 predominant s.
 psoriatic s.
spondyloarthropathy (SpA)
 seronegative s.
spondyloepiphyseal dysplasia (SED)
spondylolisthesis
 isthmic s.
spondylolysis
spondylometry
spondylosis
 s. deformans
 s. hyperostotica
spongiform
 s. pustule
 s. pustule of Kogoj
spongiosis
 eosinophilic s.
spontanea
 dactylolysis s.
spontaneous
 s. agglutination
 s. gangrene of newborn
 s. phagocytosis
 s. pseudoscar
 s. regression

spoon
s. nail
sharp s.
spora
air s.
sporangiospore
sporangium
Sporanox Oral
spore
airborne s.
mold s.
Sporidin-G
sporoagglutination
Sporobolomyces salmonicolor
Sporothrix schenckii
sporotrichosis
cutaneous s.
fixed cutaneous s.
mucocutaneous s.
visceral s.
sporotrichositic chancre
Sporotrichum schenckii
sports medicine
SPO₂T
Pocket S.
spot
ash-leaf s.
blue s.
café au lait s.
Campbell-De Morgan s.
cayenne pepper s.
cherry s.
cotton-wool s.
Filatov s.
Fordyce s.
gift s.
Horder s.
Koplik s.
liver s.
mongolian s.
mulberry s.
rose s.
Roth s.
ruby s.
shin s.
sky-blue s.
temperature s.

s. test
Trousseau s.
s. weld
SpotCheck+ handheld pulse oximeter
spotted
s. fever
s. sickness
spotted-fever tick
spray
aerosol s.
Caldecort Anti-Itch s.
Fluori-Methane Topical S.
vapocoolant s.
spreading phenomenon
spring ophthalmia
sprout
brussel s.
spruce
s. tree
sprue
celiac s.
Spumavirinae
Spumavirus
spur
calcaneal s.
sputum, pl. sputa
copious s.
purulent s.
s. viscosity and elasticity
SQ
subcutaneous
squama
squamate
squame
squamosum
eczema s.
squamous
s. cell
s. cell carcinoma (SCC)
s. cell epithelioma
s. cell layer
s. cell lung tumor
square shouldered lesion
squarrose
squash
squeeze effect

S

NOTES

SR
Deconamine S.
Respaire-120 S.
Respaire-60 S.
Sr
Congess S.
SRF-A
slow-reacting factor of anaphylaxis
SRID
single radial immunodiffusion
SRS
slow-reacting substance
SRS-A
slow-reacting substance of
anaphylaxis
SS
Sjögren syndrome
SS hemoglobin disease
Uroplus SS
SSC
suprascapular nerve compression
SSD AF
SSD Cream
SSKI
saturated solution of potassium
iodide
SSPE
subacute sclerosing panencephalitis
SSS
soluble specific substance
SSSS
staphylococcal scalded skin
syndrome
SSYA
Uroplus S.
St.
S. Joseph Adult Chewable
Aspirin
S. Louis encephalitis
S. Louis encephalitis virus
stabilate
stable
s. fly
s. fly bite
Stachybotrys atra
stacking
epidermal s.
stage
algid s.
cold s.
convalescent s.
defervescent s.
incubative s.

s. of invasion
Kellgren-Lawrence s.
latent s.
meningeal s.
patch s.
plaque s.
prodromal s.
s. 1 sleep
s. 4 sleep
tumor s.
staged abdominal repair (STAR)
staging
TNM s.
stain
alizarin red S s.
bovine rotavirus s.
calcofluor s.
Clay-Adams s.
Congo red s.
cytotoxin-positive s.
Dieterle s.
Diff-Quick s.
fluorescent antibody s. (FA)
Giemsa s.
Gram s.
immunofluorescent s.
Kinyoun s.
mucicarmine s.
PAS s.
periodic acid-Schiff s.
pneumococcal s.
port-wine s.
potassium chloride s. (KOH)
silver s. (IFA)
silver-methenamine s.
Warthin-Starry s.
Wright s.
Ziehl-Nielsen s.
staining
avidin-biotin-peroxidase s.
diffuse s.
nucleolar s.
pattern of s.
peripheral s.
speckled s.
Stallerkit
Stallerpointe needle
staminate
standard deviation (SD)
Standards
National Committee for
Clinical Laboratory S.
(NCCLS)

S. for Pediatric Immunization (SPI)
Staphcillin
StaphVAX
staphylococcal
s. abscess
s. blepharitis
s. enterotoxin
s. scalded skin syndrome (SSSS)
s. toxic shock syndrome
staphylococcal-binding assay
staphylococcolysin
staphylococcolysis
Staphylococcus
S. albus
S. aureus
S. aureus vaccine
S. epidermidis
methicillin-resistant *S. aureus* (MRSA)
S. vaccine
staphylococcus
s. antitoxin
staphyloderma
staphylodermatitis
staphylohemolysin
staphylolysin
staphylotoxin
stapling
bleb s.
STAR
staged abdominal repair
star
venous s.
starch-iodine test
starfish
s. sting
Star Sync
starvation syndrome
stasis
dermatitis s.
s. dermatitis
s. eczema
s. vascular ulcer
state
anaphylactic s.

carrier s.
excited s.
hypercoagulable s.
hyperimmune s.
static gangrene
Staticin topical
stationary phase
statistical analysis system (SAS)
Statistics
National Center for Health S. (NCHS)
stature
brittle hair, intellectual impairment, decreased fertility, short s. (BIDS)
decreased fertility, short s.
impairment, decreased fertility, short s.
photosensitivity, ichthyosis, brittle hair, intellectual impairment, decreased fertility, and short s. (PIBIDS)
status
s. asthmaticus
s. epilepticus
stavudine
S-T Cort
STD
sexually transmitted disease
stearothermophilus
Bacillus s.
steatocystoma
multiplex s.
s. multiplex
steatoma
steatorrhea
postinfectious s.
steel factor
Steinberg test
Steinbrocker
S. classification
S. criteria
stellate
s. abscess
s. ganglion block
s. ganglion blockade
s. hair

S

NOTES

stellate *(continued)*
    s. morphology
    s. pattern
    s. patterned disease
    s. pseudoscar
stem cell
Stemex
Stemphylium
    S. botryosum
    S. solani
stenosing tenosynovitis
stenosis, pl. **stenoses**
    bronchial s.
    cicatricial s.
    tracheal s.
stenothermal
Stenotrophomonas maltophilia
stent
    T-Y s.
Sterapred Oral
stercoralis
    Strongyloides s.
sterile
    s. abscess
    s. pustule
    s. technique
sterilisans
    therapia magna s.
sterility
sterilization
    discontinuous s.
    fractional s.
    intermittent s.
sterilize
sterilizer
sternoclavicular joint
sternocleidomastoid muscle
sternocostal joint
sternomastoid
steroid
    s. acne
    anabolic s.
    s. burst
    s. chalk
    s. fever
    group 5 topical s.
    s. myopathy
    Psorcon topical s.
    s. pulse
    s. sulfatase deficiency
    systemic s.
    s. taper
    topical s.
    s. ulcer
steroid-dependent asthma
sterol
Stevens-Johnson syndrome
Stewart-Treves syndrome
stibogluconate sodium
Sticker disease
Stickler syndrome
Stifcore
stiff hand syndrome
stiffness
    morning s.
stigma, pl. **stigmata**
Still disease
stimulating factor (SF)
stimulation
    alpha adrenergic s.
    beta adrenergic s.
    juxtacrine s.
    transcutaneous electrical
      nerve s. (TENS)
stimulator
    long-acting thyroid s. (LATS)
    transcutaneous electrical
      neuromuscular s. (TENS)
stimulea
    Sibine s.
stimuli
    psychological s.
stimulus, pl. **stimuli**
    chemical s.
    physical s.
sting
    Africanized honeybee s.
    ant s.
    Apis mellifera s.
    arthropod s.
    ashgray blister beetle s.
    bark scorpion s.
    bee s.
    blister beetle s.
    blue bottle s.
    Bombus s.
    box jellyfish s.
    brown moth larvae s.
    brown-tail moth s.
    bumblebee s.
    caterpillar s.
    catfish s.
    Centruroides exilicauda s.
    Centruroides sculpturatus s.
    Centruroides vittatus s.

Chironex fleckeri s.
coelenterate s.
common striped scorpion s.
Dolichorespula s.
Epicauta fabricii s.
Epicauta vitlata s.
Euproctis chrysorrhoea s.
European blister beetle s.
fire ant s.
fire coral s.
gypsy moth larva s.
honeybee s.
hornet s.
Hymenoptera s.
insect s.
io moth larva s.
jellyfish s.
Lymantria dispar s.
Lytta vesicata s.
marine animal s.
Megabombus s.
Megalopyge opercularis s.
millipede s.
Paederus gemellus s.
Paederus limnophilus s.
Paravespula s.
Polistes s.
Portuguese man-of-war s.
puss caterpillar s.
Pyrobombus s.
red imported fire ant s.
saddle back caterpillar s.
scorpion s.
sea anemone s.
sea cucumber s.
sea urchin s.
Sibine stimulea s.
Solenopsis invecta s.
Solenopsis richteri s.
Spanish fly s.
starfish s.
sting ray s.
striped blister beetle s.
Vespula s.
wasp s.
yellow jacket s.

stinger
  barbed s.
  imbedded s.
  smooth s.
stinging
  s. caterpillar
stink gland
stinkweed
STIR
  short tau inversion recovery
Stobo antigen
stock
  s. strain
  s. vaccine
stocking nevus
Stockman nodule
Stokoguard
stomatitis
  allergic s.
  angular s.
  aphthous s.
  bovine papular s.
  denture s.
  fusospirochetal s.
  gangrenous s.
  gonococcal s.
  lead s.
  s. medicamentosa
  mercurial s.
  nicotine s.
  s. papulosa
  primary herpetic s.
  ulcerative s.
  vesicular s.
stomatodynia
stomatomalacia
stomatomycosis
stomatonecrosis
stomatonoma
stomatopyrosis
Stomoxys bite
stones
  skin s.
stool
  s. culture
  mucous s.

S

NOTES

storage
    neutral lipid s.
    phytanic acid s.
strain
    BORSA s.
    carrier s.
    cell s.
    0157-H7 s.
    hypothetical mean s. (HMS)
    lysogenic s.
    pseudolysogenic s.
    rabies virus, Flury s.
    rabies virus, Kelev s.
    recombinant s.
    stock s.
    type s.
strand
    complementary s.
    homology of s.
    plus s.
    viral s.
strands
stratification
stratum
    central s.
    s. compactum
    s. corneum
    s. disjunctum
    s. germinativum
    s. granulosum
    s. lucidum
    s. malpighii
    s. mucosum
    s. spinosum
strawberry
    s. angioma
    s. birthmark
    s. hemangioma
    s. mark
    s. nevus
    s. tongue
straw itch
streak
    angioid s.
    meningitic s.
streaking
    linear s.
street virus
Strength
    Allerest Maximum S.
    Aspirin Free Anacin
      Maximum S.
    Bayer Low Adult S.

Clocort Maximum S.
Cortaid Maximum S.
Streptobacillus moniliformis
streptocerca
    Dipetalonema s.
    Mansonella s.
streptococcal
    s. balanoposthitis
    s. M1
    s. M3
    s. M antigen
    s. nephritis
    s. pharyngitis
    s. pyrogenic exotoxin (SPE)
    s. septicemia
    s. tonsillitis
    s. toxic shock syndrome
streptococci
    α-s.
    group A s.
    β-hemolytic s.
    hemolytic s.
Streptococcus
    S. agalactiae
    S. faecalis
    S. infection
    S. intermedius
    S. M antigen
    penicillin-resistant *S.*
      pneumoniae (PRSP)
    S. pyogenes
streptococcus
    s. erythrogenic toxin
    group A s. (GAS)
    group A beta-hemolytic s.
      (GABHS)
    group B s. (GBS)
    s. M antigen
streptoderma
streptodermatitis
streptokinase-streptodornase (SK-SD)
streptolysin
streptolysin O
Streptomyces
    S. somaliensis
    S. tsukubaensis
streptomycin
    G unit of s.
    L unit of s.
    s. sulfate
    S unit of s.
    s. unit
streptozyme agglutination test

stress
    emotional s.
    s. fracture
    intrapsychic s.
    redox s.
stress-generated electric potential
stretch
    s. marks
    s. reflex
stria, pl. **striae**
    s. alba
    s. albicans
    s. atrophica
    striae cutis distensae
    elastotic s.
    striae gravidarum
    s. nasi transversa
    s. rubra
    striae scleroatrophy
    Wickham s.
striata
    dermatitis pratensis s.
    melanonychia s.
striate
    s. atrophy of skin
striatum
    atrophoderma s.
striatus
    lichen s.
stricto
    sensu s.
stridor
string bean
strip
    Breathe Right nasal s.
    Nu-Hope skin barrier s.
striped
    s. blister beetle
    s. blister beetle sting
stripes
    Mees s.
stroke volume (SV)
stromal
    s. cell
stromatolysis
stromelysin
Strongyloides stercoralis

strongyloidiasis
strophulosus
    lichen s.
strophulus
    s. candidus
    s. intertinctus
    s. pruriginosus
structure
    hair-like s.
    pilosebaceous s.
    spiny s.
struma
    Riedel s.
Strümpell disease
Struthers
    ligament of S.
strychnine poisoning
Stryker
    S. arthroscope
    S. microshaver
Stryker-Halbeisen syndrome
S.T.S.
    serologic test for syphilis
stucco keratosis
Student's *t* test
study
    aerometric s.
    case control s.
    cohort s.
    meglumine diatrizoate enema s.
    metabolic s.
    nerve conduction s. (NCS)
    secretory antibody s.
    sleep s.
    T1-weighted s.
    T2-weighted s.
stupe
Sturge-Weber syndrome
sty, stye
style
Styloviridae
styptic
    s. collodion
    s. pencil
subacuta
    prurigo simplex s.

S

NOTES

subacute
  s. bacterial endocarditis (SBE)
  s. cutaneous lupus
    erythematosus (SCLE)
  s. inclusion body encephalitis
  s. lupus erythematosus
  s. migratory panniculitis
  s. nodular migratory
    panniculitis
  s. sclerosing leukoencephalitis
  s. sclerosing panencephalitis
    (SSPE)
  s. spongiform encephalopathy
subchondral
  s. cyst
  s. erosion
subclinical asthma
subcorneal
  s. blister
  s. pustular dermatitis
  s. pustular dermatosis
subcutanea
  lipogranulomatosis s.
  urticaria s.
subcutaneous (sc, SQ)
  s. calcification
  s. dirofilariasis
  s. emphysema
  s. epinephrine
  s. fat necrosis
  s. fat necrosis of newborn
  s. fungal infection
  s. granuloma annulare
  s. granulomatous nodule
  s. injection
  s. morphea
  s. mycosis
  s. myiasis
  s. necrotizing infection
  s. nodule
  s. phycomycosis
  s. rheumatoid nodule
  s. T-cell lymphoma
subcuticular
subcutis
subdermic
subepidermal
  s. abscess
  s. nodular fibrosis
  s. vesiculation
subepithelia
subepithelium

suberosis
subgallate
  bismuth s.
subglottis
subinfection
subinhibitory
subintegumental
subitum
  exanthema s.
subjective synonym
sublamina densa
subluxation
submersion reflex
submucosa
submucosal
  s. gland hypertrophy
  s. plaque
subpapular
subsalicylate
  bismuth s.
subsegmental bronchus
subset
  CD4 T cell s.
  CD4+ T cell s.
  CD8 T cell s.
substance
  amorphous s.
  bacteriotropic s.
  blood group s.
  exogenous s.
  ground s.
  nonirritating test s.
  reducing s.
  sensitizing s.
  slow-reacting s. (SRS)
  soluble specific s. (SSS)
  specific capsular s.
substance P
substitute
  saliva s.
subsulfate
  ferric s.
subsynovium
subtalar joint
subtegumental
subtilis
  Bacillus s.
subtropical
subtype
  Reston s.
  Sudan s.
  Zaire s.

subtype)
Russian spring-summer
encephalitis (Eastern s.
Russian spring-summer
encephalitis (Western s.
tick-borne encephalitis (Central
European s.
tick-borne encephalitis
(Eastern s.
subungual
s. abscess
s. exostosis
s. hematoma
s. hyperkeratosis
s. melanoma
s. wart
subungualis
hyperkeratosis s.
subunit vaccine
succinate
sumatriptan s.
succinylcholine
succulence
succussion
suction
Bowins s.
s. loose body forceps
Sudafed
S. Plus Liquid
S. Plus Tablet
sudamen
sudamina
sudaminal
Sudan
S. black
S. subtype
sudation
sudden
s. unexpected death in infants
(SUDI)
s. unexplained death in infants
(SUDI)
Sudex
SUDI
sudden unexpected death in infants
sudden unexplained death in infants

sudor
s. sanguineus
s. urinosus
sudoral
sudoresis
sudoriferous
nevus s.
sudorific
sudorikeratosis
sudoriparous
s. abscess
sudorometer
sudorrhea
Suds
Murex S.
Sufedrin
sufentanil
suffodiens
folliculitis abscedens et s.
folliculitis et perifolliculitis
abscedens et s.
perifolliculitis abscedens et s.
perifolliculitis capitis abscedens
et s.
sugar
s. beet
s. maple
s. maple tree
specific soluble s.
suggillation
suicide
procollagen s.
suid herpesvirus
suis
Actinobacillus s.
Haemophilus s.
sulbactam
ampicillin and s.
sulcatum
keratoderma plantare s.
keratolysis plantare s.
keratoma plantare s.
sulconazole
s. nitrate
Sulcosyn topical
Sulf-10 Ophthalmic

NOTES

S

383

sulfacetamide
  sodium s.
  sulfur and sodium s.
Sulfacet-R topical
sulfadiazine
  silver s.
  s., sulfamethazine, and
    sulfamerazine
sulfadoxine and pyrimethamine
sulfa drug
Sulfair Ophthalmic
sulfamerazine
  sulfadiazine, sulfamethazine,
    and s.
Sulfamethoprim
sulfamethoxazole
Sulfamylon topical
sulfapyridine
sulfate
  amikacin s.
  aminosidine s.
  atropine s.
  bleomycin s.
  Capastat s.
  capreomycin s.
  chondroitin s.
  chondroitin s. B
  chondroitin sulfate/dermatan s.
    (CS/DS)
  colistin s.
  ephedrine s.
  gentamicin s.
  heparin s.
  hydroxychloroquine s.
  indinavir s.
  kanamycin s.
  magnesium s.
  metaproterenol s.
  morphine s.
  neomycin s.
  netilmicin s.
  nickel s.
  paromomycin s.
  polymyxin b s.
  quinine s.
  streptomycin s.
  terbutaline s.
  trospectomycin s.
  vinblastine s.
  zinc s.
sulfation
Sulfatrim
  S. DS

sulfhydryl compound
sulfide
  selenium s.
sulfimycin
sulfinpyrazone
sulfisoxazole
  erythromycin and s.
  s. and phenazopyridine
sulfites
sulfonamide
sulfosalicylate
  meclocycline s.
sulfoxide
  albendazole s.
  dimethyl s.
sulfur
  s. dioxide (SO_2)
  s. flake
  s. granule
  s. and salicylic acid
  s. and sodium sulfacetamide
sulfureum
  Trichophyton s.
sulfuric acid
sulindac
Sulzberger-Bloch syndrome
Sulzberger-Garbe
  S.-G. disease
  S.-G. syndrome
sumac, sumach
  poison s.
sumatriptan succinate
summer
  s. acne
  s. asthma
  s. eruption
  s. itch
  s. prurigo
  s. rash
  s. sore
Sumycin Oral
sun
  s. and chemical combination
    damage
  s. exposure
  s. protection factor (SPF)
sunburn
  s. reactivation
sunburn-like rash
sunflower
sunscreen
  chemical s.
  physical s.

superantigen
superfatted synthetic detergent
superficial
    s. angioma
    s. basal cell carcinoma
    s. basal cell epithelioma
    s. burn
    s. corium
    s. follicular pyoderma
    s. granulomatous pyoderma
    s. hemangioma
    s. infection
    s. malignant melanoma
    s. pustular perifolliculitis
    s. spreading melanoma
superficialis
    lupus s.
superinduce
superinfection
supernatant
supernumerary digit
superoxide
superpigmentation
suppedanium
supplemental oxygen
support
    s. group
    volume-assured pressure s.
      (VAPS)
supportive therapy
Suppository
    Anucort-HC S.
    Anuprep HC S.
    Anusol-HC S.
    Truphylline S.
suppressor cell
suppressor-sensitive mutant
suppuration
suppurativa
    genital hidradenitis s.
    hidradenitis s.
suppurative arthritis
suprabasal clefting
suprascapular
    s. nerve compression (SSC)
    s. nerve entrapment
supraspinatus tendon

suprasternal reaction
Suprax
suprofen
sural nerve entrapment
SureCell Strep A test
Sure-Closure skin stretching system
surface
    s. antigen
    dorsal s.
    extensor s.
    flexor s.
    s. freezing
    RBC s.
    s. receptor
surfactant
    hydrolysis of s.
    pulmonary s.
surgery
    acne s.
    collimated bema handpiece
      (CBH-1) for laser s.
    laser s.
    microscopically controlled s.
    Mohs micrographic s.
    video-assisted thoracic s.
      (VATS)
surgical
    s. erysipelas
    s. therapy
sursanure
surveillance
    immune s.
    immunological s.
survey
    environmental s.
    human immune status s.
      (HISS)
    reduced joint s. (RJS)
susceptibility
    s. cassette
suspectum
    Heloderma s.
suspension
    AK-Spore H.C. Ophthalmic s.
    amoxicillin/clavulanate s.
    AMX/CL s.
    Aristocort Intralesional s.

S

NOTES

suspension *(continued)*
    betamethasone sodium
      phosphate and acetate s.
    cefuroxime axetil s. (CAE)
    Children's Motrin s.
    Cortisporin Ophthalmic s.
    FML-S Ophthalmic s.
    penicillin v s.
    Poly-Pred Ophthalmic s.
    Terra-Cortril Ophthalmic s.
    Vexol Ophthalmic s.
Sus-Phrine
Sustacal Plus
sustained release
Sustaire
sutilains
Sutton
    S. disease
    S. nevus
    S. ulcer
suture
    Ethilon s.
    Vicryl s.
SV
    simian virus
    stroke volume
SV40
    simian vacuolating virus No. 40
SV40-adenovirus hybrid
SVC, pl. **venae cavae**
    slow vital capacity
swamp
    s. fever
    s. fever virus
    s. itch
Swann antigen
swan-neck deformity
Sw^a antigen
swarming
sweat
    s. bee
    s. chloride
    s. chloride elimination
    colliquative s.
    s. gland
    s. gland carcinoma
    insensitive s.
    red s.
sweating
    excessive s.
sweat-retention syndrome
sweaty feet syndrome
Sween

sweet
    s. clover
    S. disease
    s. potato
    S. syndrome
    s. vernal
    s. vernal grass
sweetgum
    s. tree
swelling
    boggy s.
    Calabar s.
    cervical lymph node s.
    fugitive s.
    joint s.
    Neufeld capsular s.
    nodules, eosinophilia,
      rheumatism, dermatitis, and s.
      (NERDS)
    rhomboid s.
Swift disease
swimmer's itch
swimming pool granuloma
swine
    atrophic rhinitis of s.
    s. encephalitis virus
    s. epithelium
    s. fever
    s. fever virus
    s. influenza
    s. influenza virus
    s. pest
    transmissible gastroenteritis
      of s. (TGE)
    transmissible gastroenteritis
      virus of s.
    s. vesicular disease
swinepox
    s. virus
Swiss
    S. chard
    S. mouse leukemia virus
    S. Therapy eye mask
    S. type agammaglobulinemia
switch
    class s.
    s. region
sycamore
    s. tree
sycoma
sycondroses
sycosiform
    s. fungous infection

sycosiforme
    ulerythema s.
sycosis
    s. barbae
    s. frambesiformis
    lupoid s.
    s. nuchae
    s. nuchae necrotisans
    tinea s.
    s. vulgaris
Sydenham chorea
sydesmophytosis
sydowi
    Aspergillus s.
Syllamalt
Sylvest disease
Symadine
Symmetrel
symmetrica
    erythrokeratodermia
        progressive s.
    keratoderma s.
symmetrical gangrene
symmetric reticulonodular x-ray
    change
symmetry
    axis of s.
sympathetic nervous system
sympathomimetic
Symphony patient monitoring
    system
symphysis
symptom
    classic allergy s.
    coincidental s.
    frequency of allergy s.
    gastrointestinal s.
    neuropsychiatric s.
    prodromal s.
    severity of allergy s.
    Sklowsky s.
    Wartenberg s.
symptomatic
    s. erythema
    s. fever
    s. porphyria
    s. pruritus

    s. reaction
    s. therapy
    s. ulcer
symptomatica
    alopecia s.
    livedo reticularis s.
    purpura s.
Synacort
Synalar
    S.-HP topical
    S. topical
synanthem
synapsin I
synaptophysin
synarthroses
Sync
    Star S.
synchronized intermittent
    mechanical ventilation
synchronous intermittent mandatory
    ventilation
syncopal attack
syncope
syncytial virus
syncytium-inhibiting (SI)
syndactylia
syndactyly
syndecan
syndesmophyte
syndesmosis
syndet
    synthetic detergent
syndrome
    Achard-Thiers s.
    Achenbach s.
    acquired immune deficiency s.
        (AIDS)
    acquired immunodeficiency s.
        (AIDS)
    actinic reticuloid s.
    acute retroviral s.
    adult respiratory distress s.
        (ARDS)
    Albright s.
    Aldrich s.
    Alezzandrini s.
    aminopterin s.

S

NOTES

syndrome *(continued)*
Angelman s.
angioedema-urticaria-
eosinophilia s.
angry back s.
antibody deficiency s.
anticardiolipin antibody s.
antiphospholipid antibody s.
(APS)
antisynthetase s.
Apert s.
Arndt-Gottron s.
ataxia telangiectasia s.
atypical mole s.
auriculotemporal s.
autoerythrocyte sensitization s.
autonomic imbalance s.
Bäfverstedt s.
Bannwarth s.
Banti s.
bare lymphocyte s.
Bart s.
Bart-Pumphrey s.
basal cell nevus s.
Basan s.
Bazex s.
Behçet s.
Bernard-Soulier s.
BIDS s.
Birt-Hoff-Dubé s.
Bjornstad s.
blind loop s.
Bloch-Sulzberger s.
Bloom s.
blue rubber-bleb nevus s.
Böök s.
Brett s.
brittle nail s.
Brooke-Spiegler s.
brown-spot s.
Brugsch s.
Buckley s.
Budd-Chiari s.
Buschke-Ollendorf s.
bypass arthritis-dermatitis s.
café coronary s.
calcinosis cutis, Raynaud
phenomenon, esophageal
motility disorder,
sclerodactyly, telangiectasia s.
Caplan s.
carcinoid s.
cardiocutaneous s.

Carney s.
carpal tunnel s. (CTS)
cauda equina s.
cellular immunity deficiency s.
cervical acceleration-
deceleration s.
Chanarin-Dorfman s.
chancriform s.
Chédiak-Higashi s.
CHILD s.
Chinese restaurant s.
chondrodysplasia punctata s.
chorda tympani s.
chronic fatigue s.
chronic fatigue and immune
dysfunction s. (CFIDS)
chronic mucocutaneous
candidiasis s.
chronic pain s.
Churg-Strauss s. (CSS)
Clouston s.
Cobb s.
Cockayne s.
Coffin-Lowry s.
Coffin-Siris s.
Cogan s.
combined immunodeficiency s.
congenital rubella s.
Conradi-Hünermann s.
COPS s.
Crandall s.
CREST s.
Cronkhite-Canada s.
Cross-McKusick-Breen s.
crowned dens s.
cubital tunnel s.
Cushing s.
DaCosta s.
defibrination s.
Degos s.
dengue shock s.
dermatitis-arthritis-
tenosynovitis s.
De Sanctis-Cacchione s.
diabetic hand s.
diabetic stiff-hand s.
diffuse infiltrative
lymphocytosis s.
DiGeorge s.
disease s.
distal intestinal obstruction s.
Dorfman-Chanarin s.
double-crush s.

Down s.
drug-induced SLE s.
Duncan s.
Dunnigan s.
dysplastic nevus s.
Eaton-Lambert s.
effort s.
Ehlers-Danlos s.
eosinophilia-myalgia s. (EMS)
eosinophilic fasciitis s.
eosinophilic myalgia s.
eosinophilic pulmonary s.
erythrodysesthesia s.
excited skin s. (ESS)
Fabry s.
familial amyloidotic
  polyneuropathy s.
familial atypical multiple mole
  melanoma s. (FAMMM)
familial cholestasis s.
familial nephropathic
  amyloidosis s.
Favre-Racouchot s.
Felty s.
fibromyalgia s. (FMS)
Fitz-Hugh and Curtis s.
Fleischner s.
Flynn-Aird s.
follicular degeneration s.
Franceschetti-Jadassohn s.
Frey s.
Gardner s.
Gardner-Diamond s.
genital Reiter s.
Gianotti-Crosti s.
Gilbert s.
Giroux-Barbeau s.
glucagonoma s.
glucocorticoid withdrawal s.
Goltz s.
Goltz-Gorlin s.
Goodpasture s.
Gopalan s.
Gorlin s.
Gorlin-Chaudhry-Moss s.
Gorlin-Goltz s.
Gorman s.

Gougerot-Blum s.
Gougerot-Carteaud s.
Graham Little s.
Graham-Little-Piccardi-
  Lasseur s.
Greither s.
Guillain-Barré s.
Gulf War s.
Haber s.
Hamman-Rich s.
hand-and-foot s.
Harada s.
Harter s.
Heck s.
Heerfordt s.
Heiner s.
HELLP s.
Helweg-Larssen s.
hemangioma-
  thrombocytopenia s.
hemolytic uremic s. (HUS)
hemophagocytic s.
hemorrhagic fever with
  renal s.
Henoch-Schönlein s. (HSS)
Herlitz s.
Hermansky-Pudlak s.
Hermansky-Pudlak s. type IV
Hermansky-Pudlak s. type VI
Hirschowitz s.
Horner s.
Howell-Evans s.
Hunt s.
Hunter s.
Huriez s.
Hurler s.
Hurler-Scheie s.
Hutchinson-Gilford s.
hydralazine s.
hypereosinophilic s.
hyper IgE s.
hyper IgM s.
hyperimmunoglobulinemia D s.
hyperimmunoglobulinemia E s.
hypermobility s.
hyperviscosity s.

S

NOTES

syndrome *(continued)*
hypocomplementemic vasculitis
  urticarial s.
iatrogenic Cushing s.
IBIDS s.
idiopathic hypereosinophilic s.
  (IHES)
iliotibial band s.
immunodeficiency s.
impingement s.
inflammatory bowel s. (IBS)
irritable bowel s. (IBS)
Jadassohn-Lewandowski s.
Job s.
Kartagener s.
Kasabach-Merritt s.
Kawasaki s.
Kelley-Seegmiller s.
Kettle s.
KID s.
kinky-hair s.
Klein-Waardenburg s.
Klinefelter s.
Klippel-Trenaunay s.
Klippel-Trenaunay-Weber s.
Kostmann s.
LAMB s.
Landry s.
Landry-Guillain-Barré s.
late respiratory systemic s.
  (LRSS)
Laugier-Hunziger s.
Lawrence-Seip s.
LEOPARD s.
Lesch-Nyhan s.
Löffler s.
Lofgren s.
loose anagen hair s.
Louis-Bar s.
lupus s.
lupus-like s.
Lyell s.
lymphocytosis s.
Maffucci s.
malignant mole s.
marfamoid hypermobility s.
Marfan s.
Marinesco-Sjögren s.
Maroteaux-Lamy s.
Marshall s.
MASS s.
McCune-Albright s.
Melkersson-Rosenthal s.

MEN s.
Mendelson s.
Menkes kinky hair s.
Milwaukee shoulder s.
Morquio s.
Moynahan s.
Mucha-Habermann s.
mucocutaneous lymph node s.
Muir-Torre s.
multiple drug allergy s.
multiple hamartoma s.
multiple lentigines s.
multiple mucosal neuroma s.
multiple sulfatase deficiency s.
Munchausen s.
Muscle-Wells s.
musician's overuse s.
myelodysplastic s. (MDS)
myofascial pain s. (MPS)
Naegeli s.
nail-patella s.
nail-patella-elbow s.
NAME s.
Nelson s.
NERDS s.
nerve compression-
  degeneration s.
nerve entrapment s.
Netherton s.
neurocutaneous s.
nevoid basal cell carcinoma s.
Nezelof s.
Nieden s.
nonarticular s.
occipital horn s.
occuloglandular s.
occupation-related s.
ocular-mucous membrane s.
Ollendorf s.
Olmstead s.
Omenn s.
one hand-two foot s.
oral allergy s.
Osler-Weber-Rendu s.
overlap s.
overuse s.
painful-bruising s.
palmar fasciitis and
  polyarthritis s.
Papillon-Lèfevre s.
paraneoplastic s.
Parinaud occuloglandular s.
Parry-Romberg s.

patellofemoral pain s.
peeling-skin s.
periarticular s.
Persian Gulf s.
Peutz-Jeghers s.
pharyngeal pouch s.
PIBIDS s.
PIE s.
piriformis s.
placental sulfatase deficiency s.
plantar nerve s.
plica s.
Plummer-Vinson s.
POEMS s.
posterior interosseous nerve s.
postphlebitic s.
Prader-Willi s.
primary Sjögren s.
pronator teres s.
pseudoradicular s.
pseudo-Turner s.
psychogenic pain s.
pulmonary disease anemia s.
pulmonary sling s.
Ramsay Hunt s.
Raynaud s.
reactive airways dysfunction s.
  (RADS)
rectus abdominis s.
"red man" s.
reflex sympathetic dystrophy s.
  (RSD syndrome)
Refsum s.
Reiter s.
REM s.
Rendu-Osler-Weber s.
respiratory distress s. (RDS)
Reye s.
Richner-Hanhart s.
Richter s.
Riley-Day s.
Romberg s.
Rosai-Dorfman s.
Rothmann-Makai s.
Rothmund s.
Rothmund-Thomson s.
RSD s.

reflex sympathetic dystrophy
  syndrome
rubber man s.
Rud s.
runting s.
Ruvalcaba-Myhre-Smith s.
Sanfilippo s.
scalded skin s.
scapulocostal s.
scapulothoracic s.
Scheie s.
Schönlein-Henoch s.
secondary Sjögren s.
Secrétan s.
Senear-Usher s.
Sézary s.
Sheehan s.
shoulder-hand s.
shrinking lung s.
Shulman s.
sicca s.
sick building s.
Simmond s.
Sjögren s. (SS)
Sjögren-Larsson s.
skin disease s.
sleep apnea s.
sleep apnea/hypopnea s.
SLE-like s.
Sly s.
Smith-Riley s.
Sneddon s.
Soto s.
staphylococcal scalded skin s.
  (SSSS)
staphylococcal toxic shock s.
starvation s.
Stevens-Johnson s.
Stewart-Treves s.
Stickler s.
stiff hand s.
streptococcal toxic shock s.
Stryker-Halbeisen s.
Sturge-Weber s.
Sulzberger-Bloch s.
Sulzberger-Garbe s.
sweat-retention s.

S

NOTES

391

syndrome *(continued)*
  sweaty feet s.
  Sweet s.
  systemic inflammatory
    response s. (SIRS)
  tarsal tunnel s.
  TASS s.
    thyroiditis, Addison disease,
      Sjögren syndrome,
      sarcoidosis syndrome
  Tay s.
  third and fourth pharyngeal
    pouch s.
  Thompson s.
  thoracic outlet s.
  thyroiditis, Addison disease,
    Sjögren syndrome,
    sarcoidosis s. (TASS
    syndrome)
  Tietze s.
  TORCH s.
  Torre s.
  total allergy s.
  toxic oil s. (TOS)
  toxic shock s. (TSS)
  toxic shock-like s. (TSLS)
  trichothiodystrophy s.
  trigeminal trophic s.
  trisomy 20 s.
  Turner s.
  two feet-one hand s.
  unusual lupus erythematosus-
    like s.
  Urbach-Wiethe s.
  Verner s.
  Vogt-Koyanagi s.
  Vogt-Koyanagi-Harada s.
  Vohwinkel s.
  Waardenburg s.
  Waldenström s.
  wasting s.
  Waterhouse-Friderichsen s.
  Weber-Cockayne s.
  Wells s.
  Werner s.
  Wernicke-Korsakoff s.
  Wiskott-Aldrich s.
  Wissler s.
  Wyburn-Mason s.
  X-linked Ehlers-Danlos s.
  XYY s.
  yellow nail s.
  Zimmerman-Laband s.

syndromic
Synemol
  S. topical
Synercid
synergistic
  s. gangrene
syngeneic
  s. graft
syngenesioplasty
syngenesiotransplantation
syngenic
syngraft
synonym
  objective s.
  senior s.
  subjective s.
synophrys
synostoses
synostosis
synovectomy
synovial
  s. biopsy
  s. capillary
  s. cyst
  s. fluid (SF)
  s. fluid changes
  s. hemangioma
  s. hemosiderosis
  s. hyperplasia
  s. hypoxia
  s. lining
  s. lining cell (SLC)
  s. lining cell type A
  s. lipoma
  s. membrane
  s. membrane tophus
  s. mesenchyme
synoviocyte
synovioma
  benign giant cell s.
synoviorthesis
synovitis
  asymptomatic cricoarytenoid s.
  nodular s.
  pigmented villonodular s.
    (PVNS)
  proliferative s.
  reactive postinfectious s.
  remitting seronegative
    symmetrical s.
  silicone s.
  tuberculous s.
  villonodular s.

synovium
    fibrous s. (FS)
    hyperplastic s. (HS)
    proliferative s.
Syn-Rx
synthase
    thromboxane s.
synthesis
    cellular immunodeficiency with
      abnormal immunoglobulin s.
    s. inhibitor
    melanin s.
synthetase
    adenylosuccinic acid s.
    alanyl-tRNA s.
    aminoacyl-tRNA s.
    glycyl-tRNA s.
    histidyl-tRNA s.
    isoleucyl-tRNA s.
    threonyl-tRNA s.
    tRNA s.
synthetic
    s. depot corticosteroid
    s. detergent (syndet)
    s. pyrethroid
syphilid
    acneform s.
    acuminate papular s.
    annular s.
    bullous s.
    corymbose s.
    ecthymatous s.
    erythematous s.
    flat papular s.
    follicular s.
    frambesiform s.
    gummatous s.
    impetiginous s.
    lenticular s.
    macular s.
    miliary papular s.
    nodular s.
    nummular s.
    palmar s.
    papular s.
    papulosquamous s.
    pemphigoid s.

    pigmentary s.
    plantar s.
    pustular s.
    rupial s.
    secondary s.
    tertiary s.
    varioliform s.
syphilide
syphilionthus
syphilis
    Captia test for s.
    s. chancre
    congenital s.
    s. d'emblée
    early latent s.
    endemic s.
    gumma of tertiary s.
    s. hereditaria tarda
    late benign s.
    late latent s.
    latent s.
    nonvenereal s.
    primary s.
    quaternary s.
    secondary s.
    serologic test for s. (S.T.S.)
    tertiary s.
syphilitic
    s. alopecia
    s. dactylitis
    s. fever
    s. leukoderma
    s. roseola
    s. ulcer
syphilitica
    acne s.
    alopecia s.
syphiliticum
    tuberculum s.
syphiliticus
    lichen s.
syphiloderm
syphilology
syphiloma
syphilomatous
syphilophobia
syringadenoma

S

NOTES

syringe
    Luer-Lok s.
syringoadenoma
syringocystadenoma papilliferum
syringoma
    chondroid s.
syringomyelia
syrup
    Actagen S.
    albuterol sulfate S.
    Allerfrin S.
    Allerphed S.
    Anamine S.
    Aprodine S.
    S. of Aristocort
    Bromfed S.
    Carbodec S.
    Cardec-S S.
    Decofed S.
    Deconamine S.
    Drixoral S.
    Histalet S.
    Hydramyn S.
    Kenacort S.
    Naldecon-EX Children's S.
    Rondec S.
    Silafed S.
    Triofed S.
    Triposed S.
    Tusstat S.
system
    Accents s.
    AccuProbe s.
    Aladdin infant flow s.
    APACHE II s.
    arch-loop-whorl s. (ALW)
    Aria CPAP s.
    autonomic nervous s.
    BACTEC s.
    blood group s.
    Brasfield scoring s.
    Cardiovit AT-10
      ECG/spirometry
      combination s.
    central nervous s. (CNS)
    Circulaire aerosol drug
      delivery s.
    CMS AccuProbe 450 s.
    Coleman microinfiltration s.
    Companion 314 nasal CPAP s.
    complement s.
    DAR breathing s.
    dermal s.

    DNA-anti-DNA s.
    DPAP interactive airway
      management s.
    drug-induced depression of
      immune s.
    Dyna-Care pressure pad s.
    Dyonics Dyosite office
      arthroscopy s.
    Dyonics InteliJet fluid
      management s.
    Finger Phantom pulse oximeter
      testing s.
    Gell and Coombs
      classification s.
    genetic depression of
      immune s.
    Haversian s.
    hematopoietic s.
    hypothalamic-pituitary-adrenal s.
    HY-TEC automated allergy
      diagnostic s.
    immune s.
    indicator s.
    integumentary s.
    kinin s.
    Larsen grading s.
    s. of macrophage
    Medi-Facts s.
    monocyte-macrophage s.
    mononuclear phagocyte s.
      (MPS)
    nervous s.
    Nu-Trake Weiss emergency
      airway s.
    Oxyfil oxygen refilling s.
    Panasol II home
      phototherapy s.
    Para-Pak Ultra Ecofix s.
    peripheral nervous s. (PNS)
    PhotoGenica laser s.
    PodoSpray nail drill s.
    properdin s.
    reticuloendothelial s. (RES)
    statistical analysis s. (SAS)
    Sure-Closure skin stretching s.
    sympathetic nervous s.
    Symphony patient
      monitoring s.
    ThAIRapy vest airway
      clearance s.
    TheraPEP positive expiratory
      pressure therapy s.

Vaccine Adverse Events
Reporting S. (VAERS)
Zimmer Pulsavac wound
debridement s.
systematized nevus
systemic
  s. amyloid
  s. anaphylaxis
  s. antibacterial therapy
  s. antifungal therapy
  s. autoimmune disease
  s. candidiasis
  s. corticosteroid
  s. febrile disease
  s. fungal infection

  s. hyalinosis
  s. hypersensitivity angiitis
  s. inflammatory response
  syndrome (SIRS)
  s. juvenile rheumatoid arthritis
  s. lupus erythematosus (SLE)
  s. malignancy
  s. mastocytosis
  s. poisoning
  s. polyarteritis nodosa
  s. reaction
  s. sclerosis
  s. steroid
  s. therapy
  s. vasculitis

NOTES

S

T

T agglutinogen
T antigen
T cell
T cell-B cell collaboration
T cytotoxic cell (Tc)
T helper cell (Th)
T lymphocyte
T tubules
T zone
T zone complexion

T4

Soluble T.

t

t. score

T1-weighted study
T2-weighted study
T.A.B.

typhoid A&B
T.A.B. vaccine

Tabanidae
tabes dorsalis
tablet

Actagen T.
Actifed T.
Actifed Allergy T.
Afrin T.
Allercon T.
Allerfrin T.
Aprodine T.
Aristocort T.
BQ T.
Bromfed T.
Bromphen T.
Carbiset T.
Carbiset-TR T.
Carbodec T.
Carbodec TR T.
Cenafed Plus T.
Chlor-Trimeton 4 Hour
Relief T.
Deconamine T.
Dimaphen T.
Dimetapp T.
Fedahist T.
Genac T.
Histalet Forte T.
Hista-Vadrin T.
Kenacort T.
Klerist-D T.
Lamisil t.

Phyllocontin T.
Pseudo-Gest Plus T.
Sinutab T.
Sudafed Plus T.
terbinafine hydrochloride t.
Triposed T.
Tylenol Cold Effervescent
Medication T.
Veltane T.
Vicks DayQuil Allergy Relief
4 Hour T.

TAC

triamcinolone cream

Tac

T. antigen

Tac-3
Tacaribe

T. complex of virus
T. virus

tache

t. bleuâtre
t. cérébrale
t. méningéale
t. noire
t. spinale

tachetic
tachyarrhythmia
tachycardia
tachyphylaxis
tachypnea
tacrolimus
tactile cell of Merkel-Ranvier
TAD

transient acantholytic dermatosis

tag

cutaneous t.
identification t.
pleural t.
sentinel t.
skin t.

Tagamet

T. HB

Tahyna virus
tail sign
Takahara disease
Takayasu

T. arteritis
T. disease

TAL

triamcinolone lotion

talc
t. slurry
zinc oxide, cod liver oil, and t.
tall dock
talon noir
Tamine
Tamm-Horsfall protein
Tanafed
Tangier disease
tanned red cell
tanner's ulcer
tanning
t. bed
delayed t.
immediate t.
TAO
triamcinolone ointment
tape
Cath-Secure t.
ColorZone t.
Cordran t.
Dermicel t.
Micropore t.
Scanpor t.
taper
prednisone t.
steroid t.
tapeworm
dog t.
tar
t. acne
coal t.
DHS T.
t. keratosis
ointment of t.
t. preparation
wood t.
Tarabine PFS
tarda
familial spondyloepiphyseal dysplasia t.
osteogenesis imperfecta t.
porphyria cutanea t. (PCT)
syphilis hereditaria t.
Tardieu petechia
tardus
nevus t.
target lesion
tarsal tunnel syndrome
tartrate
belladonna, phenobarbital, and ergotamine t.

phenindamine t.
trimeprazine t.
tartrazine
TASS syndrome
thyroiditis, Addison disease, Sjögren syndrome, sarcoidosis syndrome
tattoo
amalgam t.
eyeline t.
oral t.
tattooing effect
Tavist
Tavist-1
Tavist-D
taxa
Taxol
taxon
taxonomic
taxonomy
numerical t.
Taylor disease
Tay-Sachs disease
Tay syndrome
Tazicef
Tazidime
tazobactam
TB
tuberculosis
TB test by PCR
3TC
lamivudine, Epivir
Tc
T cytotoxic cell
technetium
Tc polyphosphate scan
Tc-dimercaptosuccinic acid (DMSA)
T-cell
T.-c. antigen receptor
T.-c. defect
T.-c. growth factor
T.-c. growth factor-1
T.-c. growth factor-2
T.-c. involvement
T.-c. leukemia
T.-c. leukemia virus type 1
T.-c. lymphocytic leukemia
T.-c. lymphocytoma cutis
T.-c. lymphoma
T.-c. mediated delayed type hypersensitivity dermatitis
T.-c. pseudolymphoma
T.-c. receptor

T.-c. replacing factor
T.-c. rosette
T-cell-counter-receptor interaction
T-cell-mediated autoimmune disease
TCN
  tetracycline
Td
  tetanus-diphtheria
T-dependent antigen
T/Derm
  Neutrogena T.
TDI
  isocyanate T.
TDTH cell
tea
  Mexican t.
Tear
  T. Drop solution
TearGard Ophthalmic solution
Teargen Ophthalmic solution
Tearisol solution
tear lysozyme
tears
  artificial t.
  Liquifilm T.
  T. Naturale
  T. Naturale Free solution
  T. Naturale II solution
  T. Naturale solution
  T. Plus solution
  T. Renewed solution
tebutate
  prednisolone t.
technetium (Tc)
  t. scan
Techni-Care surgical scrub
technique
  aseptic t.
  Blenderm patch t.
  cognitive-behavioral t.
  enzyme-multiplied
    immunoassay t. (EMIT)
  fluorescent antibody t.
  Hotchkiss-McManus t.
  immunodiffusion t.
  immunofluorescence t.
  immunometric t.

Jerne t.
light scatter t.
Mancini t.
Mohs fresh-tissue t.
Ouchterlony t.
PAS t. '
periodic acid-Schiff t.
shave t.
skin window t.
sterile t.
volumetric t.
technology
  PulseDose oxygen delivery t.
tecogalen
tectate
Tectiviridae
Tedral
teeth
  Hutchinson t.
Tegaderm semipermeable dressing
Tega-Vert Oral
Tegison
Tegopen
Tegretol
Tegrin-HC
tegument
tegumentum
TEH
  theophylline, ephedrine, and
    hydroxyzine
teicoplanin
Telachlor Oral
Teladar
telangiectases (*pl. of* telangiectasis)
telangiectasia
  ataxia t.
  calcinosis cutis, Raynaud
    phenomenon, esophageal
    motility disorder,
    sclerodactyly, t. (CREST)
  cephalo-oculocutaneous t.
  dermatomal superficial t.
  essential t.
  hemorrhagic t.
  hereditary hemorrhagic t.
  t. macularis eruptiva perstans
    (TMEP)

T

NOTES

399

telangiectasia *(continued)*
  nevoid t.
  periungual t.
  primary t.
  secondary t.
  spider t., spider telangiectasis
  unilateral dermatomal
    superficial t.
  unilateral nevoid t.
  t. verrucosa
telangiectasias
  oculocutaneous t.
telangiectasis, pl. telangiectases
  hereditary hemorrhagic t.
  multiple hereditary
    hemorrhagic t.
  tortuous t.
telangiectatic
  t. erythema
  t. systemic mastocytosis
  t. wart
telangiectatica
  livedo t.
telangiectaticum
  granuloma t.
telangiectodes
  elephantiasis t.
  purpura annularis t.
Teldrin Oral
teleangiectases
  linear t.
telemetry
  multiple-parameter t. (MPT)
teletactor
teleutospore
Teline Oral
teliospore
telogen
  t. effluvium
  t. phase
telopeptide
temafloxacin
Temaril
Temovate
  T. topical
temperate
  t. bacteriophage
  t. virus
temperature
  maximum t.
  minimum t.
  optimum t.
  room t.

  t. sensitive (TS)
  t. spot
temperature-dependent dermatosis
temperature-sensitive
  t.-s. mutant
  t.-s. oculocutaneous albinism
template
temporal
  t. arteritis
  t. artery biopsy
  t. canthus
  t. giant cell arteritis
  t. relationship
**temporomandibular dysfunction
  (TMD)**
Tempra
TEN
  toxic epidermal necrolysis
tenascin
tendinitis
  bicipital t.
  t. bursitis
  calcific t.
  patellar t.
tendinosis
tendinosum
  xanthoma t.
tendinous xanthoma
tendon
  Achilles t.
  peroneal t.
  t. sheath
  supraspinatus t.
  t. xanthoma
tendonesis effect
teniposide
tennis
  t. elbow
  t. shoe foot
Tenon
  T. capsule
  T. space
tenosynovectomy
tenosynovitis
  de Quervain t.
  stenosing t.
tenoxicam
TENS
  transcutaneous electrical nerve
    stimulation
  transcutaneous electrical
    neuromuscular stimulator
  Sham TENS

tension-time index
tentacle print
tenuis
   Alternaria t.
   Nocardia t.
Terak Ophthalmic Ointment
teratogenic
Terazol
terbinafine
   t. hydrochloride cream
   t. hydrochloride tablet
terbutaline
   t. sulfate
terconazole
terebrans
   basiloma t.
terfenadine
   t. and pseudoephedrine
Terfonyl
terminal
   t. hair
   postsynaptic t.
   presynaptic t.
terpine anhydride
Terra-Cortril
   T.-C. Ophthalmic suspension
Terramycin
   T. I.M. injection
   T. Ophthalmic Ointment
   T. Oral
   T. w/Polymyxin B Ophthalmic
   Ointment
terrestrial snake
terreus
   Aspergillus t.
Terry nail
tertiary
   t. syphilid
   t. syphilis
Teschen
   T. disease
   T. disease virus
Tessalon Perles
test
   ACADERM patch t.
   adhesion t.
   Adson t.
   alkali patch t.

allergen inhalation challenge t.
Amplified Mycobacterium
   Tuberculosis Direct T.
antibiotic sensitivity t.
antiglobulin t.
antihuman globulin t.
antinuclear antibody
   screening t.
ASO t.
bacterial phagocytosis t.
basophil degranulation t.
bentonite flocculation t.
Bioclot t.
blood coagulation t.
bronchial inhalation
   challenge t.
bronchial provocation t.
broth t.
Brucella card t.
Buhler t.
C3 t.
C4 t.
Calmette t.
Candida skin t.
capillary fragility t.
capillary resistance t.
Captia t.
Casoni intradermal t.
Casoni skin t.
CF t.
challenge t.
chloride sweat t.
chrome patch t.
closed patch t.
Clostridium difficile t.
   (CLOtest)
Coamatic protein C t.
collagen vascular serologic t.
colony-stimulating factor
   fluorescent treponemal
   antibody-absorption t. (CSF-
   FTA-ABS)
colony-stimulating factor
   microhemagglutination-
   Treponema pallidum t. (CSF-
   MHA-TP)
combion t.

T

NOTES

test *(continued)*
  complement-fixation t.
  Coombs t.
  Coulter ICD-Prep t.
  CSD skin t.
  cutaneous t.
  cutaneous tuberculin t.
  cutireaction t.
  cytotropic antibody t.
  DA pregnancy t.
  diagnostic t.
  Dick t.
  dimethylgloxime spot t.
  direct agglutination t.
  direct Coombs t.
  direct fluorescent antibody t.
  DNA-binding t.
  DNA hybridization t.
  DNA probe t.
  Draize Repeat Insult patch t.
  drawer t.
  Ducrey t.
  EBNA IgG ELISA t.
  EB nuclear antigen t.
  EB-specific IgM t.
  EB viral capsid antigen t.
  ELISA t.
  ELISPOT t.
  epicutaneous t.
  epsilometric t.
  Epstein-Barr nuclear antigen t.
  Epstein-Barr virus t.
  erythrocyte adherence t.
  false-negative patch t.
  false-positive patch t.
  false-positive syphilis t.
  Farr t.
  Finkelstein t.
  First Check rapid diagnostic t.
  Fisher exact t.
  Fisher two-tailed exact t.
  flocculation t.
  fluorescent treponemal
    antibody-absorption t.
  forearm ischemic exercise t.
  Formo-Test t.
  Foshay t.
  Frei t.
  Freund complete adjuvant t.
  FTA-ABS t.
  gel diffusion precipitin t.
  Gen-Probe rapid tuberculosis t.
  Göthlin t.

HBV DNA probe t.
head compression t.
head distraction t.
Helisal rapid blood t.
hemadsorption virus t.
hemagglutination t.
Hess t.
Hinton t.
histoplasmin-latex t.
Hivagen antibody t.
HIV DNA PCR t.
hybridization t.
ice cube t.
IgE radioallergosorbent t.
IgG avidity t.
immune adhesion t.
immunologic pregnancy t.
indirect agglutination t.
indirect Coombs t.
indirect fluorescent antibody t.
indirect hemagglutination t.
insulin skin t.
intradermal skin t.
Ito-Reenstierna t.
killing t.
Kolmer t.
Kruskal-Wallis t.
Kveim t.
Lachman t.
latex agglutination t.
latex fixation t.
leishmanin t.
lepromin t.
leukocyte histamine release t.
Liatest C4b-BP t.
liver function t. (LFT)
lupus band t. (LBT)
lupus erythematosus cell t.
macrophage migration
  inhibition t.
macroscopic agglutination t.
Mann-Whitney U t.
Mantoux t.
t. material
Mazzotti t.
McKenzie t.
McNemar t.
McNemar t. of significance
Mecholyl skin t.
Meinicke t.
methacholine chloride skin t.
MHA-TP t.

microhemagglutination-
Treponema pallidum t.
microimmunofluorescence t.
(MIF)
microscopic agglutination t.
midpoint skin t.
migration inhibition t.
migration inhibitory factor t.
Mitsuda t.
mixed agglutination t.
mixed lymphocyte culture t.
MLC t.
Moloney t.
MTD T.
mucin clot t.
multiple puncture t. (MPT)
multiple puncture tuberculin t.
Multitest t.
mumps sensitivity t.
Murray t.
nasal antigen challenge t.
nasal provocation t.
negative control t.
negative patch t.
negative schick t.
neutralization t.
nitroblue tetrazolium t.
nontreponemal t.
occlusive patch t.
t. for O&P
open t.
open application t.
open epicutaneous t. (OET)
open patch t.
OsteoGram bone density t.
Osteomark urine-based t.
Ouchterlony t.
oxacillin disk diffusion t.
Pap t.
  Papanicolaou test
Papanicolaou t. (Pap test)
paracoccidioidin skin t.
passive cutaneous
  anaphylaxis t.
passive transfer t.
patch t.
Paul t.

Paul-Bunnell t.
Pearson chi square t.
pediatric infectious disease
  developmental screening t.
  (PIDDST)
percutaneous t.
pertussis agglutination t.
photo-patch t.
physiologic t.
pilocarpine iontophoresis
  sweat t.
Pirquet t.
P-K t.
platelet neutralization t.
Porges-Meier t.
PPL skin t.
Prausnitz-Küstner t.
precipitation t.
precipitin t.
predictive patch t.
prick t.
prick-prick t.
prick puncture t.
protection t.
provocative use t. (PUT)
pulmonary function t. (PFT)
pulse t.
quellung t.
radioallergosorbent t. (RAST)
radioimmunosorbent t. (RIST)
RAST t.
Recombinant HIV-1 latex
  agglutination t.
red cell adherence t.
Reiter t.
repeat open reaction
  application t.
RF t.
Rh blocking t.
Rheumatex t.
Rheumaton t.
rhinovirus challenge t.
ring precipitin t.
Rinne t.
Römer t.
rosette t.
Rose-Waaler t.

T

NOTES

403

test *(continued)*
    rub t.
    rubella HI t.
    rubella IgG ELISA t.
    Rumpel-Leede t.
    Sabin-Feldman dye t.
    Sachs-Georgi t.
    scarification t.
    Schick t.
    Schirmer t.
    Schober t.
    Scotch Tape t.
    scratch t.
    scratch chamber t.
    screen t.
    serial dilutional intradermal
      skin t.
    single-breath nitrogen
      washout t.
    skin t.
    skin-puncture t.
    spot t.
    starch-iodine t.
    Steinberg t.
    streptozyme agglutination t.
    Student's *t* t.
    SureCell Strep A t.
    TheoFAST t.
    thermostable opsonin t.
    tine t.
    tourniquet t.
    TPHA t.
    TPI t.
    transfer t.
    Trendelenburg t.
    treponemal t.
    Treponema pallidum
      hemagglutination t.
    Treponema pallidum
      immobilization t.
    T.R.U.E. T.
    T.R.U.E. allergy patch t.
    tube precipitin t.
    tuberculin t.
    tuberculin skin t.
    Tukey standardized range t.
    Tzanck t.
    use t.
    VDRL t.
    vitamin C t.
    in vitro t.
    Vollmer t.
    volume t.

    Wassermann t.
    Weber t.
    Weil-Felix t.
    Western Blot t.
    Whiff t.
    Widal t.
    Wilcoxon rank sum t.
    x-square t.
    Yates corrected chi square t.
testing
    antimicrobiology
      susceptibility t.
    battery patch t.
    conjunctival t.
    delayed hypersensitivity skin t.
    electrodermal t.
    epidermal t.
    histocompatibility t.
    human immunodeficiency virus
      antigen t.
    hypersensitivity skin t.
    p24 antigen t.
    patch t.
    population-based t.
    predictive t.
    prick t.
    provocative dose t.
    RCR t.
    Rinkle t.
    scratch t.
    skin t.
    venom t.
Testoderm patch
testosterone
TET
    tetracycline
tetanolysin
tetanospasmin
tetanotoxin
tetanus
    t. antitoxin
    t. antitoxin unit
    t. immune globulin
    t. immune globulin, human
    t. immunoglobulin
    t. toxin
    t. toxoid
    t. toxoid, adsorbed
    t. toxoid, fluid
    t. vaccine
tetanus-diphtheria (Td)
tetanus-perfringens antitoxin
Tete virus

tetracaine
    t. hydrochloride
    t. with dextrose
Tetracap Oral
tetracycline (TCN, TET)
tetrad
    acne t.
tetrahydrozoline hydrochloride
Tetralan Oral
Tetram Oral
Tetramune
    T. fish food
tetrazolium
    nitroblue t.
tetrodotoxin
tetter
    branny t.
    crusted t.
    dry t.
    honeycomb t.
    humid t.
    milk t.
    moist t.
    scaly t.
    wet t.
Texas
    T. coral snake
    T. coral snake bite
Tg cell
TGE
    transmissible gastroenteritis of swine
    TGE virus
T/Gel
TGF
    transforming growth factor
TGFα
    transforming growth factor α
TGFβ
    transforming growth factor β
TGF-induced immunosuppression
TGV
    trapped gas volume
Th
    T helper cell
ThAIRapy vest airway clearance system

thalassemia
    t. major
β-thalassemia intermedia
thalidomide
thallus
thanatophoric diastrophic chondrodysplasia
Thayer-Martin medium
Theiler
    T. disease
    T. mouse encephalomyelitis virus
    T. original strain of mouse encephalomyelitis virus (TO)
    T. original virus
    T. virus
Theo-24
Theobald Smith phenomenon
Theobid
Theochron
Theoclear L.A.
Theo-Dur
TheoFAST test
Theo-G
Theolair
Theolate
theophylline
    anhydrous t.
    t., ephedrine, and hydroxyzine (TEH)
    t., ephedrine, and phenobarbital
    t. and guaifenesin
    t. salt
theophylline-induced convulsion
theory
    Arrhenius-Madsen t.
    cellular immune t.
    clonal deletion t.
    clonal selection t.
    Ehrlich t.
    Ehrlich side-chain t.
    germ t.
    immune t.
    instructive t.
    Metchnikoff t.
    neural t.
    side-chain t.

T

NOTES

Theospan-SR
Theovent
Theo-X
thèque
TheraCys
Theramin Expectorant
TheraPEP positive expiratory
pressure therapy system
therapeutic
    t. interferon
    t. irradiation
    t. malaria
    t. ratio
therapia magna sterilisans
Theraplex Z
therapy
    ACTH t.
    adrenocorticosteroid t.
    adrenocorticotropic hormone t.
    alkylating t.
    alternate-day t.
    antibacterial t.
    antifungal t.
    anti-IIb-IIIA mAB t.
    anti-inflammatory t.
    antipruritic t.
    antituberculous t.
    antiviral t.
    around-the-clock oral
      maintenance bronchodilator t.
    augmentation t.
    autoserum t.
    biomagnetic t.
    blood transfusion t.
    calcipotriene t.
    Candida t.
    chloroquine t.
    coherence t.
    cytotoxic immunosuppressive t.
    diagnostic surgical t.
    dressing t.
    empiric t.
    factor replacement t.
    fluid t.
    foreign protein t.
    gold t.
    grenz ray t.
    heterovaccine t.
    hydroxychloroquine t.
    hyperbaric oxygen t.
    immunocompetent tissue t.
    immunosuppressive t.
    interferon t.

    medical t.
    nonspecific t.
    occlusive t.
    occupational t. (OT)
    oral iron t.
    orthomolecular t.
    penicillin t.
    pharmacologic t.
    plasma t.
    postnatal t.
    prenatal t.
    protein shock t.
    psychotropic agent t.
    replacement t.
    retinoid t.
    salvage t.
    sedative t.
    serum t.
    skin lubrication t.
    soak t.
    supportive t.
    surgical t.
    symptomatic t.
    systemic t.
    systemic antibacterial t.
    systemic antifungal t.
    topical t.
    topical antibacterial t.
    topical antifungal t.
    vitamin B t.
TheraSnore oral appliance
thermal
    t. anhidrosis
    t. burn
    t. flushing
    t. relaxation time
Thermazene
Thermoactinomyces **vulgaris**
thermoduric
thermogenic anhidrosis
thermolabile opsonin
thermolamp
thermophile
thermophilic
thermophylic
thermorisistable
    Mycobacterium t.
thermosetting resin
thermostabile
thermostable
    t. opsonin
    t. opsonin test
thermotolerant

Theroxide Wash
thesaurismosis
thesaurosis
theta antigen
thiabendazole
thiacetazone
thiamine deficiency
thiazide
thick
    t. and sticky mucus
    t. tongue
thickened skin
thickening
    disciform t.
    scleroderma-like skin t.
Thiemann disease
thimerosal
thin-layer immunoassay
thin-section CT
thioglucose
    gold sodium t.
thiomalate
    gold sodium t.
thioridazine
thiosulfate
    sodium t.
third
    t. degree burn
    t. disease
    t. and fourth pharyngeal pouch
      syndrome
third-generation cephalosporin
thistle
    Russian t.
Thompson syndrome
Thomson sign
thoracentesis
thoracic outlet syndrome
thoracoabdominal
    t. dyssynchrony
    t. paradox
thoracocardiography
thoraco-lumbar-sacral orthosis
thoracoplasty
thoracoscope
    rigid t.
thoracoscopy

thoracostomy
    tube t.
Thorazine
three-day
    t.-d. fever
    t.-d. measles
threonyl-tRNA synthetase
thresher's lung
threshold
    acoustic reflex t.
    t. audiometry
    erythema t.
thrill
thrive
    failure to t.
thrix
    t. annulata
throat
    itchy t.
thrombi
    intramural t.
thrombocytopenia
    autoimmune t. (AITP)
    autoimmune neonatal t.
    drug-induced t.
    familial t.
    immune t.
    isoimmune neonatal t.
    sepsis-induced t.
thrombocytopenic
    t. hemangiomatosis
    t. purpura
thrombogenesis
thrombolytic
thrombomodulin
thrombophlebitis
    retinal t.
thrombosis
thrombospondin
thrombotic
    t. gangrene
    t. thrombocytopenic purpura
      (TTP)
thromboxane
    t. synthase
throwing act

T

NOTES

thrush
oral t.
thylacitis
thymectomy
thymic
t. alymphoplasia
t. hormone
t. hypoplasia
t. lymphopoietic factor
thymidine
thymin
thymine
Thymoctonan
thymocyte
thymoma
thymopentin
thymopoietin
thymosin
thymus
congenital aplasia of t.
thymus-derived leukemia
thymus-independent antigen
Thyro-Block
thyroglossal cyst
thyroid
t. acropachy
t. disorder
thyroiditis
Hashimoto t.
thyroiditis, Addison disease, Sjögren syndrome, sarcoidosis syndrome (TASS syndrome)
thyroid-stimulating antibody
thyrotoxic
t. complement-fixation factor
t. serum
thyrotoxicosis
thyrotoxin
tic
habit t.
Ticar
ticarcillin
t. and clavulanic acid
t. disodium
TICE
TICE Bacillus Calmette-Guérin Live (TICE BCG)
TICE BCG
TICE Bacillus Calmette-Guérin Live
tick
t. bite
t. bite alopecia

black-legged t.
California black-legged t.
deer t.
t. fever
hard t.
Ixodes dammini t.
Ixodes pacificus t.
Ixodes ricinus wood t.
Lone Star t.
Pacific t.
t. paralysis
t. pyrexia
Rocky Mountain t.
seed t.
soft t.
spotted-fever t.
western black-legged t.
wood t.
tickborne
tick-borne
t.-b. disease
t.-b. encephalitis (Central European subtype)
t.-b. encephalitis (Eastern subtype)
t.-b. encephalitis virus
t.-b. relapsing fever
t.-b. virus
tidal volume
Tietze syndrome
tiger snake antivenom
tight asthmatic
Tilade
T. Inhalation Aerosol
Tilcotil
tilorone
TILS
tumor-infiltrating lymphocyte
tiludronate
time
activated partial thromboplastin t. (APTT)
dilute Russell viper venom t.
germinative t.
median survival t. (MST)
partial thromboplastin t. (PTT)
Russell viper venom t.
thermal relaxation t.
transit t.
Timecelles
Sinufed T.
timed intermittent rotation
Timentin

timolol
Timoptic Ophthalmic
Timoptic-XE Ophthalmic
timori
Brugia t.
timothy
t. grass
Tinactin
TINA monitor
TinBen
TinCoBen
tinctorial change
tincture
Fungoid t.
tinea
t. amiantacea
t. barbae
t. capitis
t. circinata
t. corporis
t. cruris
t. dermatitis
t. faciei
t. favosa
t. glabrosa
t. imbricata
t. incognito
t. inguinalis
t. kerion
t. manus
t. nigra
t. nodosa
t. pedis
t. pedis et manus
t. profunda
t. sycosis
t. tonsurans
t. tropicalis
t. unguium
t. versicolor
tine test
tinnitus
Tinted
Oxy-5 T.
Tinver
T. Lotion
Ti-Screen

Tisit
tissue
acellular pannus t.
autodigestion of connective t.
t. confirmation
connective t.
t. detritus
elastic t.
extra-articular t.
fibroblastic t.
t. fluke
granulation t.
gut-associated lymphoid t.
(GALT)
hemangiomatous t.
t. inhibitor
t. ligand
mesenchymal t.
mucosa-associated lymphoid t.
(MALT)
necrotic t.
neural t.
t. remodeling
t. repair
soft t.
tissue-specific antigen
titer
anti-rotavirus IgA t.
antistreptolysin O t.
ASLO t.
ASO t.
geometric mean t. (GMT)
IgG t.
indirect Coombs t.
mycoplasma IgM t.
titin
titration
Rinkel serial endpoint t.
Tj antigen
TLC
total lung capacity
T-lymphocyte
TM
tympanic membrane
Tm cell
TMD
temporomandibular dysfunction

NOTES

TMEP
 telangiectasia macularis eruptiva
  perstans
TMP
 trimethyl psoralen
TMP-SMX
 trimethoprim-sulfamethoxazole
TNF
 tumor necrosis factor
  TNF mRNA cytokine
TNM
 tumor, node, metastasis
TNM staging
TO
 Theiler original strain of mouse
  encephalomyelitis virus
  TO virus
toad skin
toasted shin
tobacco
 t. leaf extract
 t. smoke
 wild t.
TobraDex
 T. Ophthalmic
tobramycin
 t. and dexamethasone
Tobrex Ophthalmic
tocopherol
 t. deficiency
Todd-Hewitt broth
toe
 black t.
 hammer t.
 Hong Kong t.
 t. itch
 mallet t.
 sausage t.
toeweb
Tofranil
Togaviridae virus
togavirus
toilet
 bronchial t.
 pulmonary t.
Tokelau ringworm
Tolectin
 T. DS
tolerance
 high dose t.
 immunologic t.
 immunological t.
 immunologic high dose t.

 nonresponder t.
 split t.
tolerogenic
tolmetin
 t. sodium
tolnaftate
tolu
 balsam of t.
tomato
 t. tumor
tombstoning
tomography
 computed t. (CT)
 high-resolution computed t.
  (HRCT)
 single photon emission
  computed t. (SPECT)
tone
 bronchial smooth muscle t.
tongue
 black hairy t.
 burning t.
 coated t.
 fissured t.
 furrowed t.
 geographic t.
 glossy t.
 hobnail t.
 painful t.
 raspberry t.
 scrotal t.
 strawberry t.
 thick t.
 white strawberry t.
tonofibril
tonofilament
tonofilament-cytoplasmic plaque
 linker
tonsil
 absent t.
 hypertrophic t.
 small t.
tonsillectomy
tonsillitis
 streptococcal t.
tonsillopharyngitis
tonsurans
 tinea t.
 Trichophyton t.
tooth
 t. pit
 t. rash

top
　red t.
tophaceous gout
tophi
　intra-articular t.
tophus, pl. tophi
　synovial membrane t.
topical
　Aclovate t.
　Actinex t.
　Akne-Mycin t.
　Ala-Quin t.
　t. anesthetic
　t. antibacterial therapy
　t. antifungal therapy
　t. antipruritic
　Aquacare t.
　Aquaphor Antibiotic t.
　A/T/S t.
　Baciguent t.
　BactoShield t.
　Bactroban t.
　Benadryl t.
　Caldesene t.
　Carmol t.
　Carmol-HC t.
　Cloderm t.
　Cordran t.
　Cordran SP t.
　Corque t.
　t. corticosteroid
　Cortin t.
　Cruex t.
　Cutivate t.
　Cyclocort t.
　Debrisan t.
　t. decongestant
　Del-Mycin t.
　Dermacomb t.
　Derma-Smoothe/FS t.
　Desitin t.
　DesOwen t.
　Dyna-Hex t.
　Efudex t.
　Elase t.
　Elase-Chloromycetin t.
　Elocon t.

　Emgel t.
　EMLA t.
　Erycette t.
　EryDerm t.
　Erygel t.
　Erymax t.
　erythromycin t.
　E-Solve-2 t.
　ETS-2% t.
　Eurax t.
　Exelderm t.
　Florone t.
　Florone E t.
　Fluonex t.
　Fluonid t.
　Fluoroplex t.
　Flurosyn t.
　FS Shampoo t.
　Furacin t.
　Garamycin t.
　G-myticin t.
　Halog t.
　Halog-E t.
　Halotex t.
　t. hemostatic agent
　Hibiclens t.
　Hibistat t.
　Hysone t.
　Lamisil t.
　Lanaphilic t.
　Lanvisone t.
　Lida-Mantle HC t.
　Lidex t.
　Lidex-E t.
　Maxiflor t.
　Meclan t.
　Merlenate t.
　Micatin t.
　t. moisturizer
　Monistat-Derm t.
　Mycifradin Sulfate t.
　Mycitracin t.
　Mycogen II t.
　Mycolog-II t.
　Myconel t.
　Mycostatin t.
　Mytrex F t.

T

NOTES

411

topical *(continued)*
Naftin t.
Neo-Cortef t.
Neomixin t.
NGT t.
Nilstat t.
Nizoral t.
Novacet t.
Nutraplus t.
Nystex t.
Nyst-Olone II t.
t. ophthalmic vasoconstrictor
Oxistat t.
Oxsoralen t.
Pedi-Cort V t.
Pedi-Pro t.
Polysporin t.
Pontocaine t.
Psorcon t.
t. PUVA
Quinsana Plus t.
Racet t.
Retin-A t.
Spectazole t.
Staticin t.
t. steroid
Sulcosyn t.
Sulfacet-R t.
Sulfamylon t.
Synalar t.
Synalar-HP t.
Synemol t.
Temovate t.
t. therapy
Travase t.
Tridesilon t.
Triple Antibiotic t.
Tri-Statin II t.
T-Stat t.
UAD t.
Ultra Mide t.
Ultravate t.
Undoguent t.
Ureacin-20 t.
Ureacin-40 t.
Vioform t.
Vitec t.
Vytone t.
Zovirax t.
Topicort
T.-LP
Toposar injection
Toradol injection

TORCH
toxoplasmosis, other infections,
rubella, cytomegalovirus infection,
and herpes simplex
TORCH syndrome
Tornalate
Torre syndrome
torti
pili t.
torticollis
dermatogenic t.
tortuous telangiectasis
tortus
pilus t.
Torula
toruloidea
Hendersonula t.
Torulopsis glabrata
torulosis
torus
t. mandibulae
mandibular t.
t. palatinus
TOS
toxic oil syndrome
Totacillin
T.-N
total
t. allergy syndrome
t. contact cast
t. hemolytic complement
t. lung capacity (TLC)
t. serum IgE
t. serum IgE level
totalis
alopecia t.
alopecia capitis t.
toto
in t.
Touraine centrofacial lentigo
tourniquet test
Touro LA
toxemia
toxemic
toxic
t. alopecia
t. epidermal necrolysis (TEN)
t. erythema
t. nephrosis
t. oil syndrome (TOS)
t. organ damage
t. shock-like syndrome (TSLS)
t. shock syndrome (TSS)

t. systemic reaction
t. unit (TU)
toxica
alopecia t.
toxicemia
toxicity
cumulative t.
ocular t.
Toxicodendron
T. diversilobum
T. radicans
T. verniciferum
toxicodendron
Rhus t.
toxicoderma
toxicodermatitis
toxicodermatosis
toxicogenic conjunctivitis
toxicopathic
toxicosis
toxicum
erythema t.
toxigenic
toxigenicity
toxin
adenylate cyclase t.
animal t.
anthrax t.
Bacillus anthracis t.
bacterial t.
botulinus t.
cholera t.
detoxified t.
diagnostic diphtheria t.
Dick test t.
dinoflagellate t.
diphtheria t.
erythrogenic t.
extracellular t.
intracellular t.
normal t.
plant t.
RNA glycosidase t.
scarlet fever erythrogenic t.
Schick test t.
Shiga-like t.
t. spectrum

streptococcus erythrogenic t.
tetanus t.
t. unit
toxinic
toxinogenic
toxinogenicity
toxinology
toxinosis
toxins
toxipathic
toxipathy
Toxocara
T. canis
T. cati
toxocariasis
toxoid
diphtheria and tetanus t.
tetanus t.
toxon
toxonosis
toxophil
toxophore
toxophorous
Toxoplasma
T. gondii
toxoplasmosis
congenital t.
cutaneous t.
epidermotropic cutaneous t.
toxoplasmosis, other infections, rubella, cytomegalovirus infection, and herpes simplex (TORCH)
ToxR protein
TPHA test
TPI test
trabecular carcinoma
trace element
trachea
extrinsic compression of t.
tracheal
t. stenosis
t. tumor
tracheitis
tracheobronchial
t. amyloidosis
Tracheolife HME
tracheomalacia

T

NOTES

413

tracheostomy
trachoma
   t. bodies
   t. virus
trachomatis
   Chlamydia t.
trachyonychia
tracks
   tram t.
tract
   dental sinus t.
   sinus t.
traction
   t. alopecia
   t. atrophy
tragacanth
tragal
tragomaschalia
tragus, pl. tragi
   accessory t.
training
   joint protection t.
trait
   autosomal recessive t.
   sickle cell t.
tram
   t. line
   t. tracks
tramadol
tranexamic acid
Tranquility Quest
tranquilizer
transaminase
transaxillary apical bullectomy
transcapsidation
transchondral fracture
transcriptase
   t. inhibitor
   reverse t.
transcription
   gene t.
   germline t.
transcutaneous
   t. electrical nerve stimulation
   (TENS)
   t. electrical neuromuscular
   stimulator (TENS)
transdermic
Transderm Scōp Patch
transduce
transductant
transduction
   abortive t.

complete t.
general t.
high frequency t.
low frequency t.
signal t.
specialized t.
specific t.
transection
transfection
transfer
   adenovirus-mediated t.
   adenovirus-mediated gene t.
   t. factor
   t. gene
   melanin t.
   t. test
transference
   passive t.
transformant
transformation
   cell t.
   logit t.
   lymphocyte t.
   malignant t.
transformed lymphocyte
transforming
   t. agent
   t. factor
   t. gene
   t. growth factor (TGF)
   t. growth factor α (TGFα)
   t. growth factor β (TGFβ)
transfusion
   blood t.
   exchange t.
   granulocyte t.
   t. hepatitis
   t. nephritis
   packed red cell t.
   t. reaction
   reciprocal t.
transgenic mice
transient
   t. acantholytic dermatosis
   (TAD)
   t. acantholytic dyskeratosis
   t. agammaglobulinemia
   t. cerebral ischemia
   t. hypogammaglobulinemia of
   infancy
   t. migratory infiltrate
   t. neonatal pustular melanosis
   t. pulmonary infiltrate

transillumination of sinus
transin
transition mutation
transitory palsy
transit time
transjugular hepatic biopsy
translation
transmembrane linker
transmissible
    t. dementia
    t. enteritis
    t. gastroenteritis of swine
      (TGE)
    t. gastroenteritis virus of swine
    t. mink encephalopathy
    t. plasmid
    t. turkey enteritis virus
transmission
    airborne t.
    bedbug disease t.
    horizontal t.
    transovarian t.
    vertical t.
transovarian transmission
transparent facial powder
transpeptidase
transplant
    hair t.
    hematopoietic stem cell t.
Trans-Plantar Transdermal Patch
transplantation
    t. antigen
    bone marrow t.
    fetal liver t.
    fetal thymus t.
    pigment cell t.
transplantin
transport
    active t.
transpose
transposition
transposon
transthyretin
transthyretin-origin amyloid deposit
transtracheal
transubstantiation

transvalensis
    Nocardia t.
transvector
transversa
    stria nasi t.
Trans-Ver-Sal transdermal patch
    Verukan solution
transverse
    t. furrow
    t. myelitis
    t. nasal groove
transversion mutation
Trantas dots
Tr^a antigen
Tranxene
trap
    Burkard t.
    Burkard spore t.
    Hirst spore t.
    Kramer-Collins Spore t.
trapped gas volume (TGV)
trapping
    air t.
trauma
    inadvertent t.
traumatic
    t. alopecia
    t. arthritis
    t. dermatitis
    t. fat necrosis
    t. fever
    t. herpes
    t. lesion
    t. purpura
traumatically induced inflammatory
    disease
Travase topical
Traveler
    Pulmo-Aide T.
treatment
    duration of t.
    Goeckerman t.
    isoserum t.
    light t.
    nonpharmacologic measure
      of t.

T

NOTES

415

treatment *(continued)*
  preventive t.
  prophylactic t.
Trecator-SC
tree
  acacia t.
  alder t.
  American elm t.
  arbor vitae t.
  Arizona ash t.
  Arizona cypress t.
  Arizona/Fremont cottonwood t.
  ash t.
  aspen t.
  Australian pine t.
  bald cypress t.
  bayberry t.
  beech t.
  birch t.
  black locust t.
  box elder maple t.
  Brazilian rubber t.
  California peppertree t.
  Chinese elm t.
  cottonwood t.
  Douglas fir t.
  elm t.
  eucalyptus t.
  fall elm t.
  Gambel oak t.
  green ash t.
  groundsel t.
  hackberry t.
  hazelnut t.
  hickory t.
  Italian cypress t.
  Japanese cedar t.
  Japanese lacquer t.
  juniper mix t.
  lilac t.
  live oak t.
  loblolly pine t.
  lodgepole pine t.
  Lombardy poplar t.
  malaleuca t.
  maple t.
  mesquite t.
  Monterey cypress t.
  mountain cedar t.
  oak t.
  olive t.
  palm t.
  paper mulberry t.

  pecan t.
  ponderosa pine t.
  poplar t.
  privet t.
  queen palm t.
  red alder t.
  red cedar t.
  red maple t.
  red mulberry t.
  redwood t.
  Russian olive t.
  salt cedar t.
  shagbark hickory t.
  slash pine t.
  slippery elm t.
  spruce t.
  sugar maple t.
  sweetgum t.
  sycamore t.
  walnut t.
  wax myrtle t.
  weeping fig t.
  Western juniper t.
  white ash t.
  white mulberry t.
  white oak t.
  white pine t.
  white poplar t.
  willow t.
  yew t.
trefoil dermatitis
trematode
tremor
  epidemic t.
trench
  t. foot
  t. hand
  t. mouth
Trendar
Trendelenburg test
Trental
trephine
  skin t.
Treponema
  T. carateum
  T. pallidum
  T. pallidum hemagglutination
    test
  T. pallidum immobilization
    reaction
  T. pallidum immobilization test
  T. pertenue
treponema-immobilizing antibody

treponemal
t. antibody
t. test
treponemata
treponematosis
nonsyphilitic t.
treponeme
tretinoin
t. cream
triacetin
triad
aspirin t.
follicular occlusion t.
retention t.
Triam-A
triamcinolone
t. acetonide
t. cream (TAC)
t. hexacetonide
t. lotion (TAL)
nystatin and t.
t. ointment (TAO)
Triaminic
T. AM Decongestant Formula
T. Expectorant
T. Oral Infant Drops
Triamolone
triangularis
alopecia t.
Triatoma
T. *gerstaeckeri*
T. *gerstaeckeri* bite
T. *protracta*
T. *sanguisuga*
T. *sanguisuga* bite
triatoma
Triatominae
triazolam
trichatrophia
trichatrophy
trichauxis
trichiasis
trichilemmal cyst
trichilemmoma
desmoplastic t.
Trichina
T. *spiralis*

Trichinella
T. *spiralis*
trichinelliasis
trichinellosis
trichiniasis
trichinosis
trichitis
trichiura
Trichuris t.
Tri-Chlor
trichloroacetic acid
trichloromonofluoromethane
dichlorodifluoromethane and t.
trichobezoar
trichoclasia
trichoclasis
trichocryptomania
trichocryptosis
trichocryptotillomania
Trichoderma viride
trichodiscoma
trichodystrophy
trichoepithelioma
acquired t.
desmoplastic t.
hereditary multiple t.
multiple t.
trichofolliculoma
sebaceous t.
trichogen
trichogenous
trichoglossia
trichokinesis
trichokleptomania
tricholemmoma
tricholith
trichologia
trichology
trichoma
trichomatose
trichomatosis
trichomatous
trichomatrioma
trichomegaly
Trichomonas vaginalis
trichomycetosis

T

NOTES

417

trichomycosis
t. axillaris
t. axillaris nodosa
t. axillaris nodularis
t. chromatica
t. nodosa
t. palmellina
t. pustulosa
trichonocardiosis
t. axillaris
trichonodosis
trichonosis
trichonosus
t. versicolor
trichopathic
trichopathophobia
trichopathy
trichophagy
trichophobia
trichophytic
t. granuloma
trichophytica
trichophyticus
lichen t.
trichophytid
trichophytin
Trichophyton, Trichophytum
T. concentricum
T. gypseum
T. mentagrophytes
T. purpureum
T. rubrum
T. schoenleinii
T. sulfureum
T. tonsurans
trichophytosis
t. barbae
t. capitis
t. corporis
t. cruris
t. unguium
trichopoliodystrophy
trichopoliosis
trichoptilosis
trichorrhea
trichorrhexis
t. invaginata
t. nodosa
trichorrhexomania
trichoschisia
trichoschisis
trichoscopy

trichosis
t. carunculae
t. sensitiva
t. setosa
Trichosporon
trichosporonosis
trichosporosis
trichostasis spinulosa
trichothiodystrophy
t. syndrome
trichotillomania
trichotoxin
trichotrophy
trichrome
Trichuris trichiura
Tri-Clear Expectorant
triclocarban
triclosan
Tricosal
tricuspid valvular leaflet
tricyclic antidepressant
Tridesilon
T. topical
trifluridine
trigeminal trophic syndrome
Trigger
Smart T.
trigger
t. factor
t. finger
triglyceride
Tri-Immunol
Tri-Kort
trilete
Trilisate
Trilog
Trilone
trimellitic anhydride
trimeprazine tartrate
trimethoprim
t. and polymyxin b
t.-sulfamethoxazole (TMP-SMX)
trimethyl psoralen (TMP)
trimetrexate glucuronate
Trimox
Trimpex
Trinalin
Triofed Syrup
trioxide
arsenic t.
trioxsalen
Tripedia
tripelennamine

tripe palm
Tri-Phen-Chlor
Triphenyl Expectorant
triphosphate
    adenosine t. (ATP)
    guanosine t. (GTP)
    inositol t.
    purine nucleotides adenosine t.
    uridine t.
Triple
    T. Antibiotic topical
    T. Paste
triple
    t. helix
    t. response
triple-jawed pedicellaria
triplet
    nonsense t.
Triposed
    T. Syrup
    T. Tablet
triprolidine and pseudoephedrine
TripTone Caplets
triradius
trisalicylate
    choline magnesium t.
Trisoject
trisomy 21, 22
trisomy 20 syndrome
Trisoralen
    T. Oral
Tri-Statin II topical
Tritin
    Dr Scholl's Maximum
      Strength T.
trivalent oral poliovirus solution
tRNA synthetase
Trobicin injection
troche
    clotrimazole t.
    Mycelex t.
trochleo-ginglymoid joint
troleandomycin
Trombicula
    T. akamushi
    T. deliensis
    T. irritans

Trombiculidae
trombidiasis
trombidiosis
tromethamine
    fosfomycin t.
    ketorolac t.
    lodoxamide t.
Trophermyma
    T. whippleii
trophic ulcer
trophodermatoneurosis
trophoneurotic leprosy
tropica
    acrodermatitis vesiculosa t.
    Leishmania t.
    leishmaniasis t.
    phagedena t.
    pyosis t.
tropical
    t. acne
    t. anhidrotic asthenia
    t. boil
    t. disease
    t. eczema
    t. eosinophilia
    t. lichen
    t. mask
    t. measles
    t. phagedenic ulcer
    t. sloughing phagedena
    t. sore
    t. typhus
    t. ulcer
tropicalis
    acne t.
    Blomia t.
    Candida t.
    tinea t.
tropicum
    granuloma inguinale t.
    papilloma inguinale t.
    ulcus t.
tropicus
    lichen t.
tropism
    viral t.
tropomyosin

NOTES

troponin
trospectomycin sulfate
trough
    peak and t.
Trousseau spot
T.R.U.E.
    T. allergy patch test
    T. Test
true
    t. progeria
    t. skin
Truphylline Suppository
TruZone peak flow meter
trypanid
Trypanosoma
    T. brucei
    T. cruzi
trypanosomiasis
    African t.
    American t.
trypanosomid
trypsin
trypsin, balsam peru, and castor
    oil
α_1-**trypsin inhibitor**
tryptase
tryptophan
    t. dysmetabolism
TS
    temperature sensitive
T/SAL Shampoo
tsetse
    t. fly
    t. fly bite
TSLS
    toxic shock-like syndrome
TSS
    toxic shock syndrome
TSTA
    tumor-specific transplantation
    antigens
T-Stat topical
Tsukamurella paurometabolum
tsukubaensis
    Streptomyces t.
tsutsugamushi
    t. disease
    t. fever
TTP
    thrombotic thrombocytopenic
    purpura
TU
    toxic unit

tubba
tube
    eustachian t.
    t. precipitin test
    Shiley tracheostomy t.
    Softech endotracheal t.
    t. thoracostomy
tubercle
    anatomical t.
    butcher's t.
    dissection t.
    naked t.
    necrogenic t.
    postmortem t.
    prosector's t.
    sebaceous t.
tubercula dolorosa
tubercular
tuberculation
tuberculatum
    erythema t.
tuberculid
    bacillary-barren t.'s
    micropapular t.
    nodular t.
    papular t.
    papulonecrotic t.
    rosacea-like t.
tuberculin
    Koch old t.
    purified protein derivative of t.
    (PPD)
    t. skin test
    t. test
tuberculin-type hypersensitivity
tuberculization
tuberculochemotherapeutic
tuberculocidal
tuberculoderma
tuberculoid
    t. leprosy
    t. rosacea
tuberculoprotein
tuberculosis (TB)
    adult t.
    appendicular t.
    arthritic t.
    attenuated t.
    childhood type t.
    cutaneous t.
    t. cutis
    t. cutis colliquativa
    t. cutis follicularis disseminata

t. cutis indurata
t. cutis indurativa
t. cutis lichenoid
t. cutis luposa
t. cutis miliaris
t. cutis orificialis
t. cutis papulonecrotica
t. cutis verrucosa
dermal t.
extrapulmonary t.
hepatosplenic t.
t. lymphadenitis
miliary t.
multi-drug-resistant t. (MDR-TB)
Mycobacterium t. (MTB)
t. papulonecrotica
postprimary t.
primary t.
reinfection t.
RISE-resistant t.
secondary t.
t. ulcerosa
t. vaccine
vertebral t.
tuberculostat
tuberculostatic
tuberculosus
lupus t.
tuberculous
t. abscess
t. chancre
t. dactylitis
t. nephritis
t. pleurisy
t. rheumatism
t. synovitis
t. wart
tuberculum
t. sebaceum
t. syphiliticum
tuberosa
urticaria t.
tuberosum
xanthoma t.

tuberous
t. sclerosis
t. xanthoma
Tubersol
TubiFast bandage
tubing
Silastic t.
tubocurarine
tubules
T t.
tubulointerstitial nephritis
tuft of hair
tuftsin
Tukey
T. post-hoc correction
T. standardized range test
tularemia
tularemic chancre
tularensis
Francisella t.
Pasteurella t.
tumbleweed
tumbu fly
tumefaciens
Agrobacterium t.
tumefacient
tumefaction
tumentia
tumid
t. lupus erythematosus
tumor
Abrikosov t.
adnexal t.
amyloid t.
t. antigen
benign t.
Brooke t.
brown t.
Buschke-Löwenstein t.
carcinoid t.
t. cell negative selection
t. cell purging
cutaneous t.
dermal duct t.
desmoid t.
epithelial t.
Ewing t.

T

NOTES

421

tumor *(continued)*
    genital t.
    giant cell t.
    glomus t.
    granular cell t.
    haarscheibe t.
    insulin t.
    Koenen t.
    Landschutz t.
    t. lysis factor
    malignant t.
    malignant peripheral nerve
        sheath t.
    t. marker
    Merkel cell t.
    mixed t.
    t. necrosis factor (TNF)
    t. necrosis factor-beta
    neuroendocrine t.
    t., node, metastasis (TNM)
    papillary t.
    peripheral nerve sheath t.
    phantom t.
    Pinkus t.
    Pott puffy t.
    premalignant t.
    primary neuroendocrine t.
    Rous t.
    sebaceous t.
    squamous cell lung t.
    t. stage
    tomato t.
    tracheal t.
    turban t.
    villous t.
    t. virus
    Wilms t.
    Yaba t.
tumoral calcinosis
tumor-associated antigen
tumoriform
tumorigenic
tumor-infiltrating lymphocyte (TILS)
tumor-specific transplantation
    antigens (TSTA)
tuna
    t. fish
Tunga
    T. penetrans
    T. penetrans bite
tungiasis
tunica dartos
tuning fork

tunnel
    t. of Guyon
turban tumor
Turbinaire
    Decadron Phosphate T.
    Dexacort T.
turbinate
turbinates
    nasal t.
turbot
Turbuhaler
    T. inhaler
turgometer
Türk
turkey
    bluecomb disease of t.
    t. feather
    t. meningoencephalitis virus
Turlock virus
Turner syndrome
turnip
Tusibron
    T.-DM
Tussin
    Safe T.
Tussionex
Tussi-Organidin
    T.-O. NR
Tuss-LA
Tusstat Syrup
twenty-nail dystrophy
Twilite Oral
Twin Jet nebulizer
twisted
    t. chondrodysplasia
    t. hair
twitch
two-dimensional
    immunoelectrophoresis
two feet-one hand syndrome
Twort-d'Herelle phenomenon
Twort phenomenon
two-site immunoradiometric assay
two-stage reaction
Ty21a vaccine
tyle
Tylenol
    T. Cold Effervescent
        Medication Tablet
tyloma
tylosis, pl. tyloses
    t. ciliaris

t. linguae
t. palmaris et plantaris
tylotic
tyloticum
eczema t.
tympanic membrane (TM)
tympanocentesis
tympanometry
tyndallization
type
t. A acanthosis nigricans
axial t.
t. B acanthosis nigricans
blood t.
t. C acanthosis nigricans
t. 1-24 cornification
epidermolysis bullosa, dermal t.
epidermolysis bullosa,
epidermal t.
epidermolysis bullosa,
junctional t.
t. IA oculocutaneous albinism
t. IB oculocutaneous albinism
t. I collagen
t. I glycogen storage disease
t. II collagen
t. III collagen
t. I–III hypersensitivity reaction
t. III immune complex drug
reaction
t. I, II tyrosinemia
t. II ocular albinism
t. II oculocutaneous albinism
t. II osteoporosis
t. II pachyonychia congenita
t. II pneumocyte
t. I–IV immunologic drug
reaction
t. I-MP oculocutaneous
albinism
t. I ocular albinism
t. I oculocutaneous albinism
t. I osteoporosis
t. I-TS oculocutaneous albinism
t. IV collagen
t. IV collagenase

t. IV delayed hypersensitivity
reaction
t. I–VII mucopolysaccharidosis
t. IX collagen
keratosis palmaris et plantaris
of the Meleda t.
peripheral t.
skin t.
t. strain
t. V collagenase
t. VI collagen
t. VII collagen
t. VIII collagen
t. XI collagen
t. XIV collagen
type 68–72
typhi
Rickettsia t.
Salmonella t.
Typhim
T. vi
T. Vi vaccine
typhimurium
Salmonella t.
typhoid
t. A&B (T.A.B.)
t. bacteriophage
t. cholera
t. fever
provocation t.
t. septicemia
t. vaccine
**typhoid-paratyphoid A and B
vaccine**
typholysin
typhosepsis
typhous
typhus
African tick t.
endemic t.
epidemic t.
mite t.
murine t.
Queensland tick t.
recrudescent t.
scrub t.

T

NOTES

typhus *(continued)*
 tropical t.
 t. vaccine
typing
 bacteriophage t.
 HLA t.
 HLA-DRB and -DRQ DNA t.
 LCR-based HLA t.
Tyroglyphus
 T. longior
 T. siro
Tyrophagus
 T. putrescentiae
tyrosinase
tyrosinase-negative oculocutaneous
 albinism

tyrosinase-positive oculocutaneous
 albinism
tyrosinase-related oculocutaneous
 albinism
tyrosine
 t. kinase
 t. metabolism
tyrosinemia
 neonatal t.
 type I, II t.
T-Y stent
Tyzine Nasal
Tzanck
 T. preparation
 T. smear
 T. test

U1 RNP antibody
UAD topical
U-Cort
UCTD
    undifferentiated connective tissue
      disease
Udder Butter lubricant/emollient
UIP
    usual interstitial pneumonia
ulcer
    acute decubitus u.
    Aden u.
    amebic u.
    amputating u.
    aphthous genital u.
    aphthous oral u.
    arterial u.
    atonic u.
    Buruli u.
    chiclero u.
    chrome u.
    chronic u.
    cockscomb u.
    cold u.
    constitutional u.
    corneal u.
    corrosive u.
    crateriform u.
    creeping u.
    cutaneous u.
    decubitus u.
    diabetic u.
    diabetic foot u.
    diphtheritic u.
    Gaboon u.
    genital aphthous u.
    gravitational u.
    gummatous u.
    hard u.
    healed u.
    herpetic u.
    indolent u.
    inflamed u.
    inflammatory u.
    ischemic u.
    Kurunegala u.
    u. lesion
    Lipschütz u.
    lupoid u.
    Marjolin u.

Meleney u.
    nasopharyngeal u.
    necrotic u.
    neurotrophic u.
    in noma u.
    oral aphthous u.
    Oriental u.
    perambulating u.
    phagedenic u.
    phlegmonous u.
    pudendal u.
    recurrent u.
    ring u.
    rodent u.
    serpiginous u.
    sickle cell u.
    skin u.
    sloughing u.
    soft u.
    stasis vascular u.
    steroid u.
    Sutton u.
    symptomatic u.
    syphilitic u.
    tanner's u.
    trophic u.
    tropical u.
    tropical phagedenic u.
    undermining u.
    varicose u.
    vascular u.
    venereal u.
    venous stasis u.
    Zambesi u.
ulcera
ulcerans
    Mycobacterium u.
ulcerate
ulcerated
ulcerating granuloma of pudendum
ulceration
    gastrointestinal u.
    intertrigo with u.
    intestinal u.
    mucous membrane u.
    nasal mucosal u.
    oral u.
    u. of oral mucosa
    rectal u.

U

ulcerative
  u. dermatosis
  u. gingivitis
  u. lichen planus
  u. proctocolitis
  u. stomatitis
ulceroglandular
ulcerosa
  tuberculosis u.
ulcerous
ulcero-vegetating plaque
ulcus
  u. ambulans
  u. durum
  u. hypostaticum
  u. migrans
  u. tropicum
  u. venereum
  u. vulvae acutum
ulerythema
  u. ophryogenes
  u. sycosiforme
ulerythematosa
  atrophoderma u.
ulex europaeus
ulnar deviation
ulodermatitis
ulotrichous
ULR
ULR-LA
Ultra
  Grisactin U.
  U. Mide topical
  U. Tears solution
Ultracef
ultrahigh frequency ventilation
Ultram
ultrasonic nebulizer
ultrasound
  A-mode u.
  Doppler u.
ultrasound-guided bronchoscopy
ultrastructural
  u. analysis
  u. component
Ultravate
  U. topical
ultraviolet (UV)
  u. A (UVA)
  u. actinotherapy
  u. B (UVB)
  u. B-range (UVB)
  u. C (UVC)

  u. lamp
  u. light
  u. radiation
  u. recall
ultravirus
umbilicated
umbilication
Umbre virus
Unasyn
Uncinaria
uncinariasis
unclassified air cleaner
uncomplemented
uncovertebral arthrosis
unction
unctuosa
  cutis u.
undecapeptide
undecylenic
  u. acid
  u. acid and derivatives
undercover cosmetic
undermining ulcer
Underwood disease
undifferentiated
  u. connective tissue disease
  (UCTD)
  u. type fevers
Undoguent topical
undulin
ungual
unguent
unguinal
unguis
  u. incarnatus
  leukopathia u.
  lunula u.
  pterygium u.
  vallum u.
unguium
  achromia u.
  canities u.
  defluvium u.
  dystrophia u.
  fragilitas u.
  gryposis u.
  scabrities u.
  tinea u.
  trichophytosis u.
Uni-Ace
unicameral cyst
Uni-Decon
Uni-Dur

unifocal Langerhans cell
unilateral
  u. dermatomal superficial
    telangiectasia
  u. hemangiomatosis
  u. hemidysplasia
  u. hemidysplasia cornification
    disorder
  u. macular degeneration
  u. nevoid telangiectasia
unilocular cyst
uninflamed
Unipen
  U. injection
  U. Oral
Uniphyl
Uni-Pro
Uniserts
  Hemril-HC U.
unit
  Å u.
    Ångström unit
  alexin u.
  allergy u. (AU)
  amboceptor u.
  Ångström u. (Å unit)
  antigen u.
  antitoxin u.
  antivenene u.
  Bethesda u. (BU)
  biologic u. (BU)
  biological standard u.
  colony-forming u. (CFU)
  complement u.
  dermal microvascular u.
  diphtheria antitoxin u.
  ELISA u. (EI.U)
  epidermal-melanin u.
  Florey u.
  follicular melanin u.
  hemolysin u.
  inhalation breath u.
  iontophoretic u.
  musculotendinous u.
  nectary of floral u.
  noon u.
  Oxford u.

  u. of penicillin
  pilosebaceous u.
  priming renal dialysis u.
  protein nitrogen u. (PNU)
  streptomycin u.
  tetanus antitoxin u.
  toxic u. (TU)
  toxin u.
unius
univalent antibody
univariant
Uni-Vent
universal donor
universale
  angiokeratoma corporis
    diffusum u.
  melasma u.
universalis
  alopecia u.
  calcinosis u.
  hypertrichosis u.
  psoriasis u.
Unna
  U. boot
  U. comedo extractor
  U. disease
  U. mark
Unna-Thost
  U.-T. disease
  U.-T. keratoderma
  keratosis palmaris et plantaris
    of U.-T.
unusual
  u. lupus erythematosus-like
    syndrome
  u. opportunistic infection
upcurved punch
upper
  u. airway obstruction
  u. dermis
  u. respiratory infection (URI)
  u. respiratory tract infection
    (URI)
  u. respiratory tract mucosa
up-regulation
urate
  u. deposition

NOTES

urate *(continued)*
    monosodium u. (MSU)
    u. nephropathy
    u. oxidase
urate-associated inflammation
Urbach-Wiethe
    U.-W. disease
    U.-W. syndrome
urban cutaneous leishmaniasis
urchin
    sea u.
urea
    u. frost
    u. and hydrocortisone
Ureacin
Ureacin-20 topical
Ureacin-40 topical
ureae
    Actinobacillus u.
urealyticum
    Ureaplasma u.
Ureaphil injection
Ureaplasma urealyticum
urediospore, uredinospore,
  ureidospore
uredo
uremic pneumonitis
urethritis
    chlamydial u.
urhidrosis
URI
    upper respiratory infection
    upper respiratory tract infection
uric acid
uricase
uricosuric drug
uridine triphosphate
uridrosis
    u. crystallina
urinary
    u. electrophoresis
    u. tract infection (UTI)
urine
    cellular casts in u.
    mouse u.
    u. myoglobin immunoassay
urinosus
    sudor u.
Uri-Tet Oral
uritis
Urobak
Uroplus
    U. DS

U. SS
U. SSYA
uroporphyrin
urtica
urticans
    purpura u.
urticant
urticaria
    u. acuta
    acute u.
    acute allergic u.
    allergic u.
    aquagenic u.
    u. bullosa
    cholinergic u.
    chronic u.
    u. chronica
    cold u.
    cold-induced u.
    u. conferta
    congelation u.
    contact u.
    cyclic u.
    u. endemica
    u. factitia
    factitious u.
    febrile u.
    u. febrilis
    giant u.
    heat u.
    u. hemorrhagica
    idiopathic u.
    idiopathic cold u.
    immunologic contact u.
    irritant contact u.
    u. maculosa
    u. medicamentosa
    papular u.
    u. papulosa
    u. perstans
    physical u.
    u. pigmentosum
    pressure u.
    recurrent u.
    solar u.
    solaris u.
    u. subcutanea
    u. tuberosa
    u. vesiculosa
    vibratory u.
urticarial
    u. dermatographia

u. plaque
u. vasculitis
urticariogenic
urticarioides
acarodermatitis u.
urticata
acne u.
urticate
urtication
urticatus
lichen u.
urushiol
use test
U3 snRNP
ustilaginism
Ustilago
ustus
Aspergillus u.
usual interstitial pneumonia (UIP)
uta
uteri
ichthyosis u.
uterine leiomyoma
UTI
urinary tract infection

Uticort
utilization
UV
ultraviolet
UVA
long-wavelength ultraviolet light
ultraviolet A
UVB
midrange-wavelength ultraviolet
light
ultraviolet B
ultraviolet B-range
UVC
ultraviolet C
uveitis
anterior u.
lens-induced u.
phacoanaphylactic u.
uveomeningoencephalitis
uviofast
uviol lamp
uvioresistant
uviosensitive

U

V

V antigen
V gene
V-2 carcinoma
vaccae
   Mycobacterium v.
vaccina
vaccinal
vaccinate
vaccination
vaccinator
vaccinatum
   eczema v.
vaccine
   ActHIB v.
   adjuvant v.
   V. Adverse Events Reporting
      System (VAERS)
   AIDS v.
   aqueous v.
   attenuated v.
   autogenous v.
   bacillus Calmette-Guérin v.
   bacterial v.
   BCG v.
   Biken CAM v.
   brucella strain 19 v.
   Calmette-Guérin v.
   chickenpox v.
   cholera v.
   crystal violet v.
   diphtheria, tetanus toxoids, and
      acellular pertussis v.
   diphtheria, tetanus toxoids, and
      whole-cell pertussis v.
   diphtheria, tetanus toxoids, and
      whole-cell pertussis vaccine
      and haemophilus b
      conjugate v.
   diphtheria toxoid, tetanus
      toxoid, and pertussis v.
      (DTP)
   duck embryo origin v. (DEV)
   Edmonston-Zagreb v.
   Flury strain v.
   foot-and-mouth disease virus v.
   Haffkine v.
   HAVRIX v.
   HbOC v.
   HbOc/DTP v.

heat-phenol inactivated v.
hepatitis A v.
hepatitis B v.
heterogenous v.
Hib-TT v.
high-egg-passage v.
hog cholera v.
human diploid cell rabies v.
   (HDCV)
Imovax Rabies intradermal v.
Imovax Rabies intramuscularv.
inactivated poliovirus v. (IPV)
influenza virus v.
lipopolysaccharide v.
live v.
live oral polio v.
live oral poliovirus v.
low-egg-passage v.
v. lymph
measles, mumps, and
   rubella v. (MMR)
measles virus v.
Melacine v.
meningococcal v.
MMR v.
multivalent v.
mumps virus v.
oil v.
Oka v.
Pasteur v.
pertussis v.
plague v.
PncCRM v.
pneumococcal v.
pneumococcal polysaccharide v.
pneumococcal
   polysaccharide/protein
   conjugate v.
poliomyelitis v.
poliovirus v.
polyvalent v.
rabies v.
rabies virus v.
Rocky Mountain spotted
   fever v.
Sabin v.
Salk v.
Semple v.
smallpox v.
split-virus v.

vaccine *(continued)*
    Staphylococcus v.
    Staphylococcus aureus v.
    stock v.
    subunit v.
    T.A.B. v.
    tetanus v.
    tuberculosis v.
    Ty21a v.
    Typhim Vi v.
    typhoid v.
    typhoid-paratyphoid A and
      B v.
    typhus v.
    varicella v.
    variola v.
    viral v.
    v. virus
    whooping-cough v.
    yellow fever v.
vaccinia
    disseminated v.
    v. gangrenosa
    generalized v.
    v. immune globulin
    v. infection
    Orthopoxvirus v.
    progressive v.
    variola v.
    v. virus
vaccinial
vacciniform
vacciniforme
    hydroa v.
vaccinist
vaccinization
vaccinogen
vaccinogenous
vaccinoid
    v. reaction
vaccinostyle
vaccinum
Vacu-Aide
vacuolar myopathy
vacuolated
vacuolating virus
vacuole
vacuole
vacuolization
    basket-weave v.
vacutome
vacuum
    Rainbow v.

VAERS
    Vaccine Adverse Events Reporting
    System
vagabond's disease
Vaginal
    Monistat V.
vaginalis
    Trichomonas v.
vaginitis
    Gardnerella v.
    granular v.
vaginosis
vagrant's disease
vagus nerve
valacyclovir
    v. HCl
valerate
    betamethasone v.
valgum
    genu v.
valgus
    hallux v.
Valisone
Valium
    V. injection
    V. Oral
vallum unguis
valproic acid and derivatives
Valrelease Oral
Valsalva maneuver
Valtrex
valve
    Passy-Muir tracheostomy
      speaking v.
valvular disease
Vamate
vanA
    v. gene
VanA phenotype
Vancenase
    V. AQ
    V. AQ Inhaler
    V. Nasal Inhaler
    V. Pockethaler
Vanceril
    V. Oral Inhaler
Vancocin
    V. injection
    V. Oral
Vancoled injection

vancomycin
 v. hydrochloride
vancomycin-resistant enterococci (VRE)
van der Waals forces
Vanex-LA
vanH gene
vanilla
vanillism
Vanoxide
Vanoxide-HC
vanS gene
Vansil
Vantin
vapocoolant spray
Vaponefrin
VAPS
 volume-assured pressure support
variabilis
 Dermacentor v.
 erythrokeratodermia v.
 erythrokeratodermia figurata v.
variable
 v. numbers of tandem repeats (VNTR)
 v. region
variant
 dystrophic v.
 generalized morphea v.
 junctional v.
 linear scleroderma v.
 Miller-Fisher v.
 morphea v.
 v. neurofibromatosis
 simplex v.
varicella
 congenital v.
 v. disease
 v. encephalitis
 v. gangrenosa
 v. vaccine
 v. virus vaccine live
varicellation
varicella-zoster (VZ)
 v.-z. immune globulin
 v.-z. immunoglobulin (VZIG)

v.-z. infection
 v.-z. virus (VZV)
varicelliform
 v. lesion
varicelloid
varicellosus
 herpes zoster v.
varicose
 v. eczema
 v. ulcer
varicosity
 venous v.
varicosum
 lymphangioma capillare v.
variegata
 parakeratosis v.
 parapsoriasis v.
variegated
variegate porphyria (VP)
variegatum
 Hyalomma v.
variola
 v. benigna
 v. hemorrhagica
 v. major
 v. maligna
 v. miliaris
 v. minor
 v. pemphigosa
 v. sine eruptione
 v. vaccine
 v. vaccinia
 v. vera
 v. verrucosa
 v. virus
variolar
variolate
variolation
variolic
varioliform
 v. syphilid
varioliformis
 acne v.
 parapsoriasis v.
 parapsoriasis acuta et v.
variolization
varioloid

NOTES

433

variolous
variolovaccine
Varivax
varix
varus
    hallux v.
VAS
    visual analogue scale
vasa nervorum
vascular
    v. cell adhesion molecule
    v. disorder
    v. dysfunction
    v. FLPD
    v. malformation birthmark
    v. permeability
    v. reaction
    v. ulcer
vasculare
    poikiloderma atrophicans v.
vascularis
    nevus v.
vasculature
vasculitic lesion
vasculitis, pl. vasculitides
    allergic v.
    coronary v.
    cutaneous v.
    granulomatous v.
    Henoch-Schönlein v.
    hypersensitivity v.
    hypocomplementemic
      urticarial v.
    immune complex v.
    large vessel v.
    leukocytoclastic v. (LCV)
    livedo v.
    mesenteric v.
    necrotizing v.
    nodular v.
    nodular granulomatous v.
    rheumatoid v.
    rheumatoid rheumatic v.
    segmental hyalinizing v.
    small vessel v.
    systemic v.
    urticarial v.
vasculopathy
vasculosus
    nevus v.
Vaseline
    V. Intensive Care moisturizer
    V. petroleum jelly

vasoactive mediator
Vasocidin
    V. Ophthalmic
Vasocon
vasoconstriction
    hypoxic v.
vasoconstrictor
    topical ophthalmic v.
Vasodilan
vasodilatation
vasodilation
vasomotor
    v. reaction
    v. rhinitis (VMR)
vaso-occlusive
    v.-o. disease
vasopressor
vasospasm
    cold-induced v.
Vasosulf Ophthalmic
vasovagal
    v. reaction
Vater-Pacini corpuscle
VATS
    video-assisted thoracic surgery
VaxSyn
VC
    vital capacity
V-Cillin K Oral
V-Dec-M
V-D-J
    V.-D.-J. gene
    V.-D.-J. gene arrangement
VDRL
    Venereal Disease Research
    Laboratories
    VDRL test
vection
vector
    biological v.
    mechanical v.
    v. of plague
    recombinant v.
vectorial
vecuronium
VEE
    Venezuelan equine
    encephalomyelitis
    VEE virus
Veetids Oral
vegetable gum
vegetans
    dermatitis v.

keratosis v.
pemphigus v.
pyoderma v.
pyostomatitis v.
vegetative bacteriophage
vehicle
veiled cell
vein
broken v.
Vel antigen
Velban
Velcro closure
veldt sore
vellus
v. hair
velocimetry
laser Doppler v.
velocity
nerve conduction v.
velogenic
Velosef
Veltane Tablet
velvet
v. grass
venae cavae (*pl. of* SVC)
Ven antigen
venenata
acne v.
cheilitis v.
dermatitis v.
Rhus v.
venenatum
erythema v.
venereal-associated arthritis
Venereal
V. Disease Research
Laboratories (VDRL)
venereal
v. bubo
v. disease
v. sore
v. ulcer
v. wart
venereum
granuloma v.
lymphogranuloma v. (LGV,
LVG)

lymphopathia v.
papilloma v.
ulcus v.
veneris
corona v.
Venezuelan
V. equine encephalomyelitis
(VEE)
V. equine encephalomyelitis
virus
venoarterial shunting
Venoglobulin-I
Venoglobulin-S
venom
bee v.
v. extract
flea v.
v. hemolysis
Hymenoptera v.
v. immunotherapy
snake v.
spider v.
v. testing
venom-bathed nematocyst
venom-bearing spine
venomous snake
veno-occlusive
venosus
nevus v.
venous
v. gangrene
v. lake
v. malformation
v. star
v. stasis ulcer
v. varicosity
ventilated alveolus
ventilation
airway pressure release v.
(APRV)
alveolar v.
high-frequency jet v.
high frequency positive
pressure v.
intermittent mandatory v.
inverse ratio v. (IRV)
maximal v. (MV)

V

NOTES

ventilation *(continued)*
    maximal voluntary v. (MVV)
    mechanical v. (MV)
    minute v.
    pressure-controlled inverse
      ratio v.
    pressure-regulated volume
      control v.
    pressure support v. (PSV)
    proportional assist v.
    synchronized intermittent
      mechanical v.
    synchronous intermittent
      mandatory v.
    ultrahigh frequency v.
    volume-cycled decelerating-
      flow v.
ventilation-perfusion
    v.-p. lung scan
    v.-p. ratio
ventilation/perfusion lung scan (V/Q lung scan)
ventilator
    High Frequency Oscillatory v.
    mechanical v.
    volume-limited v.
ventilator-associated pneumonia
ventilatory failure
Ventolin
    V. nebules
    V. Rotacaps
VenTrak respiratory mechanics monitor
ventral
ventricosus
    dermatitis pediculoides v.
    Pediculoides v.
    Pyemotes v.
ventricular pseudoaneurysm (PVA)
ventriculography
    radionuclide v.
ventriculoperitoneal shunt (VP)
Venture demand oxygen delivery device
venular lesion
venules
    high endothelial v. (HEV)
venulitis
    cutaneous necrotizing v.
Venus
    collar of V.
    crown of V.
    necklace of V.

VePesid
    V. injection
    V. Oral
vera
    cutis v.
    polycythemia v.
    variola v.
verge
    nasal v.
vergeture
Vergogel Gel
Vergon
vermicularis
    atrophoderma v.
    Enterobius v.
    Oxyuris v.
vermiculatum
    atrophoderma v.
vermilion
    v. border
Vermizine
Vermox
vernal
    v. conjunctivitis
    v. encephalitis
    v. grass
    v. keratoconjunctivitis
    sweet v.
Verner syndrome
Verneuil
    hidradenitis axillaris of V.
    V. neuroma
verniciferum
    Toxicodendron v.
vernix
    Rhus v.
veronii
    Aeromonas v.
verruca, pl. verrucae
    v. acuminata
    v. digitata
    v. filiformis
    v. glabra
    v. mollusciformis
    v. necrogenica
    v. peruana
    v. peruviana
    v. plana
    v. plana juvenilis
    v. plana senilis
    v. planta
    v. plantaris
    seborrheic v.

v. senilis
v. simplex
v. vulgaris
verruciform
verruciformis
acrokeratosis v.
epidermodysplasia v.
verruciforms
verrucosa
v. cutis
dermatitis v.
elephantiasis nostra v.
pachyderma v.
Phialophora v.
telangiectasia v.
tuberculosis cutis v.
variola v.
verrucose
verrucosis
lymphostatic v.
verrucosum
eczema v.
erysipelas v.
molluscum v.
verrucosus
lichen planus v.
lichen ruber v.
lupus v.
nevus v.
verrucous
v. angiokeratoma
v. carcinoma
v. hemangioma
v. nevus
v. scrofuloderma
v. xanthoma
verruga
Versacaps
Versed
versican CS/DS
versicolor
Aspergillus v.
pityriasis v.
tinea v.
trichonosus v.
vertebral tuberculosis
Vertex

vertex
vertical
v. growth phase
v. section
v. transmission
Verticillium alboatrum
very late activation antigen (VLA-1 antigen)
vesica
vesicae
pachyderma v.
vesicant
vesicate
vesication
vesicatoria
Lytta v.
vesicatory
vesicle
vesicobullous
v. lesion
vesicopustular
v. eruption
vesicopustules
vesicular
v. dermatitis
v. eruption
v. exanthema
v. exanthema of swine virus
v. stomatitis
v. stomatitis virus
v. viral infection
vesiculate
vesiculated
vesiculation
creeping v.
intraepidermal v.
subepidermal v.
vesiculiform
vesiculobullous
vesiculopapular
vesiculopustular
vesiculosa
urticaria v.
vesiculose
vesiculosum
eczema v.
hydroa v.

NOTES

V

vesiculotomy
vesiculous
Vesiculovirus
vespid
    Hymenopterous v.
Vespula
    V. crabro
Vespula **sting**
vessel blockage
vestibular
    v. cyst
    v. papilla
vestimenti
    pediculosis v.
vestimentorum
    pediculosis corporis vel v.
Vexol Ophthalmic suspension
V-Gan injection
VH gene
Vi
    V. antibody
    V. antigen
vi
    Typhim v.
vibex
Vibramycin
    V. injection
    V. Oral
Vibra-Tabs
vibration
    chest percussion and v.
vibratory
    v. angioedema
    v. urticaria
Vibrio
    V. cholerae
    V. vulnificus
vibrio
    Nasik v.
Vicks
    V. DayQuil Allergy Relief 4
    Hour Tablet
    V. DayQuil Sinus Pressure &
    Congestion Relief
    V. 44D Cough & Head
    Congestion
    V. 44 Non-Drowsy Cold &
    Cough Liqui-Caps
    V. Sinex Long-Acting Nasal
    solution
Vicryl suture
Vidal disease
vidarabine

video
    Sony VHS HQ Digital
    Picture v.
video-assisted thoracic surgery
    (VATS)
Videx
    V. Oral
Vierra sign
view
    coronal v.
    Waters v.
Vigilon dressing
vigorous hydration
villi
villoma
villonodular
    v. synovitis
villous
    v. fold
    v. frond
    v. tumor
villus
vinblastine
    v. sulfate
Vinca **alkaloid**
Vincent
    V. angina
    V. infection
    V. white mycetoma
vincristine
vinyl
    v. chloride
    v. chloride exposure
vinyl-alternating air mattress
Vioform
    V. topical
violaceous
    v. plaque
violet
    gentian v.
violet-blue erythema
violin-back
    v.-b. spider
    v.-b. spider bite
Vira-A Ophthalmic
Viracept
viral
    v. arthritis
    v. conjunctivitis
    v. disease
    v. dysenteriae
    v. encephalomyelitis
    v. envelope

v. exanthema
v. gastroenteritis
v. genome
v. hemagglutination
v. hemorrhagic fever
v. hemorrhagic fever virus
v. hepatitis
v. hepatitis type A
v. hepatitis type B
v. hepatitis type C
v. hepatitis type D
v. hepatitis type E
v. immunization
v. infection
v. neutralization
v. pneumonia
v. probe
v. respiratory infection
v. sandfly fever
v. strand
v. tropism
v. vaccine
v. wart
Viramune
Virazole
V. Aerosol
viremia
Virend
viricidal
viricide
viridans hemolysis
viride
Trichoderma *v.*
virion
Virivac
viroid
virologist
virology
viropexis
Viroptic Ophthalmic
virucidal
virucide
virucopria
virulence
virulent
v. bacteriophage
viruliferous

viruria
virus
2060 v.
Abelson murine leukemia v.
adeno-associated v. (AAV)
adenoidal-pharyngeal-
conjunctival v.
adenosatellite v.
African horse sickness v.
African swine fever v.
African tick v.
v. A hepatitis
AIDS-related v. (ARV)
Akabane v.
Aleutian mink disease v.
Amapari v.
amphotropic v.
animal v.
anti-Epstein-Barr v. (anti-EBV)
A-P-C v.
Arenaviridae v.
Argentine hemorrhagic fever v.
arthropod-borne v.
Astroviridae v.
attenuated v.
attenuate vaccinia v.
Aujeszky disease v.
Australian X disease v.
avian encephalomyelitis v.
avian erythroblastosis v.
avian infectious
laryngotracheitis v.
avian influenza v.
avian leukosis-sarcoma v.
avian lymphomatosis v.
avian myeloblastosis v.
avian neurolymphomatosis v.
avian pneumoencephalitis v.
avian sarcoma v.
avian viral arthritis v.
B v.
B19 v.
bacterial v.
Bittner v.
BK v.
v. blockade
bluecomb v.

V

NOTES

virus *(continued)*
bluetongue v.
Borna disease v.
Bornholm disease v.
bovine leukemia v. (BLV)
bovine leukosis v.
bovine papular stomatitis v.
bovine virus diarrhea v.
Bunyamwera v.
Bwamba v.
CA v.
Caliciviridae v.
California v.
canarypox v.
canine distemper v.
Capim v.
Caraparu v.
cat distemper v.
cattle plague v.
Catu v.
CELO v.
Central European tick-borne
  encephalitis v.
C group v.
Chagres v.
chicken embryo lethal
  orphan v.
chickenpox v.
chikungunya v.
Coe v.
cold v.
Colorado tick fever v.
Columbia S. K. v.
common cold v.
contagious pustular
  stomatitis v.
Coronaviridae v.
cowpox v.
Coxsackie B v.
Crimean-Congo hemorrhagic
  fever v.
croup-associated v.
cytopathogenic v.
Dakar bat v.
defective v.
delta v.
dengue v.
distemper v.
DNA v.
dog distemper v.
duck hepatitis v.
duck influenza v.
duck plague v.

Duvenhaga v.
eastern equine
  encephalomyelitis v.
EB v.
Ebola v.
ECBO v.
ECHO v.
ECHO v. 28
ECMO v.
ecotropic v.
ECSO v.
ectromelia v.
EEE v.
EMC v.
emerging v.
encephalitis v.
v. encephalomyelitis
encephalomyocarditis v.
enteric v.
enteric cytopathogenic bovine
  orphan v.
enteric cytopathogenic human
  orphan v.
enteric cytopathogenic monkey
  orphan v.
enteric cytopathogenic swine
  orphan v.
enteric orphan v.
enzootic encephalomyelitis v.
ephemeral fever v.
epidemic gastroenteritis v.
epidemic keratoconjunctivitis v.
epidemic myalgia v.
epidemic parotitis v.
epidemic pleurodynia v.
Epstein-Barr v. (EBV)
equine abortion v.
equine arteritis v.
equine coital exanthema v.
equine infectious anemia v.
equine influenza v.
equine rhinopneumonitis v.
FA v.
feline leukemia v. (FeLV)
feline panleukopenia v. (FPV)
feline rhinotracheitis v.
fibrous bacterial v.
filamentous bacterial v.
Filoviridae v.
filtrable v.
fixed v.
Flury strain rabies v.
FMD v.

foamy v.
foot-and-mouth disease v.
fowl erythroblastosis v.
fowl lymphomatosis v.
fowl myeloblastosis v.
fowl neurolymphomatosis v.
fowl plague v.
fowlpox v.
fox encephalitis v.
Friend v.
Friend leukemia v.
GAL v.
gallus adeno-like v.
genital herpes simplex v.
German measles v.
Germiston v.
goatpox v.
Graffi v.
green monkey v.
Gross v.
Gross leukemia v.
Guama v.
Guaroa v.
HA1 v.
HA2 v.
hand-foot-and-mouth disease v.
Hantaan v.
hard pad v.
helper v.
hepatitis v.
hepatitis A v. (HAV)
hepatitis B v. (HBV)
hepatitis C v. (HCV)
hepatitis D v. (HDV)
hepatitis E v. (HEV)
hepatitis G v. (HGV)
herpes v.
herpes simplex v. (HSV)
herpes simplex v. type II
herpes zoster v.
hog cholera v.
horsepox v.
human immunodeficiency v.
  (HIV)
human orf v.
human T-cell leukemia v.
  (HTLV)

human T-cell
  leukemia/lymphoma v.
  (HTLV)
human T-cell lymphotrophic v.
  (HTLV)
human T-cell lymphotrophic v.
  type I (HTLV-I)
human T-cell lymphotrophic v.
  type II (HTLV-II)
human T-cell lymphotrophic v.
  type III (HTLV-III)
Ibaraki v.
IBR v.
v. III of rabbit
Ilhéus v.
inclusion conjunctivitis v.
infantile gastroenteritis v.
infectious bovine
  rhinotracheitis v.
infectious bronchitis v. (IBV)
infectious ectromelia v.
infectious hepatitis v.
infectious papilloma v.
infectious porcine
  encephalomyelitis v.
influenza v.
insect v.
iridescent v.
Jamestown Canyon v. (JCV)
Japanese B encephalitis v.
JH v.
Junin v.
K v.
Kelev strain rabies v.
v. keratoconjunctivitis
Kilham rat v.
Kisenyi sheep disease v.
Koongol v.
Korean hemorrhagic fever v.
Kotonkan v.
Kyasanur Forest disease v.
labial herpes simplex v.
La Crosse v.
lactate dehydrogenase v.
Lassa v.
latent rat v.
Lipovnik v.

V

NOTES

441

virus *(continued)*
   louping-ill v.
   Lucké v.
   Lunyo v.
   lymphadenopathy-associated v.
     (LAV)
   lymphocytic choriomeningitis v.
     (LCMV)
   lymphogranuloma venereum v.
   Machupo v.
   maedi v.
   malignant catarrhal fever v.
   Maloney leukemia v.
   Marburg v.
   Marek disease v.
   marmoset v.
   masked v.
   Mason-Pfizer v.
   Mayaro v.
   measles v.
   medi v.
   Mengo v.
   milkers' nodule v.
   mink enteritis v.
   MM v.
   Mokola v.
   molluscum contagiosum v.
   Moloney v.
   monkey B v.
   monkeypox v.
   mouse encephalomyelitis v.
   mouse hepatitis v.
   mouse leukemia v.
   mouse mammary tumor v.
   mouse parotid tumor v.
   mouse poliomyelitis v.
   mousepox v.
   mouse thymic v.
   mucosal disease v.
   Muerto Canyon v.
   mumps v.
   murine sarcoma v.
   Murray Valley encephalitis v.
   Murutucu v.
   MVE v.
   myxomatosis v.
   Nairobi sheep disease v.
   naked v.
   ND v.
   Nebraska calf scours v.
   Neethling v.
   negative strand v.
   Negishi v.

   neonatal calf diarrhea v.
   neonatal herpes simplex v.
   neurotropic v.
   Newcastle disease v.
   non-A non-B hepatitis v.
   nonoccluded v.
   Norwalk v.
   occluded v.
   Omsk hemorrhagic fever v.
   oncogenic v.
   o'nyong-nyong v.
   orf v.
   Oriboca v.
   ornithosis v.
   orphan v.
   Orthomyxoviridae v.
   Pacheco parrot disease v.
   pantropic v.
   papilloma v.
   pappataci fever v.
   parainfluenza v.
   parainfluenza v.
   Paramyxoviridae v.
   paravaccinia v.
   parrot v.
   Patois v.
   pharyngoconjunctival fever v.
   Phlebotomus fever v.
   Picornaviridae v.
   plant v.
   v. pneumonia of pigs
   poliomyelitis v.
   polymerase chain reaction-based
     detection of hepatitis G v.
   porcine hemagglutinating
     encephalomyelitis v.
   Powassan v.
   primary genital herpes
     simplex v.
   progressive pneumonia v.
   pseudocowpox v.
   pseudolymphocytic
     choriomeningitis v.
   pseudorabies v.
   psittacosis v.
   PVM v.
   quail bronchitis v.
   Quaranfil v.
   rabbit fibroma v.
   rabbit myxoma v.
   rabbitpox v.
   rabies v.
   Rauscher v.

Rauscher leukemia v.
recurrent genital herpes
  simplex v.
recurrent intraoral herpes
  simplex v.
recurrent labial herpes
  simplex v.
REO v.
respiratory enteric orphan v.
respiratory syncytial v. (RSV)
Rida v.
Rift Valley fever v.
rinderpest v.
RNA v.
RNA tumor v.
Ross River v.
Rous-associated v. (RAV)
Rous sarcoma v. (RSV)
Rous sarcoma v. immune
  globulin intravenous (RSV-
  IGIV)
Rs v.
Rubarth disease v.
rubella v.
rubella vaccine v.
rubeola v.
Russian autumn encephalitis v.
Russian spring-summer
  encephalitis v.
Salisbury common cold v.
salivary v.
salivary gland v.
sandfly fever v.
San Miguel sea lion v.
Semliki Forest v.
Sendai v.
serum hepatitis v.
v. shedding
sheep-pox v.
shipping fever v.
Shope fibroma v.
Shope papilloma v.
Simbu v.
simian v. (SV)
Sindbis v.
slow v.
smallpox v.

snowshoe hare v.
soremouth v.
Spondweni v.
St. Louis encephalitis v.
street v.
swamp fever v.
swine encephalitis v.
swine fever v.
swine influenza v.
swinepox v.
Swiss mouse leukemia v.
syncytial v.
Tacaribe v.
Tacaribe complex of v.
Tahyna v.
temperate v.
Teschen disease v.
Tete v.
TGE v.
Theiler v.
Theiler mouse
  encephalomyelitis v.
Theiler original v.
Theiler original strain of
  mouse encephalomyelitis v.
  (TO)
tick-borne v.
tick-borne encephalitis v.
TO v.
Togaviridae v.
trachoma v.
transmissible turkey enteritis v.
tumor v.
turkey meningoencephalitis v.
Turlock v.
Umbre v.
vaccine v.
vaccinia v.
vacuolating v.
varicella-zoster v. (VZV)
variola v.
VEE v.
Venezuelan equine
  encephalomyelitis v.
vesicular exanthema of
  swine v.
vesicular stomatitis v.

NOTES

virus *(continued)*
   viral hemorrhagic fever v.
   visceral disease v.
   visna v.
   VS v.
   WEE v.
   Wesselsbron disease v.
   western equine encephalitis v.
   western equine
    encephalomyelitis v.
   West Nile v.
   West Nile encephalitis v.
   v. X disease
   xenotropic v.
   Yaba v.
   Yaba monkey v.
   yellow fever v.
   Zika v.
virus-1
   human immunodeficiency v.
    (HIV-1)
virus-2
   human immunodeficiency v.
    (HIV-2)
virusoid
virus-transformed cell
visage
   Hippocratic v.
viscera
visceral
   v. disease virus
   v. larva migrans
   v. leishmaniasis
   v. lymphomatosis
   v. sporotrichosis
viscosity
visna
   v. virus
Vistaquel
Vistaril
Vistazine
Vistide
visual analogue scale (VAS)
VitaCuff
vitae
   arbor v.
vital capacity (VC)
vitamin
   v. A
   v. A deficiency
   antioxidant v.
   v. A and Vitamin D
   v. B_1 deficiency

v. B_5 deficiency
v. B_6
v. B_6 deficiency
v. B_{12} deficiency
v. B deficiency
v. B therapy
v. C
v. C deficiency
v. C test
v. D deficiency
v. E
v. E deficiency
v. K deficiency
microbial v.
vitamin-related obesity
Vitec topical
vitiligines
vitiliginous
vitiligo
   acral v.
   acrofacial v.
   v. capitis
   Cazenave v.
   Celsus v.
   facial v.
   generalized v.
   localized v.
   segmental v.
vitiligoidea
vitlata
   Epicauta v.
Vitrasert
   V. intraocular device
vitreitis
vitreous body
vitro
   in v.
vitronectin
vittatus
   Centruroides v.
Viva-Drops solution
vivax
   Plasmodium v.
viviparus
   Dictyocaulus v.
vivo
   in v.
Vivotif Berna Oral
VK
   pen V.
   Penicillin V.
VLA-1 antigen
Vmax

VMR
    vasomotor rhinitis
VNTR
    variable numbers of tandem repeats
VO$_2$
    oxygen consumption per minute
        VO$_2$ max
Voerner disease
Vogt-Koyanagi-Harada syndrome
Vogt-Koyanagi syndrome
Vohwinkel
    mutilating keratoderma of V.
    V. syndrome
Voigt line
volar
    v. skin
volatile odor
volcanic border
vole bacillus
Volkmann cheilitis
Vollmer test
Volmax
Voltaren Oral
volume
    expiratory residual v. (ERV)
    forced expiratory v. (FEV)
    high lung v.
    residual v.
    stroke v. (SV)
    v. test
    v. thickness index (VTI)
    tidal v.
    trapped gas v. (TGV)
volume-assured pressure support (VAPS)
volume-cycled decelerating-flow ventilation
volume-limited ventilator
volumetric
    v. method
    v. technique
volutrauma
volvae
volvulosis
volvulus
    Onchocerca v.

vomiting
    epidemic v.
von
    v. Economo disease
    v. Economo encephalitis
    v. Gierke glycogen storage disease
    v. Recklinghausen disease
    v. Zumbusch disease
    v. Zumbusch pustular psoriasis
Vontrol
Vorner variant of Unna-Thost keratoderma
VoSol
    V. HC Otic
    V. Otic
VP
    variegate porphyria
    ventriculoperitoneal shunt
V/Q lung scan
VRE
    vancomycin-resistant enterococci
VS virus
VTI
    volume thickness index
vulgaris
    acne v.
    apple jelly papule of lupus v.
    Faba v.
    ichthyosis v.
    impetigo v.
    lupus v.
    pemphigus v.
    Proteus v.
    sycosis v.
    Thermoactinomyces v.
    verruca v.
    xerosis v.
vulnificus
    Vibrio v.
vulva, pl. vulvae
    kraurosis v.
    leukoplakia v.
    pruritus v.
vulvar
    v. intraepithelial neoplasia

NOTES

vulvar *(continued)*
   v. lesion
   v. wart
vulvitis
   chronic atrophic v.
   follicular v.
   leukoplakic v.
   plasma cell v.
vulvodynia
vulvovaginal candidiasis (VVC)
vulvovaginitis
Vumon injection

VVC
   vulvovaginal candidiasis
Vw antigen
Vytone topical
VZ
   varicella-zoster
VZIG
   varicella-zoster immunoglobulin
VZV
   varicella-zoster virus
    VZV retinitis

W-135
meningococcal polysaccharide vaccine, groups A, C, Y and W.
Waardenburg syndrome
Wagner potion
Waldenström
hypergammaglobulinemia of W.
W. macroglobulinemia
W. purpura
W. syndrome
Walker-Murdoch sign
wall
nail w.
w. pellitory
shaggy thick w.
walnut
black w.
w. tree
Walter Reed classification
wandering
w. erysipelas
w. rash
waning
waxing and w.
warble
Wardrop disease
warehouseman's itch
warfarin
w. sodium
warm
w. agglutinin
w. autoantibody
warm-cold hemolysin
wart
acuminate w.
anatomical w.
asbestos w.
cattle w.
common w.
digitate w.
fig w.
filiform w.
flat w.
fugitive w.
genital w.
infectious w.
moist w.
mosaic w.
myrmecia w.

necrogenic w.
paronychial w.
periungual w.
Peruvian w.
pitch w.
plane w.
plantar w.
pointed w.
postmortem w.
prosector's w.
seborrheic w.
seed w.
senile w.
soft w.
soot w.
subungual w.
telangiectatic w.
tuberculous w.
venereal w.
viral w.
vulvar w.
Wartenberg symptom
Warthin-Finkeldey cell
Warthin-Starry stain
Warthin-Starry-staining bacillus
wart-like excrescence
wartpox
warty
w. dyskeratoma
w. horn
w. keratotic plaques
Wash
Benzac AC W.
Sastid Plain Therapeutic Shampoo and Acne W.
Theroxide W.
washed maternal platelets
washerman's mark
washerwoman's itch
wasp
paper w.
w. sting
Wassermann
W. antibody
W. reaction (W.r.)
W. test
wasting
w. disease
w. syndrome

W

water
    w. canker
    w. itch
    w. moccasin snake
    w. sore
water-based
    w.-b. facial foundation
    w.-b. mascara
water-free facial foundation
Waterhouse-Friderichsen syndrome
water-impermeable, non-silicone-based occlusive dressing
watermelon
Waterpik
waterpox
Waters view
wave splash
wax
    w. myrtle
    w. myrtle tree
waxing and waning
waxy finger
4-Way Long Acting Nasal solution
WCS-90
    Clorpactin W.
weakness
    generalized w.
    motor neuron w.
    muscle w.
weal
wean-ling diarrhea
Webb antigen
webbed pattern
Weber-Christian disease
Weber-Cockayne
    W.-C. disease
    W.-C. syndrome
Weber test
web formation
WEE
    western equine encephalomyelitis
    WEE virus
weed
    careless w.
    poverty w.
weeping
    w. dermatitis
    w. eczema
    w. fig
    w. fig tree
    w. lesion
    w. willow
Wegener granulomatosis

weight loss
Weil disease
Weil-Felix
    W.-F. reaction
    W.-F. test
Weinberg reaction
weld
    spot w.
Wellcovorin
    W. injection
    W. Oral
well-demarcated skin reaction
Well disease
Wells syndrome
welt
    indurated w.
wen
Werlhof
    W. disease
    W. purpura
werneckii
    Cladosporium w.
    Exophiala w.
Werner syndrome
Wernicke-Korsakoff syndrome
Werther
    W. disease
    W. nevus
Wesselsbron
    W. disease
    W. disease virus
    W. fever
Wessely ring
West
    W. African fever
    W. Indian smallpox
    W. Nile encephalitis virus
    W. Nile fever
    W. Nile virus
Westcort
Westergren sedimentation rate
westermani
    Paragonimus w.
Western
    W. blot
    W. blot infection
    W. Blot test
    W. blot vaccine profile
    W. juniper
    W. juniper tree
    W. ragweed
    W. red cedar

western
  w. black-legged tick
  w. equine encephalitis virus
  w. equine encephalomyelitis (WEE)
  w. equine encephalomyelitis virus
  w. poison oak
  w. water hemp
Westrim LA
wet
  w. cutaneous leishmaniasis
  w. dressing
  w. flush
  w. gangrene
  w. smear
  w. tetter
whale finger
Whatman 3MM
wheal
  w. and flare
  skin w.
wheal-and-erythema reaction
wheal-and-flare reaction
whealing
wheat
  w. flour
  w. grain dust mite
  whole w.
wheeze
  monophonic w.
wheezing
  intractable w.
  nocturnal w.
wheezy bronchitis
Whiff test
whiplash injury
Whipple
  W. bacillus
  W. disease
whippleii
  Trophermyma w.
white
  w. ash
  w. ash tree
  w. blood cell count
  w. burrobrush

  w. dermatographia
  w. dermographism
  w. finger
  w. frontal forelock
  w. gangrene
  w. graft
  w. lesion
  w. line
  w. line response
  w. melanin
  w. mulberry
  w. mulberry tree
  w. oak
  w. oak tree
  w. petrolatum
  w. piedra
  w. pine
  w. pine tree
  w. poplar tree
  w. scar
  w. sponge nevus
  w. spot disease
  w. strawberry tongue
white-faced hornet
whitegraft reaction
whitehead
whitepox
Whitfield Ointment
whitlow
  herpes w.
  herpetic w.
  melanotic w.
WHO
  World Health Organization
  WHO Class IV
  WHO criteria
whole
  w. blood
  w. wheat
whole-body extract
whooping cough
whooping-cough vaccine
whorl
  digital w.
whorled
Wickham stria

NOTES

W

449

Widal
- W. reaction
- W. test

wide
- w. excision
- w. spectrum

widow's peak
Wigraine
Wilcoxon rank sum test
wild
- w. rye
- w. rye grass
- w. tobacco

wildfire rash
Willan disease
willow
- w. tree
- weeping w.

Wilms tumor
Wilson
- W. disease
- W. lichen

windborne pollen
windburn
window
- nasoantral w.

Winer
- dilated pore of W.

wingscale
Winkler disease
WinRho SD
winter
- w. dysentery of cattle
- w. eczema
- w. itch
- w. vomiting disease

Wiskott-Aldrich syndrome
Wissler syndrome
Wistar rats
witch hazel
witkop
Wohlfahrtia
Wood
- W. glass
- W. lamp
- W. light
- W. light examination

wood
- pao ferro w.

- w. tar
- w. tick

woodcutter's encephalitis
wool
- sheep w.
- w. wax alcohol

woolly hair
woolly-hair nevus
Wor Ditchling agent
Woringer-Kolopp disease
World Health Organization (WHO)
worm
- biting reef w.
- blood w.
- Guinea w.

worm-like
wormwood
Woronoff ring
wound
- w. botulism
- w. contraction
- w. fever
- w. healing
- w. myiasis
- puncture w.

W.r.
- Wassermann reaction

Wr^a
- Wright antigen
- Wr^a antigen

wrap
- elastic w.

Wright
- W. antigen (Wr^a)
- W. nebulizer
- W. stain

wrinkle
wrinkling
- cigarette-paper w.

writing
- skin w.

wucher atrophy
Wuchereria
- *W. bancrofti*

Wyburn-Mason syndrome
Wycillin injection
Wyeth bifurcated needle
Wymox

Xanax
xanchromatic
xanthelasma
    generalized x.
    x. palpebrarum
xanthelasmoidea
xanthine
    x. inhibition
    x. stone excretion
xanthinuria
xanthism
xanthochroia
xanthochromatic
xanthochromia
    x. striata palmaris
xanthochromic
xanthochroous
xanthoderma
xanthogranuloma
    juvenile x.
    necrobiotic x.
xanthoma, pl. xanthomata
    x. diabeticorum
    diffuse plane x.
    x. dissemination
    x. disseminatum
    eruptive x.
    fibrous x.
    hypercholesteremic x.
    hyperlipemic x.
    x. multiplex
    normocholesteremic x.
    x. palpebrarum
    palpebrarum x.
    x. planum
    x. striata palmaris
    x. striatum palmare
    x. tendinosum
    tendinous x.
    tendon x.
    x. tuberosum
    tuberous x.
    verrucous x.
xanthomatosis
    cerebrotendinous x.
    normolipemic x.
xanthomatous
Xanthomonas maltophilia
xanthopathy
xanthopsydracia

X chromosome
Xe
    xenon
xenogeneic
    x. graft
xenogenic
xenogenous
xenograft
xenon (Xe)
xenoparasite
xenopi
    Mycobacterium x.
Xenopsylla
    X. cheopis
    X. cheopis bite
xenotropic virus
Xerac AC
xerasia
xerochilia
xeroderma, xerodermia
    x. pigmentosum
Xero-Lube
xeronosus
xerophthalmia
xerosis
    x. vulgaris
xerostomia
xerotes
xerotic
    x. eczema
xerotica
xerotripsis
Xg antigen
xinafoate
    salmeterol x.
X-linked
    X.-l. agammaglobulinemia
    X.-l. Ehlers-Danlos syndrome
    X.-l. hypogammaglobulinemia
    X.-l. ichthyosis
x-radiation
X-ray
x-ray
    x.-r. dermatitis
    x.-r. finding
X-seb T
x-square test
XT
    Contuss X.

X

XXMEN-OE5
    X.-O. antiendotoxin
Xylocaine
    X. with epinephrine
xylose

xylosoxidans
    Achromobacter x.
    Alcaligenes x.
XYY syndrome

Yaba
    Y. monkey virus
    Y. tumor
    Y. virus
YAG
    yttrium-aluminum-garnet
    YAG laser
Yangtze edema
Yates corrected chi square test
yaw
    mother y.
yaws
    bosch y.
    bush y.
    crab y.
    foot y.
    forest y.
    guinea corn y.
    ringworm y.
yeast
    y. form
    y. infection
Yeast-Gard Medicated Douche
yellow
    y. albinism
    y. disease
    y. dock
    y. fever

    y. fever vaccine
    y. fever virus
    y. hornet
    y. jacket
    y. jacket sting
    y. lesion
    y. mustard
    y. nail
    y. nail syndrome
    y. oculocutaneous albinism
    y. skin
Yergason supination sign
Yersinia
    Y. enterocolitica
    Y. pestis
    Y. pestis bite
    Y. pseudotuberculosis
Yersinia
    Yersinia arthritis
    Yersinia pseudotuberculosis
        agglutinin
yew tree
YF-VAX
ylang-ylang oil
Yodoxin
Yt^a antigen
yttrium-aluminum-garnet (YAG)

Zaditen
zafirlukast
Zagam
Zaire subtype
zalcitabine (ddC)
Zambesi ulcer
Zambusch (*See* Zumbusch)
Zantac
    Z. injection
    Z. Oral
Zartan
ZDV
    zidovudine
Zeasorb-AF
    Z.-A. Powder
ZEEP
    zero end-expiratory pressure
Zefazone
Zeis gland
Zephrex
Zephrex LA
Zerit (d4T)
zero end-expiratory pressure
    (ZEEP)
Zetar
Zetran injection
zidovudine (ZDV)
Ziehl-Neelsen smear
Ziehl-Nielsen stain
Zika
    Z. fever
    Z. virus
zileuton
Zimmerman-Laband syndrome
Zimmer Pulsavac wound
    debridement system
Zinacef injection
zinc
    z. deficiency
    DHS z.
    z. gluconate lozenge
    z. oxide, cod liver oil, and
      talc
    z. pyrithione
    z. sulfate
Zincon
    Z. Shampoo
ZIP
    zoster immune plasma
zirconium granuloma

zit
Zithromax
ZNP Bar
zoacanthosis
Zolicef
Zoloft
zona
    z. corona
    z. dermatica
    z. facialis
    z. ignea
    z. ophthalmica
    z. serpiginosa
Zonalon
    Z. cream
zonal type reaction
zone
    barrier z.
    basement membrane z. (BMZ)
    equivalence z.
    floristic z.
    T z.
zoograft
Zoon
    balanitis of Z.
    Z. disease
    Z. erythroplasia
zoonosis
zoonotic
    z. cutaneous leishmaniasis
    z. infection
    z. potential
zootoxin
ZORprin
zoster
    acute herpes z.
    z. encephalomyelitis
    herpes z. (HZ)
    z. immune globulin
    z. immune plasma (ZIP)
    z. sine herpetic
zosteriform
    z. pattern
zosteroid
Zostrix
Zostrix-HP
Zosyn
Zovirax
    Z. injection

Z

455

Zovirax *(continued)*
    Z. Oral
    Z. topical
Zoysia
Z-plasty procedure
z score
Zumbusch
    Z. disease

generalized pustular psoriasis
    of von Z.
Zygomycetes
zygospore
Zyloprim
zymosan
zymotic papilloma
Zyrtec

Appendix 1
Anatomical Illustrations

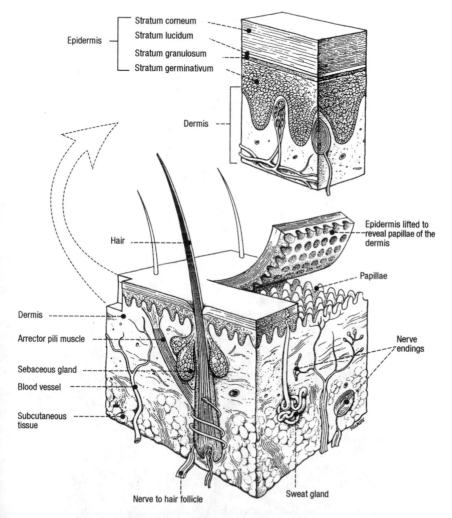

Figure 1. *The skin components and layers.* ·

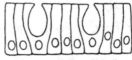

Columnar epithelium of intestines

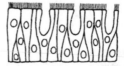

Pseudostratified ciliated columnar epithelium

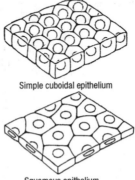

Simple cuboidal epithelium

Squamous epithelium

Figure 2. *Types of epithelial cells.*

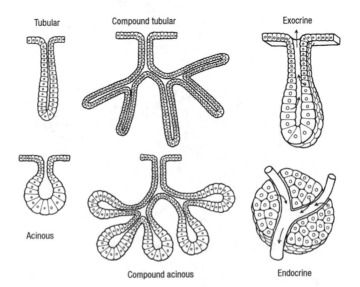

Figure 3. *Types of glands.*

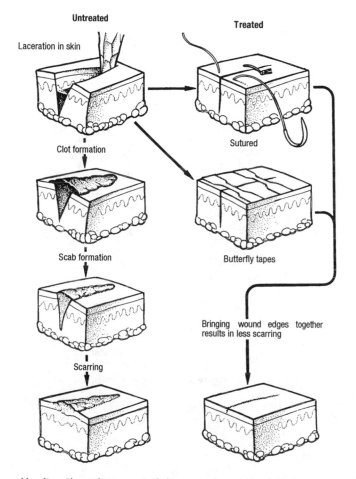

Figure. 4. *Wound healing.* Shows how a typical skin wound would heal if left untreated versus treated.

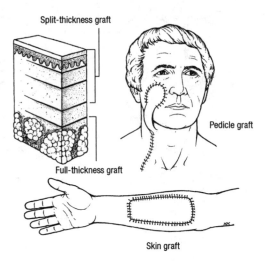

Split-thickness graft

Pedicle graft

Full-thickness graft

Skin graft

Figure 5. *Types of skin grafts.*

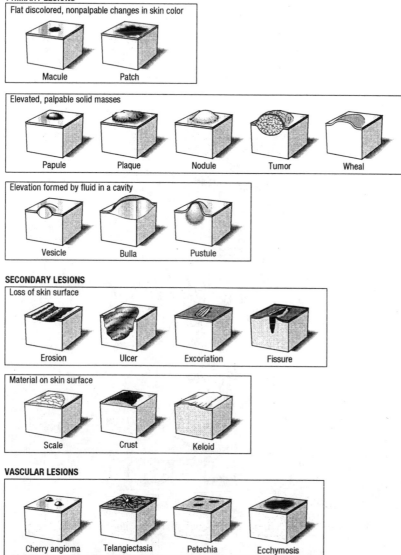

Figure 6. *Types of primary, secondary, and vascular lesions.* From Willis MC. Medical Terminology, Baltimore: Williams & Wilkins, 1996.

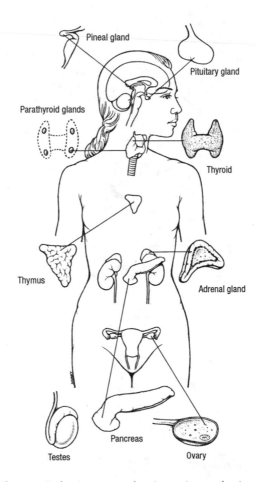

Figure 7. *Endocrine system showing various endocrine organs.*

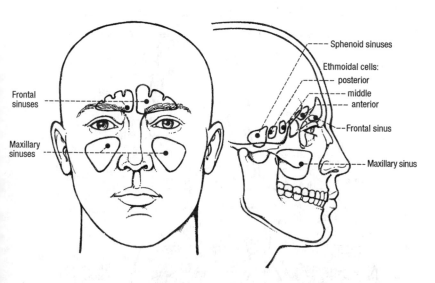

Figure 8. *Anterior and lateral view of head showing the paranasal sinuses.*

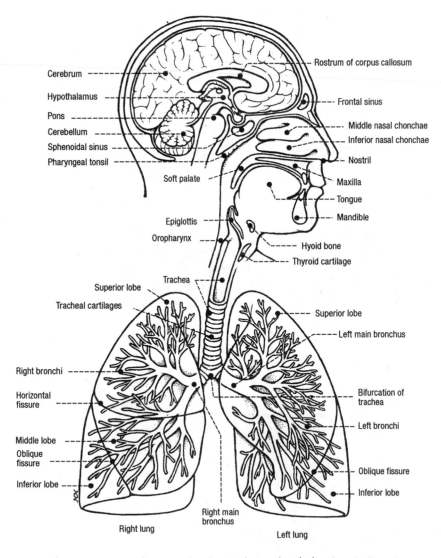

Cerebrum

Hypothalamus

Pons

Cerebellum

Sphenoidal sinus

Pharyngeal tonsil

Soft palate

Epiglottis

Oropharynx

Rostrum of corpus callosum

Frontal sinus

Middle nasal chonchae

Inferior nasal chonchae

Nostril

Maxilla

Tongue

Mandible

Hyoid bone

Thyroid cartilage

Trachea

Superior lobe

Tracheal cartilages

Superior lobe

Left main bronchus

Right bronchi

Horizontal fissure

Middle lobe

Oblique fissure

Inferior lobe

Bifurcation of trachea

Left bronchi

Oblique fissure

Inferior lobe

Right main bronchus

Right lung

Left lung

Figure 9. *Anterior (thorax) and mid-sagittal view (head) showing respiratory anatomy.*

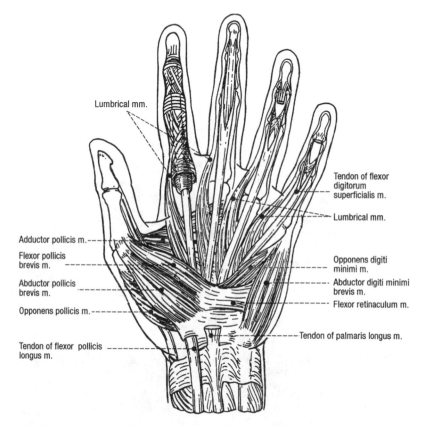

Figure 10. *Superficial muscles of the hand.* From Chung KW. Gross anatomy, 2nd ed. Baltimore: Williams & Wilkins, 1991.

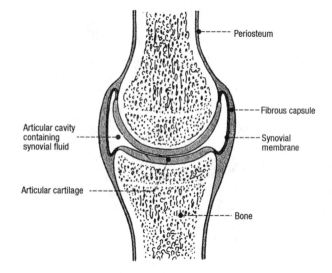

Figure 11. *The features of a typical synovial joint.* From Hall-Craggs ECB. Anatomy, 3rd ed. Baltimore: Williams & Wilkins, 1995.

Dermatology Drugs by Indication

ACNE
Accutane
Akne-Mycin Topical
Ambi 10
A/T/S Topical
azelaic acid
Azelex
Ben-Aqua
Benoxyl
Benzac AC Gel
Benzac AC Wash
Benzac W
Benzamycin
Benzashave
benzoyl peroxide
benzoyl peroxide and hydrocortisone
Brevoxyl
Clear By Design
Clearsil
Cleocin T
clindamycin
Declomycin
Del-Mycin Topical
demeclocycline hydrochloride
Dermoxyl
Desquam-X
Emgel Topical
Erycette Topical
EryDerm Topical
Erygel Topical
Erymax Topical
erythromycin and benzoyl peroxide
erythromycin, topical
E-Solve-2 Topical
ETS-2% Topical
Exact
isotretinoin
Loroxide
Meclan Topical
meclocycline sulfosalicylate

Neutrogena Acne Mask
Novacet Topical
Oxy-5
Oxy-5 Tinted
PanOxyl
PanOxyl-AQ
Peroxin A5
Peroxin A10
Persa-Gel
Retin-A Topical
Staticin Topical
Sulfacet-R Topical
sulfur and sodium sulfacetamide
Theroxide Wash
tretinoin
T-Stat Topical
Vanoxide
Vanoxide-HC

ALOPECIA
Amcort
Aristocort Tablet
Aristospan
Delta-Tritex
Duralutin Injection
hydroxyprogesterone caproate
Hy-Gestrone Injection
Hylutin Injection
Hyprogest Injection
Kenacort Syrup
Kenacort Tablet
Kenalog Injection
minoxidil
Pro-Depo Injection
Prodrox Injection
Rogaine
triamcinolone

AMYLOIDOSIS
acetylcysteine
Mucomyst
Mucosol

ANESTHESIA, INFILTRATION

Anestacon
bupivacaine hydrochloride
Carbocaine Injection
chloroprocaine hydrochloride
Citanest Forte
Citanest Plain
Duranest Injection
etidocaine hydrochloride
Isocaine HCl Injection
lidocaine hydrochloride
mepivacaine hydrochloride
Nervocaine
Nesacaine
Nesacaine-MPF
Novocain Injection
Octocaine
Polocaine Injection
prilocaine
procaine hydrochloride
Sensorcaine
Sensorcaine-MPF
Xylocaine

ANESTHESIA, LOCAL

Anestacon
bupivacaine hydrochloride
Carbocaine Injection
chloroprocaine hydrochloride
Dermaflex Gel
Dilocaine
Duo-Trach
Duranest Injection
etidocaine hydrochloride
Isocaine HCl Injection
lidocaine and epinephrine
lidocaine hydrochloride
LidoPen
Marcaine
mepivacaine hydrochloride
Nervocaine
Nesacaine

Nesacaine-MPF
Novocain Injection
Octocaine
Octocaine Injection
Polocaine Injection
Pontocaine Injection
Pontocaine Topical
procaine hydrochloride
Sensorcaine
Sensorcaine-MPF
tetracaine hydrochloride
tetracaine with dextrose
Xylocaine
Xylocaine With Epinephrine

ANESTHESIA, TOPICAL

benzocaine, butyl aminobenzoate,
    tetracaine, and benzalkonium
    chloride
benzocaine, gelatin, pectin, and
    sodium carboxymethylcellulose
Cetacaine
dichlorodifluoromethane and
    trichloromonofluoromethane
EMLA Topical
ethyl chloride and
    dichlorotetrafluoroethane
Fluori-Methane Topical Spray
Fluro-Ethyl Aerosol
lidocaine and prilocaine
Orabase With Benzocaine

ANTHRAX

Achromycin V Oral
Beepen-VK Oral
Betapen-VK Oral
Bio-Tab Oral
chloramphenicol
Chloromycetin
Crysticillin A.S. Injection
Doryx Oral
Doxychel Injection
Doxychel Oral
doxycycline

Doxy Oral
E.E.S. Oral
E-Mycin Oral
Eryc Oral
EryPed Oral
Ery-Tab Oral
Erythrocin Oral
erythromycin
Ilosone Oral
Ledercillin VK Oral
Monodox Oral
Nor-tet Oral
Panmycin Oral
PCE Oral
penicillin g, parenteral, aqueous
penicillin g procaine
penicillin v potassium
Pen.Vee K Oral
Pfizerpen-AS Injection
Pfizerpen Injection
Robicillin VK Oral
Robitet Oral
Sumycin Oral
Teline Oral
Tetracap Oral
tetracycline
Tetralan Oral
Tetram Oral
V-Cillin K Oral
Veetids Oral
Vibramycin Injection
Vibramycin Oral
Vibra-Tabs
Wycillin Injection

BITES (INSECT)

Aclovate Topical
Aeroseb-Dex
A-hydroCort
Ala-Cort
Ala-Scalp
alclometasone dipropionate
Alphatrex

amcinonide
Amcort
Ana-Kit
Anestacon
Anusol HC-1
Anusol HC-2.5%
Anusol-HC Suppository
betamethasone
Betatrex
Beta-Val
Caldecort
Caldecort Anti-Itch Spray
clobetasol dipropionate
Clocort Maximum Strength
clocortolone pivalate
Cloderm Topical
Cordran SP Topical
Cordran Topical
CortaGel
Cortaid Maximum Strength
Cortaid with Aloe
Cort-Dome
Cortef Feminine Itch
Cortizone-5
Cortizone-10
Cutivate Topical
Cyclocort Topical
Decaspray
Delcort
Deltasone Oral
Delta-Tritex
Dermacort
Dermaflex Gel
Dermarest Dricort
Dermatop
DermiCort
Dermolate
Dermtex HC with Aloe
desonide
DesOwen Topical
desoximetasone
dexamethasone
diflorasone diacetate

Dilocaine
Diprolene
Diprolene AF
Diprosone
Duo-Trach
Eldecort
Elocon Topical
Florone E Topical
Florone Topical
fluocinolone acetonide
fluocinonide
Fluonex Topical
Fluonid Topical
flurandrenolide
Flurosyn Topical
fluticasone propionate
FS Shampoo Topical
Gynecort
halcinonide
Haldrone
halobetasol propionate
Halog-E Topical
Halog Topical
Hi-Cor-1.0
Hi-Cor-2.5
Hycort
Hydrocort
hydrocortisone
Hydrocortone Acetate
HydroSKIN
Hydro-Tex
Hytone
insect sting kit
LactiCare-HC
Lanacort
Lidex-E Topical
Lidex Topical
lidocaine hydrochloride
LidoPen
Liquid Pred Oral
Locoid
Maxidex
Maxiflor Topical

Maxivate
methylprednisolone
Meticorten Oral
mometasone furoate
Neo-Cortef Topical
neomycin and hydrocortisone
Nervocaine
Nutracort
Octocaine
Orabase HCA
Orasone Oral
paramethasone acetate
Penecort
prednicarbate
Prednicen-M Oral
prednisone
Procort
Proctocort
Psorcon Topical
Psorion Cream
Scalpicin
Selestoject
Solurex
S-T Cort
Stemex
Sterapred Oral
Synacort
Synalar-HP Topical
Synalar Topical
Synemol Topical
Tac-3
Tegrin-HC
Teladar
Temovate Topical
Topicort
Topicort-LP
triamcinolone
Tridesilon Topical
Tri-Kort
Trilog
Trilone
Trisoject
U-Cort

Ultravate Topical
Uticort
Valisone
Westcort
Xylocaine

BITES (SPIDER)
antivenin, black widow spider
  (equine)
antivenin (crotalidae) polyvalent
calcium gluconate
Delaxin
diazepam
Dizac Injection
Kalcinate
Marbaxin
methocarbamol
Robaxin
Robomol
Valium Injection
Valium Oral
Valrelease Oral
Zetran Injection

BULLOUS SKIN DISEASE
Auralate
aurothioglucose
azathioprine
cyclophosphamide
Cytoxan Injection
Cytoxan Oral
Deltasone Oral
Folex PFS
gold sodium thiomalate
Imuran
Liquid Pred Oral
methotrexate
Meticorten Oral
Myochrysine
Neosar Injection
Orasone Oral
Prednicen-M Oral
prednisone
Rheumatrex

Silvadene
silver sulfadiazine
Solganal
SSD AF
SSD Cream
Sterapred Oral
Thermazene

BURNS
A and D Ointment
Desitin Topical
Furacin Topical
mafenide acetate
nitrofurazone
Silvadene
silver sulfadiazine
SSD AF
SSD Cream
Sulfamylon Topical
sutilains
Thermazene
Travase Topical
vitamin a and vitamin d
zinc oxide, cod liver oil, and talc

CANDIDIASIS (CUTANEOUS)
ciclopirox olamine
clotrimazole
Dermacomb Topical
econazole nitrate
Fungoid Creme
Fungoid HC Creme
Fungoid Tincture
Gyne-Lotrimin
ketoconazole
Loprox
Lotrimin
Lotrimin AF Cream
Lotrimin AF Lotion
Lotrimin AF Powder
Lotrimin AF Solution
Lotrimin AF Spray Liquid
Lotrimin AF Spray Powder

Maximum Strength Desenex
  Antifungal Cream
Micatin Topical
miconazole
Monistat-Derm Topical
Mycelex
Mycelex-7
Mycelex-G
Mycogen II Topical
Mycolog-II Topical
Myconel Topical
Mycostatin Oral
Mycostatin Topical
Mytrex F Topical
NGT Topical
Nilstat Topical
Nizoral Topical
nystatin
nystatin and triamcinolone
Nystat-Rx
Nystex Topical
Nyst-Olone II Topical
Pedi-Dri
Spectazole Topical
Tri-Statin II Topical
Zeasorb-AF Powder

CANDIDIASIS (MUCOCUTANEOUS)
amphotericin B
Diflucan Oral
fluconazole
Fungizone
ketoconazole
Mycostatin Topical
Nilstat Topical
Nizoral Oral
nystatin
Nystat-Rx
Nystex Topical
Pedi-Dri

CARCINOMA (SKIN)
Adrucil Injection
Blenoxane

bleomycin sulfate
Efudex Topical
Fluoroplex Topical
fluorouracil
Retin-A Topical
tretinoin

CHROMO-BLASTOMYCOSIS
amphotericin B
Fungizone
Fungizone Intravenous
ketoconazole
Nizoral Oral

CRYPTOCOCCOSIS
amphotericin B
Ancobon
Diflucan Injection
Diflucan Oral
fluconazole
flucytosine
Fungizone
Fungizone Intravenous

DANDRUFF
AquaTar
Aveeno Cleansing Bar
Balnetar
Capitrol
chloroxine
coal tar
coal tar and salicylic acid
coal tar, lanolin, and mineral oil
Denorex
DHS Tar
DHS Zinc
Duplex T
Estar
Exsel
Fostex
Fototar
Head & Shoulders
Metasep

Neutrogena T/Derm
parachlorometaxylenol
Pentrax
Pernox
Polytar
psoriGel
pyrithione zinc
Sastid Plain Therapeutic Shampoo
  and Acne Wash
Sebulex
Sebulon
selenium sulfide
Selsun
Selsun Blue
Selsun Gold for Women
sulfur and salicylic acid
T/Gel
Theraplex Z
X-seb T
Zetar
Zincon Shampoo
ZNP Bar

DEBRIDE CALLOUS TISSUE
Tri-Chlor
trichloroacetic acid

DEBRIDEMENT OF ESCHAR
Granulex
trypsin, balsam peru, and castor oil

DECUBITUS ULCERS
Biozyme-C
collagenase
Debrisan Topical
dextranomer
Elase-Chloromycetin Topical
Elase Topical
fibrinolysin and desoxyribonuclease
Granulex
Santyl
sutilains

Travase Topical
trypsin, balsam peru, and castor oil

DERMATOMYCOSIS
amphotericin B
Fulvicin P/G
Fulvicin-U/F
Fungizone
Fungizone Intravenous
Fungoid Creme
Fungoid HC Creme
Fungoid Tincture
Grifulvin V
Grisactin
Grisactin Ultra
griseofulvin
Gris-PEG
ketoconazole
Lotrimin AF Powder
Lotrimin AF Spray Liquid
Lotrimin AF Spray Powder
Maximum Strength Desenex
  Antifungal Cream
Micatin Topical
miconazole
Monistat-Derm Topical
naftifine hydrochloride
Naftin Topical
Nizoral Oral
Nizoral Topical
oxiconazole nitrate
Oxistat Topical
Zeasorb-AF Powder

DERMATOSIS
Aclovate Topical
Aeroseb-Dex
A-hydroCort
Ala-Cort
Ala-Scalp
alclometasone dipropionate
Alphatrex
amcinonide
betamethasone

Betatrex
Beta-Val
Caldecort
Carmol-HC Topical
clobetasol dipropionate
Clocort Maximum Strength
clocortolone pivalate
Cloderm Topical
Cordran SP Topical
Cordran Topical
CortaGel
Cortaid Maximum Strength
Cortaid with Aloe
Cort-Dome
Cortizone-5
Cortizone-10
Cutivate Topical
Cyclocort Topical
Decaspray
Delcort
Delta-Tritex
Dermacort
Dermarest Dricort
Dermatop
DermiCort
Dermolate
Dermtex HC with Aloe
desonide
DesOwen Topical
desoximetasone
dexamethasone
diflorasone diacetate
Diprolene
Diprolene AF
Diprosone
Eldecort
Elocon Topical
Florone E Topical
Florone Topical
fluocinolone acetonide
fluocinonide
Fluonex Topical
Fluonid Topical

flurandrenolide
Flurosyn Topical
fluticasone propionate
Gynecort
halcinonide
halobetasol propionate
Halog-E Topical
Halog Topical
Hi-Cor-1.0
Hi-Cor-2.5
Hycort
Hydrocort
hydrocortisone
Hydrocortone Acetate
HydroSKIN
Hydro-Tex
Hytone
LactiCare-HC
Lanacort
Lida-Mantle HC Topical
Lidex-E Topical
Lidex Topical
lidocaine and hydrocortisone
Locoid
Maxidex
Maxiflor Topical
Maxivate
methylprednisolone
mometasone furoate
Neo-Cortef Topical
neomycin and hydrocortisone
Nutracort
Penecort
prednicarbate
Procort
Proctocort
Psorcon Topical
Psorion Cream
Scalpicin
Solurex
S-T Cort
Synacort
Synalar-HP Topical

Synalar Topical
Synemol Topical
Teladar
Temovate Topical
Topicort
Topicort-LP
triamcinolone
Tridesilon Topical
Trisoject
U-Cort
Ultravate Topical
urea and hydrocortisone
Uticort
Valisone
Westcort

DISCOID LUPUS ERYTHEMATOSUS (DLE)

Aclovate Topical
alclometasone dipropionate
Alphatrex
amcinonide
Amcort
Aralen Phosphate
betamethasone
Betatrex
Beta-Val
chloroquine phosphate
clobetasol dipropionate
clocortolone pivalate
Cloderm Topical
Cordran SP Topical
Cordran Topical
CortaGel
Cort-Dome
Cutivate Topical
Cyclocort Topical
Dermacort
Dermatop
DermiCort
Dermolate
desonide
DesOwen Topical

desoximetasone
dexamethasone
diflorasone diacetate
Diprolene
Diprolene AF
Diprosone
Eldecort
Elocon Topical
Florone E Topical
Florone Topical
fluocinolone acetonide
fluocinonide
Fluonex Topical
Fluonid Topical
flurandrenolide
Flurosyn Topical
fluticasone propionate
Gynecort
halcinonide
halobetasol propionate
Halog-E Topical
Halog Topical
Hycort
Hydrocort
hydrocortisone
Hydrocortone Acetate
HydroSKIN
Hydro-Tex
hydroxychloroquine sulfate
Hytone
LactiCare-HC
Lanacort
Lidex-E Topical
Lidex Topical
Locoid
Maxidex
Maxiflor Topical
Maxivate
methylprednisolone
mometasone furoate
Neo-Cortef Topical
neomycin and hydrocortisone
Nutracort

Orabase HCA
Penecort
Plaquenil
prednicarbate
Procort
Proctocort
Psorcon Topical
Psorion Cream
Scalpicin
Selestoject
Solurex
S-T Cort
Synacort
Synalar-HP Topical
Synalar Topical
Synemol Topical
Tegrin-HC
Teladar
Temovate Topical
Topicort
Topicort-LP
triamcinolone
Tridesilon Topical
U-Cort
Ultravate Topical
Uticort
Valisone
Westcort

DRY SKIN

Amino-Opti-E Oral
Aquacare Topical
Aquasol E Oral
camphor, menthol and phenol
Carmol Topical
Gormel Creme
Lac-Hydrin
lactic acid and sodium-PCA
lactic acid with ammonium hydroxide
LactiCare
Lanaphilic Topical
lanolin, cetyl alcohol, glycerin, and
    petrolatum
Lubriderm

Nutraplus Topical
Rea-Lo
Sarna
Ultra Mide Topical
urea
Ureacin-20 Topical
Ureacin-40 Topical
Ureaphil Injection
vitamin e
Vitec Topical

ECZEMA

Aclovate Topical
Aeroseb-Dex
A-hydroCort
Ala-Cort
Ala-Quin Topical
Ala-Scalp
alclometasone dipropionate
Alphatrex
amcinonide
Amcort
AquaTar
Baldex
betamethasone
Betatrex
Caldecort
Cel-U-Jec
clioquinol and hydrocortisone
clobetasol dipropionate
Clocort Maximum Strength
clocortolone pivalate
Cloderm Topical
coal tar
coal tar and salicylic acid
Cordran SP Topical
Cordran Topical
Corque Topical
CortaGel
Cortaid Maximum Strength
Cortaid with Aloe
Cort-Dome
Cortin Topical
Cortizone-5

Cortizone-10
Cutivate Topical
Cyclocort Topical
Dalalone
Decadron
Delcort
Delta-Tritex
Denorex
Dermacort
Dermarest Dricort
Derma-Smoothe/FS Topical
Dermatop
DermiCort
Dermolate
Dermtex HC with Aloe
desonide
DesOwen Topical
desoximetasone
dexamethasone
DHS Tar
diflorasone diacetate
Diprolene
Diprolene AF
Diprosone
Duplex T
Eldecort
Elocon Topical
Estar
Florone E Topical
Florone Topical
fluocinolone acetonide
fluocinonide
Fluonex Topical
Fluonid Topical
flurandrenolide
Flurosyn Topical
fluticasone propionate
Fototar
FS Shampoo Topical
Gynecort
halcinonide
halobetasol propionate
Halog-E Topical

Halog Topical
Hi-Cor-1.0
Hi-Cor-2.5
Hycort
Hydrocort
hydrocortisone
HydroSKIN
Hydro-Tex
Hysone Topical
Hytone
I-Methasone
iodoquinol and hydrocortisone
Kenonel
Lanvisone Topical
Lidex-E Topical
Lidex Topical
Locoid
Maxiflor Topical
Maxivate
methylprednisolone
mometasone furoate
Neo-Cortef Topical
neomycin and hydrocortisone
Neutrogena T/Derm
Nutracort
Orabase HCA
Pedi-Cort V Topical
Penecort
Pentrax
Polytar
prednicarbate
Procort
Proctocort
Psorcon Topical
psoriGel
Psorion Cream
Racet Topical
Scalpicin
Synacort
Synalar-HP Topical
Synalar Topical
Synemol Topical
Tegrin-HC

Teladar
Temovate Topical
T/Gel
Topicort
Topicort-LP
triamcinolone
Tridesilon Topical
UAD Topical
Ultravate Topical
Uticort
Valisone
Vytone Topical
Westcort
X-seb T
Zetar

EPIDERMOLYSIS BULLOSA
Dilantin
Diphenylan Sodium
phenytoin

EPITHELIOMATOSIS
Pod-Ben-25
Podocon-25
Podofin
podophyllum resin

ERYSIPELAS
Beepen-VK Oral
Betapen-VK Oral
Crysticillin A.S. Injection
E.E.S. Oral
E-Mycin Oral
Eryc Oral
EryPed Oral
Ery-Tab Oral
Erythrocin Oral
erythromycin
Ilosone Oral
Ledercillin VK Oral
PCE Oral
penicillin g, parenteral, aqueous
penicillin g procaine

penicillin v potassium
Pen.Vee K Oral
Pfizerpen-AS Injection
Pfizerpen Injection
Robicillin VK Oral
V-Cillin K Oral
Veetids Oral
Wycillin Injection

ERYSIPELOID
Ancef
cefazolin sodium
Cleocin HCl
Cleocin Pediatric
Cleocin Phosphate
clindamycin
Kefzol
penicillin g, parenteral, aqueous
Pfizerpen Injection
Zolicef

ERYTHROPOIETIC PROTOPORPHYRIA (EPP)
beta-carotene
Max-Caro
Provatene
Solatene

FANCONI SYNDROME
Bicitra
Oracit
sodium bicarbonate
sodium citrate and citric acid

FURUNCULOSIS
Bactocill Injection
Bactocill Oral
Cleocin HCl
Cleocin Pediatric
Cleocin Phosphate
clindamycin
dicloxacillin sodium
Dycill
Dynapen
E.E.S. Oral

E-Mycin Oral
Eryc Oral
EryPed Oral
Ery-Tab Oral
Erythrocin Oral
erythromycin
Ilosone Oral
Nafcil Injection
nafcillin sodium
Nallpen Injection
oxacillin sodium
Pathocil
PCE Oral
Prostaphlin Injection
Prostaphlin Oral
Unipen Injection
Unipen Oral

GRANULOMA (INGUINALE)

Achromycin V Oral
ampicillin
Bactrim
Bactrim DS
Bio-Tab Oral
Cotrim
Cotrim DS
co-trimoxazole
Doryx Oral
Doxychel Injection
Doxychel Oral
doxycycline
Doxy Oral
Garamycin Injection
gentamicin sulfate
Jenamicin Injection
Marcillin
Monodox Oral
Nor-tet Oral
Omnipen
Omnipen-N
Panmycin Oral
Polycillin

Polycillin-N
Principen
Robitet Oral
Septra
Septra DS
streptomycin sulfate
Sulfamethoprim
Sulfatrim
Sulfatrim DS
Sumycin Oral
Teline Oral
Tetracap Oral
tetracycline
Tetralan Oral
Tetram Oral
Totacillin
Totacillin-N
Uroplus DS
Uroplus SS
Vibramycin Injection
Vibramycin Oral
Vibra-Tabs

HARTNUP DISEASE

Niacels
niacin
niacinamide
Nicobid
Nicolar
Nicotinex
Slo-Niacin

HERPES SIMPLEX

acyclovir
Cytovene
foscarnet
Foscavir Injection
ganciclovir
Herplex Ophthalmic
idoxuridine
trifluridine
vidarabine
Vira-A Ophthalmic
Viroptic Ophthalmic

Zovirax Injection
Zovirax Oral
Zovirax Topical

HERPES ZOSTER
acyclovir
capsaicin
Capsin
Capzasin-P
famciclovir
Famvir
No Pain-HP
R-Gel
valacyclovir
Valtrex
vidarabine
Vira-A Ophthalmic
Zostrix
Zostrix-HP
Zovirax Injection
Zovirax Oral
Zovirax Topical

ICHTHYOSIS
Duofilm Solution
Keralyt Gel
salicylic acid and lactic acid
salicylic acid and propylene glycol

IMPETIGO
bacitracin, neomycin, and
    polymyxin b
Bactroban Topical
Beepen-VK Oral
Betapen-VK Oral
Crysticillin A.S. Injection
E.E.S. Oral
E-Mycin Oral
Eryc Oral
EryPed Oral
Ery-Tab Oral
Erythrocin Oral
erythromycin
Ilosone Oral

Ledercillin VK Oral
Medi-Quick Topical Ointment
mupirocin
Mycitracin Topical
Neomixin Topical
Neosporin Topical Ointment
Ocutricin Topical Ointment
PCE Oral
penicillin g procaine
penicillin v potassium
Pen.Vee K Oral
Pfizerpen-AS Injection
Robicillin VK Oral
Septa Topical Ointment
Triple Antibiotic Topical
V-Cillin K Oral
Veetids Oral
Wycillin Injection

KALA-AZAR
amphotericin B
Fungizone
Fungizone Intravenous
NebuPent Inhalation
Pentacarinat Injection
Pentam-300 Injection
pentamidine isethionate

KAWASAKI DISEASE
Anacin
Arthritis Foundation Pain Reliever
A.S.A.
Ascriptin
aspirin
Asprimox
Bayer Aspirin
Bayer Buffered Aspirin
Bayer Low Adult Strength
Bufferin
Easprin
Ecotrin
Empirin
Extra Strength Bayer Enteric 500
    Aspirin

Gamastan
Gamimune N
Gammagard S/D
Gammar
Gensan
Halfprin 81
immune globulin, intramuscular
immune globulin, intravenous
Measurin
pentoxifylline
Polygam S/D
Sandoglobulin
St. Joseph Adult Chewable Aspirin
Trental
Venoglobulin-I
Venoglobulin-S
ZORprin

KERATOSIS (ACTINIC)

Actinex Topical
masoprocol

KERATOSIS PALMARIS

Duofilm Solution
Keralyt Gel
salicylic acid and lactic acid
salicylic acid and propylene glycol

LEPROSY

Avlosulfon
clofazimine palmitate
dapsone
Lamprene

LICE

A-200 Pyrinate
Elimite Cream
End Lice
G-well Lotion
G-well Shampoo
Kwell Cream
Kwell Lotion
Kwell Shampoo
Lice-Enz
lindane

Nix Creme Rinse
permethrin
pyrethrins
Pyrinyl II
RID
Scabene Lotion
Scabene Shampoo
Tisit

LYMPHOGRANULOMA (VENEREUM)

Achromycin V Oral
Bactrim
Bactrim DS
Bio-Tab Oral
Cotrim
Cotrim DS
co-trimoxazole
Doryx Oral
Doxychel Injection
Doxychel Oral
doxycycline
Doxy Oral
E.E.S. Oral
E-Mycin Oral
Eryc Oral
EryPed Oral
Ery-Tab Oral
Erythrocin Oral
erythromycin
Ilosone Oral
Monodox Oral
Nor-tet Oral
Panmycin Oral
PCE Oral
Robitet Oral
Septra
Septra DS
Sulfamethoprim
Sulfatrim
Sulfatrim DS
Sumycin Oral
Teline Oral

Tetracap Oral
tetracycline
Tetralan Oral
Tetram Oral
Uroplus DS
Uroplus SS
Vibramycin Injection
Vibramycin Oral
Vibra-Tabs

MELANOMA

Blenoxane
bleomycin sulfate
CeeNU Oral
cisplatin
Cosmegen
dacarbazine
dactinomycin
DTIC-Dome
Hydrea
hydroxyurea
interferon alfa-2a
interferon alfa-2b
Intron A
lomustine
Platinol
Platinol-AQ
Roferon-A
teniposide
Vumon Injection

MYCOSIS (FUNGOIDES)

Adlone Injection
Alkaban-AQ
A-methaPred Injection
Articulose-50 Injection
betamethasone
Celestone Soluspan
Cel-U-Jec
Cortef
cortisone acetate
Cortone Acetate Injection
Cortone Acetate Oral
cyclophosphamide

Cytoxan Injection
Cytoxan Oral
Dalalone
Dalalone D.P.
Dalalone L.A.
Decadron
Decadron-LA
Decadron Phosphate
Decaject
Decaject-LA
Delta-Cortef Oral
Deltasone Oral
depMedalone Injection
Depoject Injection
Depo-Medrol Injection
Depopred Injection
dexamethasone
Dexasone
Dexasone L.A.
Dexone
Dexone LA
D-Med Injection
Duralone Injection
Florinef Acetate
fludrocortisone acetate
Folex PFS
Hexadrol
Hexadrol Phosphate
Hydeltrasol Injection
Hydeltra-T.B.A. Injection
hydrocortisone
Hydrocortone Acetate
Hydrocortone Phosphate
I-Methasone
Key-Pred Injection
Key-Pred-SP Injection
Liquid Pred Oral
mechlorethamine hydrochloride
Medralone Injection
Medrol Oral
methotrexate
methoxsalen
methylprednisolone

Meticorten Oral
M-Prednisol Injection
Mustargen Hydrochloride
Neosar Injection
Nutracort
Orasone Oral
Oxsoralen Topical
Oxsoralen-Ultra Oral
Pediapred Oral
Predaject Injection
Predalone Injection
Predcor Injection
Predicort-50 Injection
Prednicen-M Oral
prednisolone
Prednisol TBA Injection
prednisone
Prelone Oral
Rheumatrex
Selestoject
Solu-Cortef
Solu-Medrol Injection
Solurex
Solurex L.A.
Sterapred Oral
Teladar
Velban
vinblastine sulfate

OILY SKIN
Aveeno Cleansing Bar
Fostex
Pernox
Sastid Plain Therapeutic Shampoo
    and Acne Wash
Sebulex
sulfur and salicylic acid

ONYCHOMYCOSIS
Fulvicin P/G
Fulvicin-U/F
Grifulvin V
Grisactin
Grisactin Ultra
griseofulvin

Gris-PEG
Lamisil tablet
terbinafine hydrochloride tablet

OTITIS EXTERNA, SEVERE (MALIGNANT)
ceftazidime
Ceptaz
ciprofloxacin hydrochloride
Cipro Injection
Cipro Oral
Fortaz
Pentacef
Tazicef
Tazidime

PAPILLITIS
Acthar
Adlone Injection
Amcort
A-methaPred Injection
Aristocort Forte
Aristocort Intralesional Suspension
Aristocort Tablet
Aristospan
Articulose-50 Injection
betamethasone
Celestone
Celestone Soluspan
Cortef
corticotropin
cortisone acetate
Cortone Acetate Injection
Cortone Acetate Oral
Decadron
Decadron Phosphate
Decaject
Decaject-LA
Delta-Cortef Oral
Deltasone Oral
depMedalone Injection
Depoject Injection
Depo-Medrol Injection
Depopred Injection
dexamethasone

Dexasone
Dexasone L.A.
Dexone
Dexone LA
D-Med Injection
Duralone Injection
Haldrone
Hexadrol
Hexadrol Phosphate
H.P. Acthar Gel
Hydeltrasol Injection
Hydeltra-T.B.A. Injection
hydrocortisone
Hydrocortone Acetate
Hydrocortone Phosphate
I-Methasone
Kenacort Syrup
Kenacort Tablet
Kenalog Injection
Key-Pred Injection
Key-Pred-SP Injection
LactiCare-HC
Liquid Pred Oral
Medralone Injection
Medrol Oral
methylprednisolone
Meticorten Oral
M-Prednisol Injection
paramethasone acetate
Pediapred Oral
Predaject Injection
Predalone Injection
Predcor Injection
Predicort-50 Injection
Prednicen-M Oral
prednisolone
Prednisol TBA Injection
prednisone
Prelone Oral
Procort
Selestoject
Solu-Cortef
Solu-Medrol Injection

Solurex
Solurex L.A.
Sterapred Oral
Tac-3

PARACOC-CIDIOIDOMYCOSIS
ketoconazole
Nizoral Oral

PELLAGRA
Niacels
niacin
Nicobid
Nicolar
Nicotinex
Slo-Niacin

PEMPHIGUS
Acthar
Adlone Injection
Amcort
A-methaPred Injection
Aralen Phosphate
Aristocort Forte
Aristocort Intralesional Suspension
Aristocort Tablet
Aristospan
Articulose-50 Injection
betamethasone
Celestone
Celestone Soluspan
chloroquine phosphate
Cortef
corticotropin
cortisone acetate
Cortone Acetate Injection
Cortone Acetate Oral
Decadron
Decadron Phosphate
Decaject
Decaject-LA
Delta-Cortef Oral
Deltasone Oral

depMedalone Injection
Depoject Injection
Depo-Medrol Injection
Depopred Injection
dexamethasone
Dexasone
Dexasone L.A.
Dexone
Dexone LA
D-Med Injection
Duralone Injection
Haldrone
Hexadrol
Hexadrol Phosphate
H.P. Acthar Gel
Hydeltrasol Injection
Hydeltra-T.B.A. Injection
hydrocortisone
Hydrocortone Acetate
Hydrocortone Phosphate
I-Methasone
Kenacort Syrup
Kenacort Tablet
Kenalog Injection
Key-Pred Injection
Key-Pred-SP Injection
LactiCare-HC
Liquid Pred Oral
Medralone Injection
Medrol Oral
methylprednisolone
Meticorten Oral
M-Prednisol Injection
paramethasone acetate
Pediapred Oral
Predaject Injection
Predalone Injection
Predcor Injection
Predicort-50 Injection
Prednicen-M Oral
prednisolone
Prednisol TBA Injection
prednisone

Prelone Oral
Procort
Selestoject
Solu-Cortef
Solu-Medrol Injection
Solurex
Solurex L.A.
Sterapred Oral
Tac-3

PHYCOMYCOSIS
amphotericin B
Fungizone
Fungizone Intravenous

PINTA
Bicillin L-A Injection
Crysticillin A.S. Injection
penicillin g benzathine
penicillin g procaine
Permapen Injection
Pfizerpen-AS Injection
Wycillin Injection

PLANTAR WARTS
Duofilm Solution
salicylic acid and lactic acid
silver nitrate

PROTECTANT (SKIN)
AeroZoin
benzoin
TinBen
TinCoBen

PRURITUS
Aller-Chlor Oral
AllerMax Oral
Antihist-1
Anxanil
astemizole
Atarax
Atozine
azatadine maleate
Banophen Oral

Belix Oral
Benadryl Oral
Benadryl Topical
Bromarest
Bromphen Elixir
brompheniramine maleate
Chlo-Amine Oral
Chlorate Oral
Chlorphed
chlorpheniramine maleate
Chlor-Trimeton Oral
Claritin
clemastine fumarate
crotamiton
cyproheptadine hydrochloride
Dexchlor
dexchlorpheniramine maleate
Diamine T.D. Oral
Dimetane Oral
diphenhydramine hydrochloride
Dormin Oral
Durrax
Efidac 24 Chlorpheniramine
Eurax Topical
E-Vista
Genahist Oral
Hismanal
Hydramyn Syrup
hydroxyzine
Hy-Pam
Hyzine-50
loratadine
Neucalm
Nidryl Oral
Nolahist
Nordryl Oral
Optimine
PBZ
PBZ-SR
Periactin
Phenameth Oral
Phendry Oral
Phenergan Oral

Phenetron Oral
phenindamine tartrate
Poladex
Polaramine
promethazine hydrochloride
Prothazine Oral
Quiess
Rezine
Seldane
Sleep-eze 3 Oral
Sleepinal
Sominex Oral
Tavist
Tavist-1
Telachlor Oral
Teldrin Oral
Temaril
terfenadine
trimeprazine tartrate
tripelennamine
Veltane Tablet
Vistaril

PSORIASIS

Aclovate Topical
Aeroseb-Dex
A-hydroCort
Ala-Cort
Ala-Scalp
alclometasone dipropionate
Alphatrex
amcinonide
Amcort
Anthra-Derm
anthralin
Balnetar
betamethasone
Betatrex
Beta-Val
Caldecort
Clear Away Disc
clobetasol dipropionate
Clocort Maximum Strength

clocortolone pivalate
Cloderm Topical
coal tar, lanolin, and mineral oil
Cordran SP Topical
Cordran Topical
CortaGel
Cortaid Maximum Strength
Cortaid with Aloe
Cort-Dome
Cortizone-5
Cortizone-10
Cutivate Topical
Cyclocort Topical
Decaspray
Delcort
Delta-Tritex
Dermacort
Dermarest Dricort
Dermatop
DermiCort
Dermolate
Dermtex HC with Aloe
desonide
DesOwen Topical
desoximetasone
dexamethasone
diflorasone diacetate
Diprolene
Diprolene AF
Diprosone
Drithocreme
Dritho-Scalp
Eldecort
Elocon Topical
etretinate
Florone E Topical
Florone Topical
fluocinolone acetonide
fluocinonide
Fluonex Topical
Fluonid Topical
flurandrenolide
Flurosyn Topical

fluticasone propionate
Folex PFS
Freezone Solution
FS Shampoo Topical
Gordofilm Liquid
Gynecort
halcinonide
halobetasol propionate
Halog-E Topical
Halog Topical
Hi-Cor-1.0
Hi-Cor-2.5
Hycort
Hydrocort
hydrocortisone
Hydrocortone Acetate
HydroSKIN
Hydro-Tex
Hytone
Keralyt Gel
LactiCare-HC
Lanacort
Lidex-E Topical
Lidex Topical
Locoid
Maxiflor Topical
Maxivate
Mediplast Plaster
methotrexate
methoxsalen
methylprednisolone
mometasone furoate
Neo-Cortef Topical
neomycin and hydrocortisone
Nutracort
Occlusal-HP Liquid
Orabase HCA
Oxsoralen Topical
Oxsoralen-Ultra Oral
Panscol Lotion
Panscol Ointment
PediaPatch Transdermal Patch
Penecort

prednicarbate
Procort
Proctocort
Psorcon Topical
Psorion Cream
P&S Shampoo
Rheumatrex
Salacid Ointment
Sal-Acid Plaster
salicylic acid
salicylic acid and propylene glycol
Scalpicin
Synacort
Synalar-HP Topical
Synalar Topical
Synemol Topical
Tac-3
Tegison
Tegrin-HC
Teladar
Temovate Topical
Topicort
Topicort-LP
Trans-Plantar Transdermal Patch
Trans-Ver-Sal Transdermal Patch
   Verukan Solution
triamcinolone
Tridesilon Topical
Tri-Kort
Trilog
Trilone
U-Cort
Ultravate Topical
Uticort
Valisone
Vergogel Gel
Westcort

SCABIES
crotamiton
Elimite Cream
Eurax Topical
G-well Lotion
G-well Shampoo

Kwell Cream
Kwell Lotion
Kwell Shampoo
lindane
Nix Creme Rinse
permethrin
Scabene Lotion
Scabene Shampoo

SEBORRHEIC DERMATITIS
AquaTar
Aveeno Cleansing Bar
Balnetar
Capitrol
chloroxine
Clear Away Disc
coal tar
coal tar and salicylic acid
coal tar, lanolin, and mineral oil
Denorex
DHS Tar
DHS Zinc
Duplex T
Estar
Exsel
Fostex
Fototar
Freezone Solution
Gordofilm Liquid
Head & Shoulders
Mediplast Plaster
Neutrogena T/Derm
Novacet Topical
Occlusal-HP Liquid
Panscol Lotion
Panscol Ointment
PediaPatch Transdermal Patch
Pentrax
Pernox
Polytar
psoriGel
P&S Shampoo
pyrithione zinc

Salacid Ointment
Sal-Acid Plaster
salicylic acid
Sastid Plain Therapeutic Shampoo
  and Acne Wash
Sebulex
Sebulon
selenium sulfide
Selsun
Selsun Blue
Selsun Gold for Women
Sulfacet-R Topical
sulfur and salicylic acid
sulfur and sodium sulfacetamide
T/Gel
Theraplex Z
Trans-Plantar Transdermal Patch
Trans-Ver-Sal Transdermal Patch
  Verukan Solution
Vergogel Gel
X-seb T
Zetar
Zincon Shampoo
ZNP Bar

SKIN INFECTION (TOPICAL THERAPY)

Aeroaid
Aquaphor Antibiotic Topical
Baciguent Topical
bacitracin
bacitracin and polymyxin b
bacitracin, neomycin, and polymyxin b
bacitracin, neomycin, polymyxin b,
  and hydrocortisone
bacitracin, neomycin, polymyxin B,
  and lidocaine
BactoShield Topical
Bactroban Topical
Betadine
Betadine First Aid Antibiotics +
  Moisturizer
Campho-Phenique

camphor and phenol
chlorhexidine gluconate
Clomycin
Clorpactin WCS-90
Cortisporin Topical Cream
Cortisporin Topical Ointment
Dyna-Hex Topical
Efodine
Exidine Scrub
Garamycin Topical
gentamicin sulfate
G-myticin Topical
hexachlorophene
Hibiclens Topical
Hibistat Topical
Iodex Regular
Isodine
Medi-Quick Topical Ointment
merbromin
Mercurochrome
Mersol
Merthiolate
mupirocin
Mycifradin Sulfate Topical
Mycitracin Topical
Neomixin Topical
neomycin and polymyxin b
neomycin, polymyxin b, and
  hydrocortisone
neomycin sulfate
Neosporin Cream
Neosporin Topical Ointment
Ocutricin Topical Ointment
oxychlorosene sodium
pHisoHex
polymyxin b sulfate
Polysporin Topical
povidone-iodine
Septa Topical Ointment
Septisol
thimerosal
Triple Antibiotic Topical
Yeast-Gard Medicated Douche

A33

SKIN ULCER
Biozyme-C
collagenase
Debrisan Topical
dextranomer
Elase-Chloromycetin Topical
Elase Topical
fibrinolysin and desoxyribonuclease
Santyl
sutilains
Travase Topical

SPOROTRICHOSIS
amphotericin B
Fungizone
Fungizone Intravenous

SUN OVEREXPOSURE
methoxycinnamate and oxybenzone
PreSun 29
Ti-Screen

TINEA
Absorbine Jr. Antifungal
Absorbine Jock Itch
Aftate
benzoic acid and salicylic acid
betamethasone and clotrimazole
Blis-To-Sol
Breezee Mist Antifungal
Caldesene Topical
carbol-fuchsin solution
ciclopirox olamine
clioquinol
clotrimazole
Cruex Topical
Desenex
Dr Scholl's Athlete's Foot
Dr Scholl's Maximum Strength Tritin
econazole nitrate
Exelderm Topical
Fulvicin-U/F
Fulvicin P/G
Fungoid

Fungoid Tincture
Fungoid Creme
Fungoid HC Creme
Fungoid Tincture
Fungoid Topical Solution
Genaspor
Grifulvin V
Gris-PEG
Grisactin
Grisactin Ultra
griseofulvin
Gyne-Lotrimin
haloprogin
Halotex Topical
ketoconazole
Lamisil topical cream
Loprox
Lotrimin
Lotrimin AF Cream
Lotrimin AF Lotion
Lotrimin AF Powder
Lotrimin AF Solution
Lotrimin AF Spray Liquid
Lotrimin AF Spray Powder
Lotrisone
Maximum Strength Desenex
    Antifungal Cream
Merlenate Topical
Micatin Topical
miconazole
Monistat-Derm Topical
Monistat Vaginal
Mycelex
Mycelex-G
Mycelex-7
naftifine hydrochloride
Naftin Topical
Nizoral Topical
NP-27
Ony-Clear Nail
oxiconazole nitrate
Oxistat Topical
Pedi-Pro Topical

Quinsana Plus Topical
sodium hypochlorite solution
Spectazole Topical
sulconazole nitrate
Sulcosyn Topical
terbinafine hydrochloride cream
Tinactin
tolnaftate
triacetin
undecylenic acid and derivatives
Undoguent Topical
Vioform Topical
Whitfield's Ointment
Zeasorb-AF
Zeasorb-AF Powder

TINEA (VERSICOLOR)

ciclopirox olamine
clotrimazole
econazole nitrate
Exsel
Gyne-Lotrimin
haloprogin
Halotex Topical
ketoconazole
Loprox
Lotrimin
Micatin Topical
miconazole
Mycelex
Nizoral Topical
selenium sulfide
Selsun
Selsun Blue
Selsun Gold for Women

sodium thiosulfate
Spectazole Topical
sulconazole nitrate
Sulcosyn Topical
Tinver Lotion
tolnaftate

TISSUE GRAFT

muromonab-CD3
Orthoclone OKT3

VITILIGO

Benoquin
methoxsalen
monobenzone
Oxsoralen Topical
Oxsoralen-Ultra Oral
trioxsalen
Trisoralen Oral

YAWS

Achromycin V Oral
Bicillin L-A Injection
chloramphenicol
Chloromycetin
Nor-tet Oral
Panmycin Oral
penicillin g benzathine
Permapen Injection
Robitet Oral
Sumycin Oral
Teline Oral
Tetracap Oral
tetracycline
Tetralan Oral
Tetram Oral

Common Related Combining Forms

aden/o a gland, glandular
adip/o fat, fatty
adren/o adrenal gland
andr/o masculine
ankyl/o bent, crooked, stiff
arthr/o a joint, an articulation
articul/o relating to the joint
blast/o budding by cells or tissue
brachi/o arm
cervic/o neck
chondr/o cartilage
chrom/o color
chyl/o juice
cost/o rib
crani/o cranium (skull)
crin/o to secrete
cutane/o skin
dactyl/o the fingers, the toes
dermat/o skin
derm/o skin
diaphor/o profuse sweating
dips/o thirst
erythr/o red, redness
fasci/o fascia (a band)
femor/o femur
fibr/o fiber
gluc/o glucose (sugar)
glyc/o sugars
hemat/o blood
hem/o blood
hidr/o sweat, sweat glands
hist/o tissue
histi/o tissue
hormon/o hormone
immun/o immune, safe
kerat/o hard
ket/o ketone bodies
keton/o ketone bodies
kyph/o humped
lei/o smooth
leuk/o white, white blood cells

lip/o fatty, lipid
lord/o bent
lumb/o loin (lower back)
lymph/o lymph (clear fluid)
melan/o black
muscul/o muscle
myc/o fungus
myel/o bone marrow or spinal cord
my/o muscle
onych/o fingernail, toenail
oste/o bone
pancreat/o pancreas
patell/o kneecap
pelv/i pelvis
phag/o eating, devouring
plas/o formation
plasm/o formative, organized
purpur/o purple
radi/o radius
reticul/o reticulum, a net
rhabd/o rod, rod shaped
sarc/o muscular substance, flesh
scoli/o twisted
seb/o sebum (oil), sebaceous
splen/o the spleen
spondyl/o the vertebrae
squam/o scale
steat/o fat
stern/o the sternum
tendin/o tendon
tend/o tendon
ten/o tendon
thorac/o the chest, the thorax
thromb/o blood clot
thym/o thymus gland
thyr/o thyroid gland
ton/o tone, tension, pressure
trich/o hair
uln/o ulna
vertebr/o vertebra
xanth/o yellow, yellowish
xer/o dry

Common Allergens

Dander (epithelia)
cat
cattle
chicken feather
cockatiel feather
cow
deer hair
dog
duck feather
ferret
French poodle
gerbil
goat
goose feather
guinea pig
hamster
horse hair
mixed feathers
mohair
monkey
moth
mouse
rabbit
rat
sheep
silk
swine
turkey feather

Environmental
acacia
Acarus
aerosol sprays
automobile exhaust
barn dust
Bermuda smut
cat
cigarette smoke
cotton linters
cottonseed

Dermatophagoides
dog
elevator grain dust mite
flaxseed
grain dust
house dust
house dust mite F (Dermatophagoides farinae)
house dust mite P (Dermatophagoides pteronyssinus)
jute
kapok
karaya
mite
newsprint
nylon
orris root
parakeet feather
parrot feather
pigeon feather
perfume
pyrethrum
silk
soybean grain dust mite
tobacco
tragacanth
Tyrophagus
wheat grain dust mite
wool

Foods
almond
apple
apricot
arrowroot
artichoke
asparagus
banana
barley
bass

beef
beet
blackberry
black mulberry
black pepper
Brazil nut
broccoli
Brussel sprouts
buckwheat
cabbage
cantaloupe
carrot
cashew
cauliflower
celery
cheese
cherry
chicken
chive
chocolate
cinnamon
clam
cocoa
coconut
codfish
coffee
corn
cornmeal
cottonseed
cow milk
crab
cucumber
currant
date
duck
eggplant
egg white
egg yolk
garlic
gelatin
ginger
goat milk
gooseberry

grape
grapefruit
green bean
green pepper
hazelnut
kale
Karaya gum
kidney bean
lamb
leek
lemon
lettuce
lentil
licorice
lima bean
lobster
malt
mustard
navy bean
oat
onion
orange
parsley
parsnip
pea
peach
peanut
pear
perch
pineapple
pistachio
plum
pork
potato
prune
pumpkin
radish
raisin
rhubarb
rice
rye meal
salmon
sardine

sesame seed
shrimp
sole
soybean meal
spinach
squash
strawberry
string bean
sweet potato
Swiss chard
Swiss cheese
tea
tomato
tuna fish
turkey
turnip
vanilla
walnut
watermelon
whole wheat
yeast

Grasses
alfalfa
annual bluegrass
Bahia
Bermuda
bromegrass
Canada bluegrass
canary
common reed
crab grass
cultivated barley smut
cultivated corn smut
cultivated oat smut
cultivated rye smut
cultivated wheat smut
grama
Johnson
June
Kentucky bluegrass
meadow fescue
meadow foxtail

oat
orchard
perennial rye
redtop A
reed canary
rye
salt
sorghum grass
sweet vernal
timothy
velvet
wild rye
Zoysia

Insects
American cockroach
bee venom
black ant
black fly
blood worm
bumblebee
cockroach
cricket
deer fly
fire ant
flea
flea venom
German cockroach
honeybee
horsefly
housefly
Hymenopterous vespid
louse
mayfly
mosquito
moth
nimitti midge
paper wasp
red ant
sweat bee
wasp
white-faced hornet
yellow hornet
yellow jacket

Molds and Fungi
Alternaria
Aspergillus
Aureobasidium
Botryomyces
Candida
Cephalosporium
Chaetomium
Chrysosporium
Cladosporium
Curvularia
Dermatiaceae mix
Drechslera
Epicoccum
Epidermophyton
Fusarium
Gliocladium
Helminthosporium
Hormodendrum
Micropolyspora
Microsporum
Monilia
Mucor
Neurospora
Nigrospora
Paecilomyces
Penicillium
Phoma
Phycomycetes
Pullularia
Rhizopus
Rhodotorula
Saccharomyces
Spondylocladium
Sporobolomyces
Sporotrichum
Stemphylium
Torulopsis
Trichoderma
Trichophyton
Verticillium
Zygomycetes

Preservatives
formaldehyde
quaternium-15
hydantoi/EDTA
Kathon-CG

Occupational
chicken feathers
Effersyl
green coffee bean
Ispaghula (laxative)
Metamucil
MSP (mouse serum protein)
MUP (mouse urine protein)
pigeon droppings
PSP (pigeon serum protein)
RSP (rat serum protein)
RUP (rat urine protein)
Sof-Cil
Syllamalt

Trees and Shrubs
acacia
alder
arbor vitae
American elm
Arizona ash
Arizona cypress
Arizona/Fremont cottonwood
aspen
Australian pine
bald cypress
bayberry
beech
birch
black locust
black walnut
box elder maple
Brazilian rubber
California peppertree
Chinese elm
cottonwood
cypress

elm
eucalyptus
Douglas fir
fall elm
Gambel oak
green ash
groundsel
hackberry
hazelnut
hickory
Italian cypress
Japanese cedar
jasmine
juniper mix
lilac
liquidambar
live oak
loblolly pine
lodgepole pine
Lombardy poplar
malaleuca
maple
marsh elder
mesquite
Monterey cypress
mountain cedar
mulberry
oak
olive
orange blossom
Oregon ash
palm
paper mulberry
pecan
pepper
poison oak
poison sumac
ponderosa pine
poplar
privet
queen palm
red alder
red birch

red cedar
red maple
red mulberry
redwood
river birch
rough marsh elder
Russian olive
Russian thistle
saltbush
salt cedar
saltwort
shagbark hickory
slash pine
slippery elm
spruce
sugar maple
sweetgum
sycamore
walnut
wax myrtle
weeping fig
weeping willow
Western juniper
white ash
white mulberry
white oak
white pine
white poplar
willow

Weeds

bitter dock
burrobrush
burweed
careless
canyon ragweed
castor bean
Chenopodium
coast sage
cocklebur
dandelion
desert ragweed
dog fennel

elder
English plantain
false ragweed
firebush
fireweed
giant ragweed
goldenrod
greasewood
green amaranth
hops
iodine bush
kochia
lamb's quarter
mugwort
mustard
nettle
oxeye daisy
pigweed
poverty weed
rabbit bush
ragweed
ragwort

redroot pigweed
rough marsh elder
Russian thistle
sagebrush
scale
seneca snakeroot
sheep sorrel
short ragweed
slender ragweed
smotherweed
spiney pigweed
sugar beet
tall dock
tumbleweed
Ustilago
Western ragweed
western water hemp
white burrobrush
wild tobacco
wormwood
yellow dock
yellow mustard

Notes

Notes